Surgical Treatment for Advanced Heart Failure

Jeffrey A. Morgan • Yoshifumi Naka
Editors

Surgical Treatment for Advanced Heart Failure

Springer

Editors
Jeffrey A. Morgan, MD
Division of Cardiothoracic Surgery
Henry Ford Hospital
Detroit, MI, USA

Yoshifumi Naka, MD, PhD
Department of Cardiothoracic Surgery
New York Presbyterian Hospital
New York, NY, USA

ISBN 978-1-4614-6918-6 ISBN 978-1-4614-6919-3 (eBook)
DOI 10.1007/978-1-4614-6919-3
Springer New York Heidelberg Dordrecht London

Library of Congress Control Number: 2013937180

Printed on acid-free paper

Springer is part of Springer Science+Business Media (www.springer.com)

Preface

The treatment of end-stage heart failure with advanced surgical therapies has evolved significantly over the years and is a growing subspecialty within cardiac surgery. Our text reviews various surgical therapies for these patients, including coronary artery revascularization, mitral valve repair, aortic valve replacement, ventricular remodeling, cardiac resynchronization, mechanical circulatory support with short-term devices for acute stabilization, long-term mechanical support as a bridge to transplant and for destination therapy, complete cardiac replacement with the total artificial heart, and cardiac transplantation. When possible, efforts were made to include diagrams, cartoons, and intraoperative photos to illustrate the operations being described. It is our hope that this text will serve as a foundation for cardiac surgeons involved with the surgical management of patients with advanced heart failure.

Detroit, MI, USA — Jeffrey A. Morgan, MD
New York, NY, USA — Yoshifumi Naka, MD, PhD

Contents

Contributors

William T. Abraham Division of Cardiovascular Medicine, The Ohio State University, Columbus, OH, USA

Sanjeev Aggarwal Department of Cardiothoracic Surgery, Saint Luke's Mid America Heart Institute, Kansas City, MO, USA

Mehmet Hakan Akay Department of Mechanical Circulatory Support, Heart Transplantation, Texas Heart Institute at St. Luke's Episcopal Hospital, Houston, TX, USA

Mrudula R. Allareddy Division of Cardiology, David Geffen School of Medicine, Ronald Reagan UCLA Medical Center, Los Angeles, CA, USA

Leora B. Balsam Department of Cardiothoracic Surgery, New York University Langone Medical Center, New York, NY, USA

Paul Chacko Division of Cardiology, Department of Internal Medicine, The Ohio State University College of Medicine, Columbus, OH, USA

Jonathan M. Chen Departments of Pediatrics and Cardiothoracic Surgery, New York Presbyterian Hospital, New York, NY, USA

Richard K. Cheng Division of Cardiology, David Geffen School of Medicine, Ronald Reagan UCLA Medical Center, Los Angeles, CA, USA

John V. Conte Department of Cardiac Surgery, Johns Hopkins Hospital, Baltimore, MD, USA

Hannah Copeland Division of Cardiovascular and Thoracic Surgery, Loma Linda University Medical Center, Loma Linda, CA, USA

Jack G. Copeland Division of Cardiovascular and Thoracic Surgery, University of California, San Diego, La Jolla, CA, USA

Mario C. Deng Division of Cardiology, David Geffen School of Medicine, Ronald Reagan UCLA Medical Center, Los Angeles, CA, USA

Eugene C. DePasquale Division of Cardiology, David Geffen School of Medicine, Ronald Reagan UCLA Medical Center, Los Angeles, CA, USA

Niloo M. Edwards Department of Cardiothoracic Surgery, University of Wisconsin School of Medicine Hospitals, Madison, WI, USA

O.H. Frazier Department of Transplant/Mechanical Circulatory Support, Texas Heart Institute at St. Luke's Episcopal Hospital, Houston, TX, USA

Aubrey Galloway Department of Cardiothoracic Surgery, New York University Langone Medical Center, New York, NY, USA

Igor D. Gregoric Center of Advanced Heart Failure, University of Texas Health Science Center Houston at Memorial Hermann Hospital, Houston, TX, USA

Eugene A. Grossi Department of Cardiothoracic Surgery, New York University Langone Medical Center, New York, NY, USA

Benjamin Hirsh Department of Medicine, New York Presbyterian-Columbia University Medical Center, New York, NY, USA

Ulrich P. Jorde New York Presbyterian Hospital, Columbia University Medical Center, New York, NY, USA

Farhana Latif Division of Cardiology, Department of Medicine, New York-Presbyterian Hospital, New York, NY, USA

Lucian Lozonschi Department of Cardiothoracic Surgery, University of Wisconsin School of Medicine Hospitals, Madison, WI, USA

S. Chris Malaisrie Department of Cardiac Surgery, Northwestern Memorial Hospital, Chicago, IL, USA

Abeel A. Mangi Department of Cardiac Surgery, Yale New Haven Hospital/Yale University School of Medicine, New Haven, CT, USA

Patrick M. McCarthy Division of Cardiac Surgery, Northwestern Memorial Hospital, Chicago, IL, USA

Jeffrey A. Morgan Division of Cardiothoracic Surgery, Henry Ford Hospital, Detroit, MI, USA

Yoshifumi Naka Department of Cardiothoracic Surgery, New York Presbyterian Hospital, New York, NY, USA

Steven M. Parnis Center for Cardiac Support, Texas Heart Institute at St. Luke's Episcopal Hospital, Houston, TX, USA

Khurram Shahzad Division of Cardiology, Department of Medicine, New York-Presbyterian Hospital, New York, NY, USA

Mark S. Slaughter Division Thoracic and Cardiovascular Surgery, University of Louisville, Louisville, KY, USA

Carter T. Smith Department of Cardiothoracic Surgery, University of Wisconsin School of Medicine Hospitals, Madison, WI, USA

Richard G. Smith Artificial Heart Program, University of Arizona Medical Center, Tucson, AZ, USA

Robert A. Sorabella Division of Cardiothoracic Surgery, Department of Surgery, New York-Presbyterian Hospital, New York, NY, USA

Benjamin C. Sun Department of Cardiothoracic Surgery, Minneapolis Heart Institute, Allina Health System, Minneapolis, MN, USA

Principles of Heart Failure

1

Benjamin Hirsh and Ulrich P. Jorde

Epidemiology

Heart failure (HF) is the common end point to nearly every form of progressive cardiovascular disease. It is estimated to affect 5.7 million Americans today. For persons older than 65, it carries an incidence of 10 per 1,000 and this rate continues to rise. Risk factors for the development of HF include hypertension, coronary artery disease, diabetes mellitus, obesity, and a family history of cardiomyopathy [1]. The prognosis for patients with HF is poor, and 20 % of those diagnosed with systolic HF will die within 1 year of diagnosis, with an annual mortality rate thereafter of 10 %. Moreover, HF heralds substantial morbidity and is associated with significant declines in physical and mental health, resulting in a markedly decreased quality of life [2].

Furthermore, HF continues to pose a tremendous economic burden on the American health-care system. In 2009, it accounted for $37.2 billion in estimated direct and indirect costs for the United States. In patients older than 65 years, it currently accounts for 20 % of all hospitalizations. Accordingly, there have been considerable efforts by insurance companies, federal agencies, and hospital administrators to reduce the rate of patients admitted to hospitals with this diagnosis [3].

Physiology of Heart Failure

In its normal state, the heart's ventricles undergo filling at low pressures during diastole. The ventricles eject a percentage of this volume forward to the rest of the circulation during systole. HF occurs when either (1) the heart is unable to maintain its normal ejection fraction (EF), known as left ventricular systolic dysfunction, or (2) the heart maintains a normal EF but does so in the setting of elevated filling pressures, known as diastolic HF or HF with normal/preserved ejection fraction.

Left- and right-sided HF can occur independently. However, in advanced stages of HF, elevated pressures from the left side of the heart transmit pressure to the right side, precipitating right-sided HF. Despite their interdependence in advanced HF, this chapter will focus on a discussion of left-sided HF to provide the clearest understanding of the physiology involved.

B. Hirsh, M.D. (✉)
Department of Medicine, New York Presbyterian-Columbia University Medical Center, 622 W. 168th St., New York, NY 10023, USA
e-mail: benjamin.hirsh@gmail.com

U.P. Jorde, M.D.
New York Presbyterian Hospital, Columbia University Medical Center, 622 W. 168th St., PH 12-Stem, New York, NY 10032, USA
e-mail: upj1@columbia.edu

J.A. Morgan and Y. Naka (eds.), *Surgical Treatment for Advanced Heart Failure*, DOI 10.1007/978-1-4614-6919-3_1, © Springer Science+Business Media New York 2013

Left Ventricular Systolic Dysfunction/ Left-Sided HF

Failure of the left ventricle to generate sufficient cardiac output results either from (a) processes that directly affect ventricular myocytes or secondarily from (b) hemodynamic stress on the myocardium.

(a) Direct Injury to Ventricular Myocardium

Direct injury to ventricular myocytes with subsequent loss of contractile function is observed most often in the case of myocardial infarction. After an extensive myocardial infarction, the infarcted tissue is no longer able to generate contractile activity, and therefore overall cardiac output is decreased. Furthermore, the myocardium adjacent to the infarcted area attempts to compensate for the loss of contractile tissue by undergoing remodeling [4]. In this process, a programmed remodeling of the non-infarcted tissue is generated by both an increased hemodynamic strain and the activation of local cytokines and systemic neurohormones (the steps of remodeling will be discussed in subsequent sections). Although remodeling allows the myocardium to compensate in some measure initially, over time these changes transmit further stress to the adjacent tissue, ultimately, propagating worsening HF (Fig. 1.1).

Direct injury to the myocardium with subsequent loss of contractile function can also be seen with infiltrative processes such as toxins, infections, and genetic abnormalities (these will be discussed further in the section on "Heart Failure with Normal/Preserved Ejection Fraction").

(b) Hemodynamic Stress on the Ventricular Myocardium

Left ventricular systolic dysfunction also develops secondarily to the hemodynamic

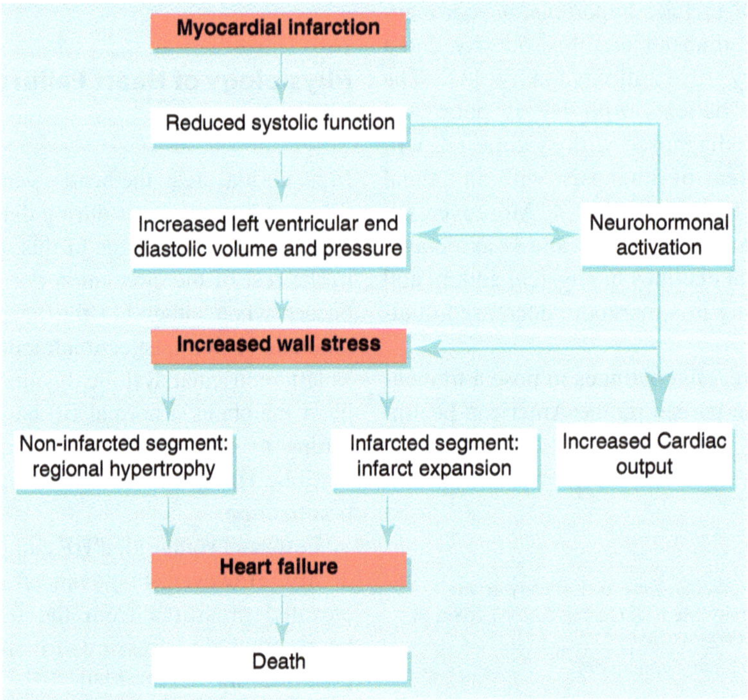

Fig. 1.1 Myocardial infarction culminating in heart failure; the direct consequences of myocardial infarction and the subsequent local and peripheral responses designed to protect the body from the effects of the failing heart (Adapted from McKay RG, Pfeffer MA, Pasternak RC, Markis JE, Come PC, Nakao S, et al. Left ventricular remodeling after myocardial infarction: a corollary to infarct expansion. Circulation. 1986;74(4):693–702)

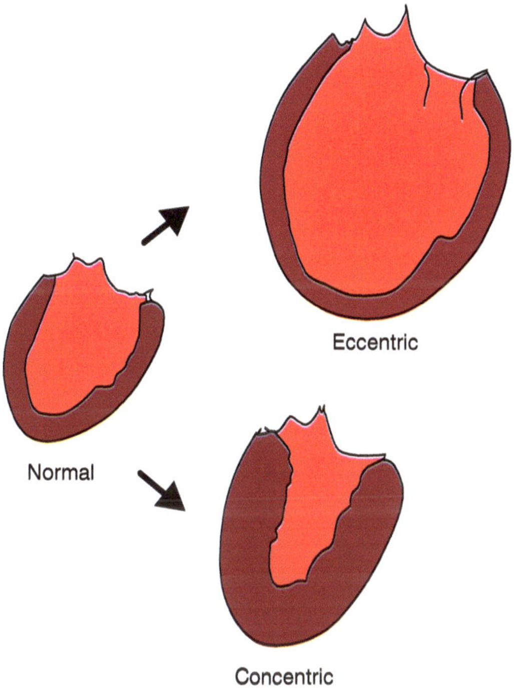

Fig. 1.2 Maladaptive cardiac hypertrophy: concentric and eccentric hypertrophy compared to a normal heart (Adapted from Katz AM. Physiology of the Heart. 3rd ed. Philadelphia, PA: Lippincott Williams & Wilkins; 2001])

stress of a chronic pressure load (termed "afterload") or volume load (termed "preload") on the ventricular wall. Increased afterload is observed in patients with aortic stenosis and in patients with uncontrolled hypertension. Similarly, increased preload is seen in patients with chronic mitral and/or aortic insufficiency, intracardiac shunts, and arteriovenous fistulas. In response to these disease processes, which impose sustained hemodynamic stress on the ventricular wall, the heart muscle undergoes a pathological hypertrophy (Fig. 1.2). This is the early phase of remodeling. In cases of increased afterload, the ventricle undergoes concentric hypertrophy, which is characterized by an increased ventricular wall thickness in comparison to wall cavity size. In cases of increased preload, the ventricle undergoes eccentric hypertrophy, characterized by an increase in chamber volume with normal or reduced wall thickness [5].

Whereas cardiac hypertrophy can be a normal physiologic response to exercise, allowing for an increase in mass and improvement in contractility, pathologic hypertrophy involves no improvement in contractility. Rather, it allows the ventricle to maintain contractile force temporarily until it can no longer overcome the increased hemodynamic stress. As mentioned, the increased wall stress also promotes the production of inflammatory cytokines. These cytokines have been shown to have deleterious effects on contractile proteins by altering their expression and by triggering pathways involved in myocyte apoptosis. Cytokine and neurohormonal production have been shown to occur in later phases of remodeling. Eventually the muscle fibers accumulate collagen and fibrose [6]. This eventually leads to left ventricular dilatation, further loss of contractile function, and thus reduced systolic function (Fig. 1.3).

Heart Failure with Normal/Preserved Ejection Fraction

Diastolic dysfunction and diastolic HF have different meanings. In both cases, the ventricle becomes less compliant, leading to impaired/abnormal ventricular filling, as measured by echocardiography or other imaging modalities. Diastolic dysfunction refers only to impaired/abnormal filling by imaging; diastolic HF instead refers to diastolic dysfunction with clinical symptoms and signs of HF. To more clearly make a distinction between these two entities, the term "diastolic HF" is now substituted by a relatively new construct referred to as Heart Failure with Normal/Preserved Ejection Fraction (HFNEF). Approximately 50 % of the overall HF population has a normal left ventricular ejection fraction (LVEF). In comparison to patients with HF and low LVEF, these individuals are more likely to be women and more likely to be older. They also have a higher likelihood of obesity, hypertension, renal failure, atrial fibrillation, and anemia [7]. The clinical syndrome of HF in these individuals can be as profound as those patients with HF

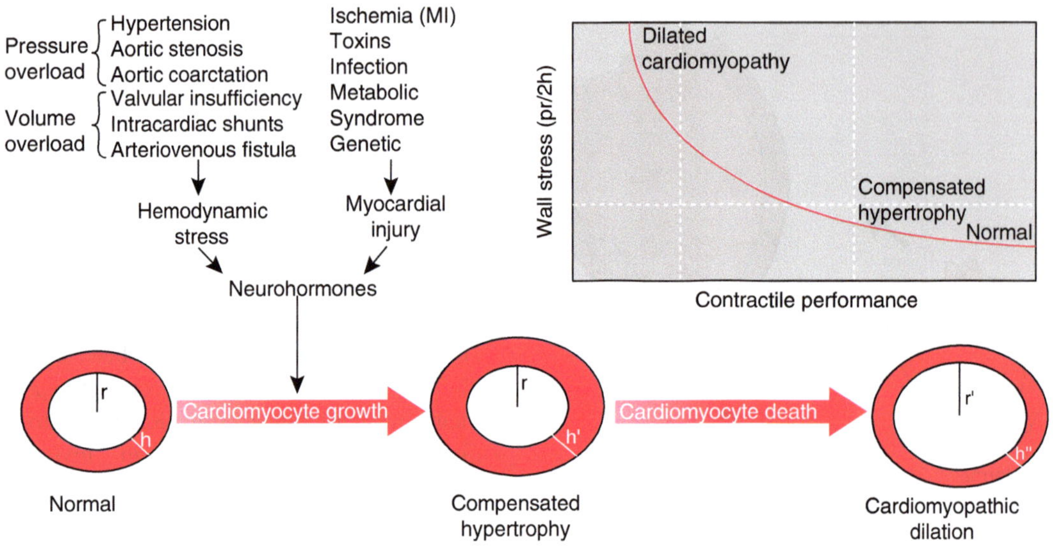

Fig. 1.3 The response of the heart muscle to stress. Hypertrophy of the cardiac muscle preserves contractile function initially, but eventually, the hypertrophied muscle fibroses and gives way to dilatation and loss of contractile function (Adapted from Diwan A, Dorn GW 2nd. Decompensation of cardiac hypertrophy: cellular mechanisms and novel therapeutic targets. Physiology (Bethesda). 2007;22(1):56–64)

symptoms and low LVEF [8]. Similarly, the prognosis of patients with clinical HF and normal LVEF is only minimally better in comparison to those with patients with a low LVEF [9].

These two entities also share common etiologies. As mentioned, aortic stenosis and poorly controlled hypertension often lead secondarily to left-sided heart failure. Prior to the development of left-sided HF, the ventricle remodels via a mechanism of concentric hypertrophy, known as left ventricular hypertrophy (LVH), as it works to preserve cardiac output. With LVH, there is often impaired ventricular relaxation and thus higher ventricular filling pressures. LVH is therefore a common cause of HFNEF since higher ventricular filling pressures can cause "backup" of fluid into the lungs despite normal LV contractility. The other major causes of HFNEF are also attributable to impaired ventricular relaxation and include transient myocardial ischemia, infiltrative processes that deposit into the myocardial architecture creating a restrictive cardiomyopathy, and hypertrophic cardiomyopathy [10]. Infiltrative processes involve the intercalation of toxins, diseases, or infections into the myocardium. The following are examples of common infiltrative sources: chemotherapy, amyloidosis and other connective tissue diseases, alcohol from long-term abuse, and human immunodeficiency virus (HIV) and other viruses. Genetic and myopathic disorders such as Duchenne Muscular Dystrophy can also produce a restrictive cardiomyopathy [11].

As mentioned, patients with left-sided HF and HFNEF not only share similar etiologies but often have similar clinical presentations. However, the mechanisms by which the left ventricle acts to maintain stroke volume in these two groups of patients are different. In HF with low LVEF, the eccentric or dilated left ventricle acts to maintain stroke volume via the Frank-Starling mechanism (Fig. 1.4). By this mechanism, the left ventricle's increased compliance accommodates for greater ventricular filling and thus a greater end-diastolic volume (EDV). This permits a greater stroke volume with each subsequent contraction and thus a way to preserve forward cardiac output, although only to a certain degree. Comparatively, in HFNEF, the left ventricle is in a remodeling phase and is able to maintain contractile function and normal stroke volume but must do so at

	HF with impaired LVEF	HFNEF
LV morphology	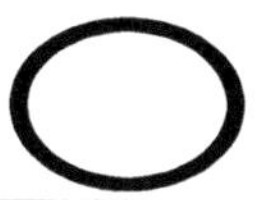	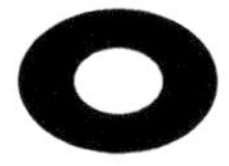
Pressure-volume loop	LV pressure 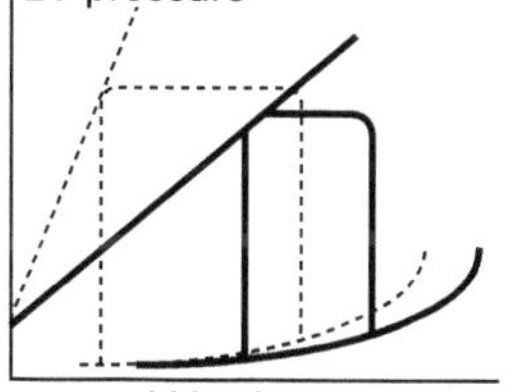 LV volume	LV pressure 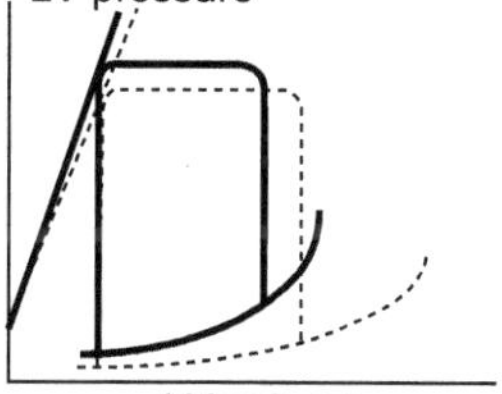 LV volume
LVEDV	↑	normal
LV mass	eccentric LV hypertrophy	concentric LV hypertrophy or concentric LV remodeling
Left atrium	dilated	dilated
LVEF	↓	normal

Fig. 1.4 Pressure and volume changes throughout different stages of ventricular remodeling in heart failure (Adapted from Maeder MT, Kaye DM. Heart failure with normal left ventricular ejection fraction. J Am Coll Cardiol. 2009;53(11):905–918)

elevated ventricular filling pressures. As a result of the elevated pressures, the EDV will be normal or reduced (Fig. 1.4).

Although their adaptive mechanisms are different, HFNEF actually exists in a continuum with left ventricular systolic dysfunction. A good example of this continuum is the ventricle's response to afterload. As described in earlier sections, in response to an afterload like aortic stenosis, the heart will undergo remodeling likely via concentric hypertrophy or LVH. During this period, the patient will often present with HFNEF, prior to the loss of contractile myocytes and left-sided HF. Conversely, patients with left-sided HF may also present with a significant component of diastolic dysfunction, owing to impaired ventricular filling from a greater EDV [12].

Compensatory Mechanisms/ Neurohormonal Alterations

In HF, the body utilizes both central and peripheral actions to mitigate the fall in cardiac output and to increase organ perfusion. These actions include (1) remodeling and ventricular hypertrophy, (2) the Frank-Starling mechanism, and (3) neurohormonal changes. The first two methods (as described in previous sections) act centrally to sustain stroke volume. Neurohormonal mechanisms acting both centrally and peripherally include (1) the adrenergic/sympathetic nervous system and (2) the renin-angiotensin-aldosterone system (RAAS). Each compensatory mechanism acts either directly or indirectly to increase cardiac output (CO) or systemic vascular resistance (SVR). Both of these terms increase arterial blood pressure, according to the equation $BP = CO \times SVR$.

Modulation of the Adrenergic/ Sympathetic Nervous System

Neurohormonal activation modulates SVR primarily via its actions on the adrenergic nervous system. To recall, the functions of the adrenergic nervous system on the heart include stimulation of inotropic and chronotropic beta receptors and alpha-receptor-mediated vascular tone. Neurohormonal modulation of this system relies on feedback from baroreceptors embedded in the smooth muscle of the arterial walls, primarily in the carotid sinus and aortic arch. Baroreceptors relay information about

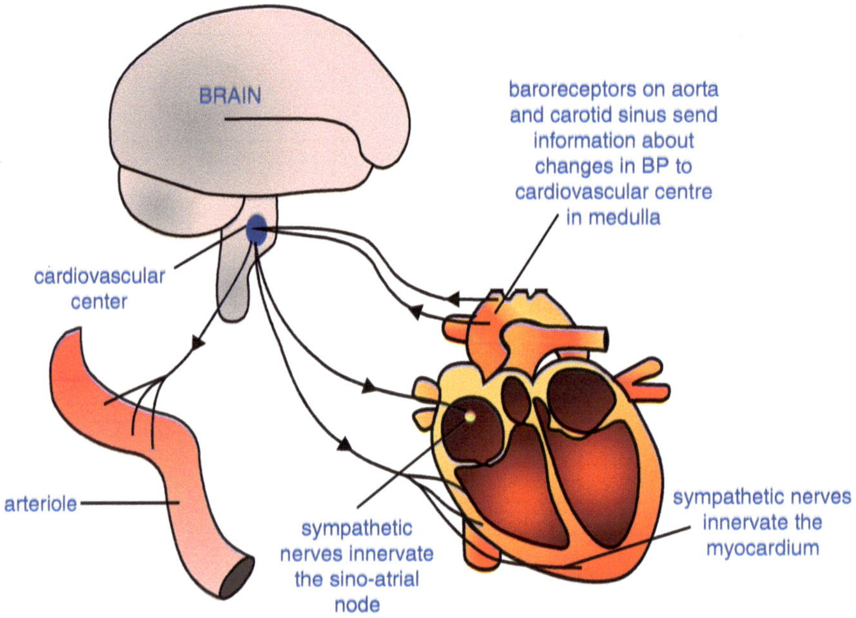

Fig. 1.5 The peripheral effects of the hyperadrenergic state in heart failure (Adapted from the Department of Physiology at Birmingham City University, United Kingdom. http://www.hcc.uce.ac.uk/physiology/images/baroreceptor.gif. Accessed October 18, 2012)

the arterial peripheral resistance to the neuroendocrine system, which then adjusts its stimulation of the adrenergic system accordingly. For example, reduced CO leads to a reduction in blood volume and thus a drop in tension of the arterial wall. The baroreceptor senses the decreased tension and sends this information to the brain's medullary vasomotor center. The vasomotor sensor processes this information and increases adrenergic output via the production of hormones or catecholamines, such as norepinephrine, from the adrenal gland [6]. The catecholamine then binds to adrenergic receptors on the heart, arteries, and veins increasing the heart rate, heart contractility, vascular tone, and venous return (Fig. 1.5).

Modulation of the RAAS

While the effects of adrenergic modulation occur rapidly, the activation of the RAAS provides a more robust, long-term response to reduced CO. The RAAS is complex and involves numerous hormones and target organs, but its greatest effect derives from its ability to resorb sodium, expand the intravascular volume, and increase SVR. The RAAS system is activated by three primary stimuli that occur in the setting of HF and other low-flow states: (1) a decrease in perfusion of the renal artery, (2) a decrease in sodium delivery to an area of the kidney known as the macula densa, and (3) stimulation of beta receptors in the juxtaglomerular apparatus (JGA) of the kidney by the adrenergic nervous system. In response to these stimuli, the kidney releases renin, which enzymatically converts angiotensinogen to angiotensin I. Angiotensin I is then converted by the angiotensin converting enzyme (ACE) to angiotensin II (AII).

AII acts as a vasoconstrictor on arteries, thereby increasing SVR, and centrally on the myocardium to promote ventricular hypertrophy in early phases of remodeling. It is AII's release of aldosterone that is responsible for its greatest effect on volume expansion. Once released from the adrenal cortex, aldosterone binds to the distal convoluted tubule of the

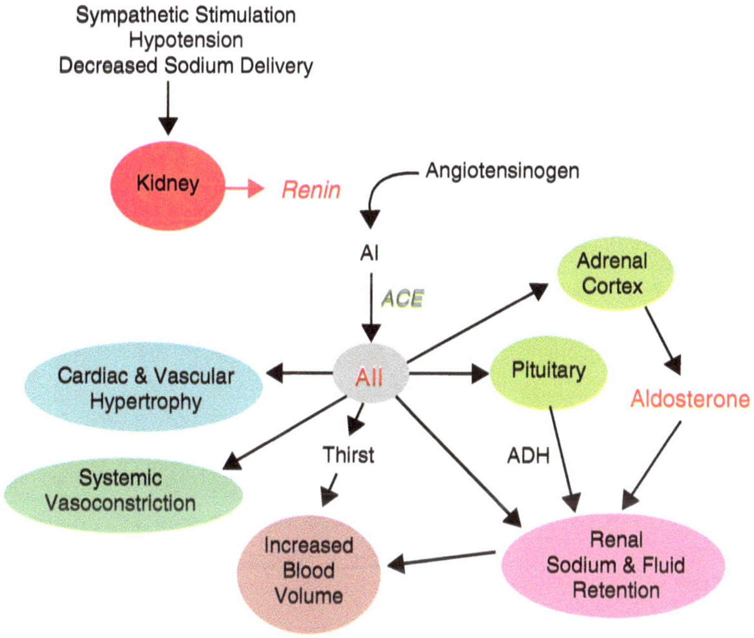

Fig. 1.6 The effects of the renin-angiotensin system in heart failure (Adapted from Klabunde RE. Cardiovascular Physiology Concepts. Philadelphia, PA: Lippincott, Williams & Wilkins; 2005)

kidney activating sodium reabsorption. The subsequent rise in intravascular volume allows for increases in preload and thus increases in CO via the Frank-Starling mechanism. AII's binding to the hypothalamus triggers the release of ADH from the posterior pituitary [13]. ADH increases CO in a similar mechanism to aldosterone; however, it does so by activating aquaporins in the distal nephron, which in turn promotes water reabsorption (Fig. 1.6).

Counterregulatory Responses

These complex physiological responses buffer the effects of reduced CO initially, but their continued use becomes a detriment to the failing heart. Beta receptors, which play a major role in ventricular remodeling, become desensitized to further stimuli and fail to respond to appropriate adrenergic signaling. Further dilatation of the LV by chronic RAAS-induced volume expansion becomes deleterious. This occurs when the ability of the LV to produce increases in CO via the Frank-Starling mechanism is exceeded. Additionally, increases in SVR and volume via the adrenergic system and RAAS further augment afterload, thus reducing CO [14].

To curtail the adverse effects of prolonged RAAS and adrenergic activation, counterregulatory forces in the form of natriuretic peptides are called into action. Ventricular and atrial wall distension from volume overload serves as the stimulus for the release of brain natriuretic peptide (BNP) and atrial natriuretic peptide (ANP) into circulation. These forces directly counteract the actions of the RAAS by promoting sodium and water loss, suppressing thirst, and dilating peripheral vessels (Fig. 1.7). Additionally, BNP in particular serves as a useful marker to measure severity of acute HF exacerbations [15]. Unfortunately, these safeguards can only temporize the continued activation of the neuroendocrine system and are eventually overcome by the latter process. Therefore, current medical and surgical management of HF patients endeavors to further moderate these compensatory mechanisms.

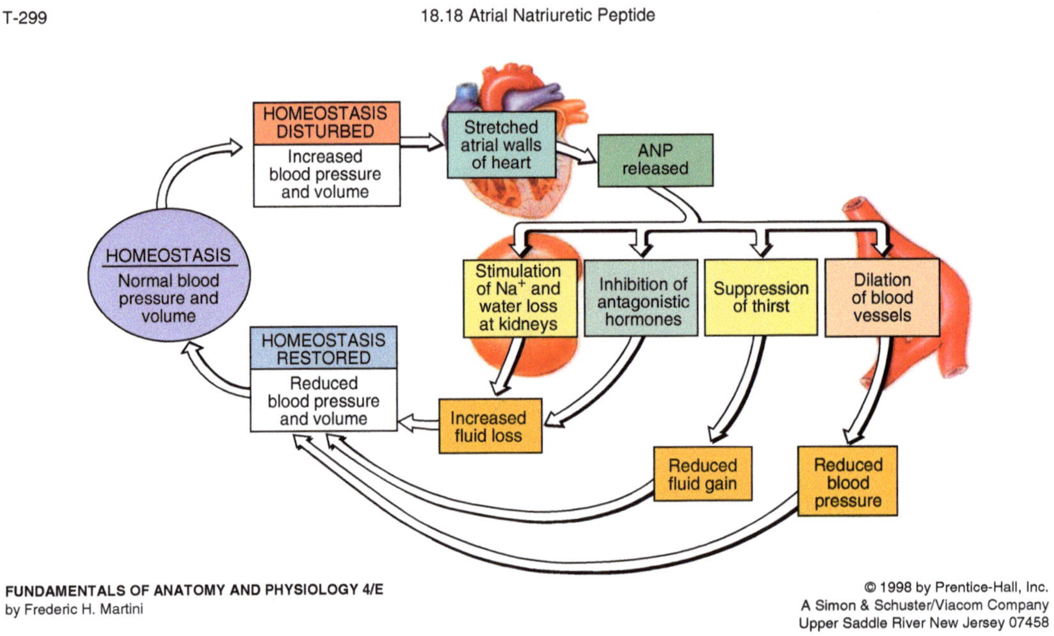

Fig. 1.7 Fluid homeostasis in heart failure—coordinated efforts of the heart and kidney (Adapted from Martini FH, Welch K. Fundamentals of Anatomy and Physiology. Upper Saddle River, NJ: Prentice Hall; 1998)

References

1. Jessup M, Brozena S. Heart failure. N Engl J Med. 2003;348:2007–18.
2. Hunt SA, Abraham WT, Chin MH, Feldman AM, Francis GS, Ganiats TG, et al. ACC/AHA 2005 Guideline Update for the Diagnosis and Management of Chronic Heart Failure in the Adult: a report of the American College of Cardiology/American Heart Association Task Force on Practice Guidelines (Writing Committee to Update the 2001 Guidelines for the Evaluation and Management of Heart Failure): developed in collaboration with the American College of Chest Physicians and the International Society for Heart and Lung Transplantation: endorsed by the Heart Rhythm Society. Circulation. 2005;112:e154–235.
3. Lloyd-Jones D, Adams R, Carnethon M, De Simone G, Ferguson TB, Flegal K, et al. Heart disease and stroke statistics 2009 update. A report From the American Heart Association Statistics Committee and Stroke Statistics Subcommittee. Circulation. 2009;119:e1–e161.
4. McKay RG, Pfeffer MA, Pasternak RC, Markis JE, Come PC, Nakao S, et al. Left ventricular remodeling after myocardial infarction: a corollary to infarct expansion. Circulation. 1986;74(4):693–702.
5. Neubauer S. The failing heart—an engine out of fuel. N Engl J Med. 2007;356(11):114–51.
6. Diwan A, Dorn GW. Decompensation of cardiac hypertrophy: cellular mechanisms and novel therapeutic targets. Physiology. 2007;22(1):56–64.
7. Hogg K, Swedburg K, McMurray J. Heart failure with preserved left ventricular systolic function; epidemiology, clinical characteristics, and prognosis. J Am Coll Cardiol. 2004;43:317–27.
8. Hobbs FD, Kenkre JF, Roalfe AK, Davis RC, Hare R, Davies MK. Impact of heart failure and left ventricular systolic dysfunction on quality of life: a cross-sectional study comparing common chronic cardiac and medical disorders and a representative adult population. Eur Heart J. 2002;23(23):1867–76.
9. Klapholz M, Maurer M, Lowe AM, Messineo F, Meisner JS, Mitchell J, et al. Hospitalization for heart failure in the presence of a normal left ventricular ejection fraction: results of the New York Heart Failure Registry. J Am Coll Cardiol. 2004;43(8):1432–8.
10. Owan TE, Hodge DO, Herges RM, Jacobsen SJ, Roger VL, Redfield MM. Trends in prevalence and outcome of heart failure with preserved ejection fraction. N Engl J Med. 2006;355:251–9.
11. McMurray JJ, Carson PE, Komajda M, McKelvie R, Zile MR, Ptaszynska A, et al. Heart failure with preserved ejection fraction: clinical characteristics of 4133 patients enrolled in the I-PRESERVE trial. Eur J Heart Fail. 2008;10:149–56.
12. Maeder MT, Kaye DM. Heart failure with normal left ventricular ejection fraction. J Am Coll Cardiol. 2009;53:905–18.
13. Paul M, Poyan Mehr A, Kreutz R. Physiology of local renin-angiotensin systems. Physiol Rev. 2006;86(3):747–803.
14. Farrell MH, Foody JM, Krumholz HM. Beta blockers in heart failure: clinical applications. JAMA. 2002;287(7):890–7.
15. McFarlane S, Winer N, Sowers JS. Role of the natriuretic peptide system in cardiorenal protection. Arch Intern Med. 2003;163:2696–704.

2 Algorithm for Treatment of Advanced Heart Failure

Richard K. Cheng, Mrudula R. Allareddy, Eugene C. DePasquale, Farhana Latif, Khurram Shahzad, and Mario C. Deng

Introduction

Epidemiology

Heart failure (HF) is a growing epidemic in the United States with steadily increasing prevalence. According to the American Heart Association (AHA) Heart Disease and Stroke Statistics 2012 update, HF prevalence was 5.7 million in the United States based on the National Health and Nutrition Examination Survey (NHANES) 2005–2008 data for Americans ≥20 years, with projected crude prevalence of 6.6 million (2.8 %) in 2010 for adults ≥18 years. Further, it is estimated that by 2030, an additional 3 million people will have HF, which is a 25 % increase in prevalence compared to 2010. HF incidence approaches 10 per 1,000 after 65 years of age with a lifetime risk of developing HF of 1 in 5 at 40 years of age in both genders [1].

Hospital discharges for HF were only mildly increased from 1999 to 2009, with first-listed diagnoses of 975,000 and 1,094,000, respectively. In 2009, HF resulted in 3,041,000 office visits, 668,000 emergency room visits, and 293,000 outpatient department visits [1]. In 2008, any mention of HF in mortality was 281,437, and death directly attributable to HF was 56,830. Currently, one in nine deaths in the United States mentions HF on the death certificate. Even though survival after HF diagnosis has improved, the death rate remains unacceptably high at approximately 50 % within 5 years from time of index diagnosis. It is a major public health concern due to its tremendous societal and economic burden, with a projected direct and indirect cost in the United States of $37.2 billion in 2009 [2], which is expected to further increase to $44.6, $57.0, $74.1, and $97.0 billion by 2015, 2020, 2025, and 2030, respectively [1].

In the international community, the epidemiological transition in less industrialized countries is associated with a reduced risk of mortality from communicable diseases and increased risk of death from cardiovascular diseases including HF [3]. As a consequence of improved management in acute coronary syndromes and improved longevity of the population, the number of patients with HF is growing. The prevalence and incidence in industrialized countries are estimated

R.K. Cheng, M.D. (✉) • M.R. Allareddy, M.D.
E.C. DePasquale, M.D.
M.C. Deng, M.D., FAAC, FESC
Division of Cardiology, David Geffen School of Medicine, Ronald Reagan UCLA Medical Center, 100 UCLA Medical Plaza, Suite 630 East, Los Angeles, CA 90095, USA
e-mail: richardkcheng@gmail.com; mallareddy@mednet.ucla.edu; edepasquale@mednet.ucla.edu; mdeng@mednet.ucla.edu

F. Latif, M.D. • K. Shahzad, M.D., M.S.
Division of Cardiology, Department of Medicine, New York-Presbyterian Hospital,
622 West 168th Street, New York, NY 10032, USA
e-mail: fl2203@columbia.edu; ks2736@columbia.edu

J.A. Morgan and Y. Naka (eds.), *Surgical Treatment for Advanced Heart Failure*,
DOI 10.1007/978-1-4614-6919-3_2,

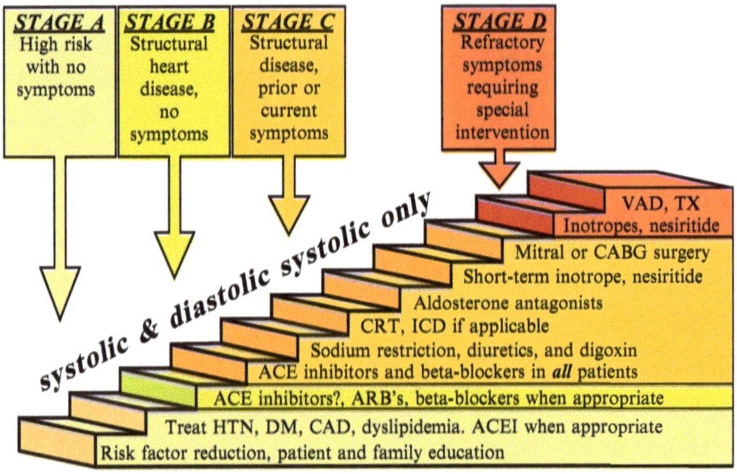

Fig. 2.1 Heart failure staging system (Adapted from Hunt SA, Abraham WT, Chin MH, Feldman AM, Francis GS, Ganiats TG, et al. ACC/AHA 2005 Guideline Update for the Diagnosis and Management of Chronic Heart Failure in the Adult: a report of the American College of Cardiology/American Heart Association Task Force on Practice Guidelines (Writing Committee to Update the 2001 Guidelines for the Evaluation and Management of Heart Failure): developed in collaboration with the American College of Chest Physicians and the International Society for Heart and Lung Transplantation: endorsed by the Heart Rhythm Society. Circulation. 2005 Sep 20;112(12):e154–235)

to be approximately 1.5 % and 0.15 % of the population, respectively [4, 5]. An estimated 10 % of persons with HF have advanced disease. In the United States and Europe alone, with ≥700 million inhabitants and ≥7 million patients with HF, the prevalence of advanced HF, constituting between 1 % and 10 % of the HF population, is estimated to total between 70,000 and 700,000 patients [6].

Definition of Heart Failure

The clinical syndrome of HF is defined as the final common pathway that results from any structural or functional cardiac disorder that impairs the ventricle from either filling with (diastolic dysfunction) or ejecting blood (systolic dysfunction). The diverse causes of HF range from disorders of the pericardium, myocardium, endocardium, or great vessels. Despite the fact that the majority of patients with HF have symptoms secondary to impaired systolic function, it is important to recognize that symptoms may also arise due to abnormal filling [7]. The overall prognosis of HF with preserved ejection fraction (HF-PEF) is less well defined, with certain observational series suggesting improved outcomes compared to HF with reduced ejection fraction (HF-REF) [8–10], while other series have shown similar mortality for HF-PEF and HF-REF [11, 12].

Stages of Heart Failure

The terminology of HF in its advanced stages is not very precise. The terms advanced, severe, congestive, refractory, and end-stage HF are used in largely exchangeable ways. The term end-stage HF reflects the impaired prognosis associated with it and has been incorporated into the recent staging system for HF (Fig. 2.1) [4], which complements the New York Heart Association (NYHA) classification of HF. This staging system has the advantage of including asymptomatic stages (risk factors, structural heart disease), thereby underscoring the importance of preventive medicine and reflecting the progressive nature of the HF syndrome. It bears resemblance with the classification of tumors, a similarly malignant group of conditions. In other words, a HF patient may progress from stage A to stage D but cannot reverse to stage A again. However, treatment may result in a patient reversing from NYHA class IV to class III due to improved symptoms.

Importance of Algorithms

In order to define and guide the optimal management of HF patients in varying clinical scenarios, treatment algorithms have become an essential cornerstone of clinical practice. These modalities are valued for their ability to help streamline clinical decision making based on disease severity. However, oversimplification of an algorithm may lead to its inapplicability in complex clinical situations. Therefore, treatment algorithms should be based on current guidelines derived from large randomized controlled clinical trials and individualized based on the assessment of a clinical situation.

In the field of heart failure, there are five main sets of guidelines developed by (1) European Society of Cardiology (ESC 2012), (2) American College of Cardiology/American Heart Association (ACC/AHA 2009), (3) Heart Failure Society of America (HFSA 2010), (4) Canadian Cardiovascular Society (CCS 2012), and (5) International Society of Heart and Lung Transplantation (ISHLT 2007). The algorithm described in Fig. 2.2 is based on these guidelines as well as current randomized controlled trials.

Initial Assessment

The algorithm starts with the encounter between the HF patient and the primary medical team, consisting of cardiologist, general internist, and nurse, who have exhausted all lifestyle and medical options without success. In this setting of acute decompensation and progression towards advanced heart failure, a phase known to be associated with a

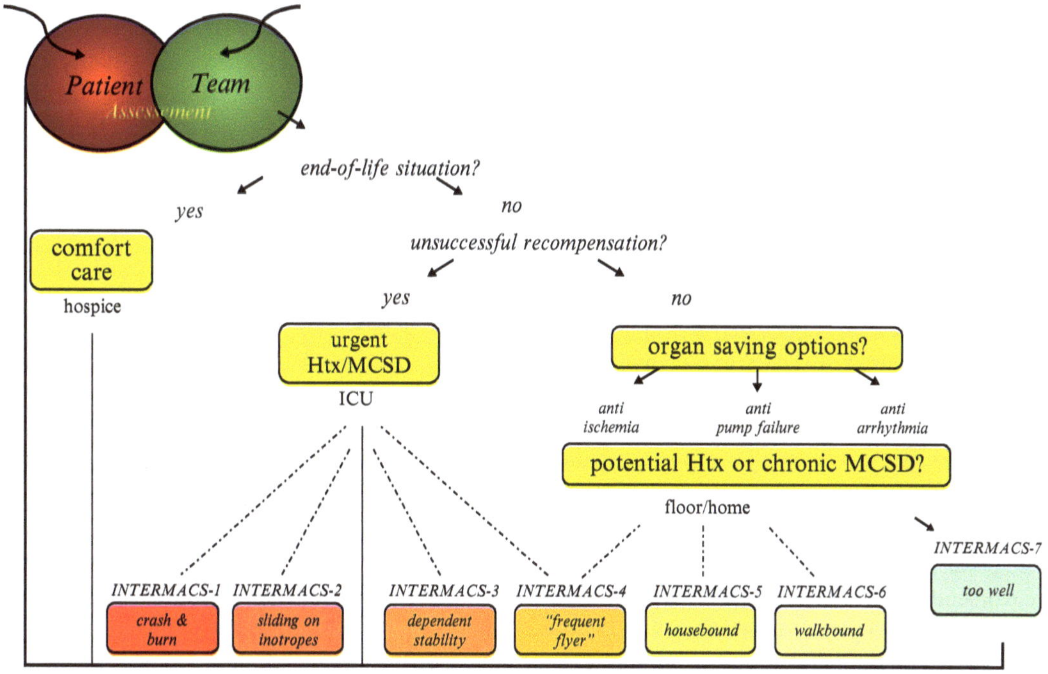

Fig. 2.2 Management algorithm in heart failure (Adapted from Deng MC, Naka Y. Mechanical Circulatory Support Therapy for Advanced Heart Failure. London: Imperial College Press; 2007)

high risk of death, a referral to a designated cardiac transplantation center for evaluation is undertaken. The initial assessment is not a complete cardiac transplantation evaluation but rather addresses the following main questions:

- How severe is the heart failure condition?
- Are there reversible causes?
- Are there risk factors limiting the overall prognosis?

After the initial assessment, a structured management algorithm (Fig. 2.2) is applied in order to recompensate the patient. If recompensation cannot be achieved, cardiac transplantation evaluation is initiated with the option of mechanical circulatory support device (MCSD) as either bridge to recovery (BTR), transplant (BTT), or destination therapy (DT). At anytime during management, a situation may arise in which the patient may not benefit from any of the modern therapies because of multiorgan failure or other conditions, leading to a patient preference for *comfort care* facilitating a humane form of death instead of prolongation of suffering [13, 14].

Risk Stratifiers

In order to plan effective treatment strategies and transplant programs, it is important to be able to objectively measure the prognosis of patients. An ideal test needs to be accurate (i.e., have a high specificity and sensitivity), reproducible, safe, and inexpensive.

The 6-min walk test can be performed by almost all patients with chronic heart failure without the need for specialized equipment. This test was first used in heart failure patients by Guyatt and colleagues in 1985 [15] and has subsequently gained widespread acceptance as a measure of exercise capacity in clinical trials and transplant programs. Zugck et al. showed that the walk test provided information on the combined end point of death and/or hospital admission due to worsening heart failure that was similar to peak oxygen uptake in patients with dilated cardiomyopathy [16]. The authors concluded the test correlated closely with peak oxygen uptake (pVO_2) and could predict individual pVO_2 when determined serially in the same patient. Opasich and colleagues also compared the prognostic role of the 6-min walk test to pVO_2 and NYHA functional class. Although the test was found to be able to predict survival in univariate analysis, this was not the case when pVO_2 or NYHA class were included in multivariate models, indicating that the walk test is not an independent prognostic indicator [17]. Whether the test is an accurate and independent predictor of prognosis in chronic heart failure, however, is the subject of some debate [18].

Peak Oxygen Uptake

Based on the groundbreaking work of Mancini and coworkers [19], a team at UCLA assessed the role of pVO_2 in reevaluation of candidates awaiting heart transplantation. All ambulatory transplant candidates with initial pVO_2 ≤14 mL/kg/min were identified. Of 107 such patients listed, 68 survived without early deterioration or transplantation to undergo repeat exercise. In 38 of the 68 patients, pVO_2 increased by ≥2 mL/kg/min to a level ≥12 mL/kg/min after 6±5 months, together with an increase in anaerobic threshold, peak oxygen pulse, and exercise heart rate reserve and a decrease in heart rate at rest. Increased pVO_2 was accompanied by stable clinical status without congestion in 31 of 38 patients, and these 31 were taken off the active waiting list. At 2 years, actuarial survival rate was 100 %, and survival rate without relisting for transplantation was 85 %. The authors concluded that an algorithm with scheduled reevaluation of exercise capacity and clinical status allowed identification of patients who became "too well" during follow-up. They estimate that 29 % of ambulatory transplant candidates could be removed from the waiting list with excellent early survival despite low pVO_2 on initial testing, allowing deferral of transplantation in favor of more compromised candidates [20].

In order to refine risk stratification in ambulatory cardiac transplantation candidates and estimate their survival probability without transplantation and thus the potential benefit from transplantation, the group at the University of Pennsylvania and Columbia University between

1987 and 1995 developed the first independently validated prognostication tool, entailing high-, medium-, and low-risk stratum [21]. The multivariable proportional hazards survival model was developed with the use of data on 80 clinical characteristics from 268 ambulatory patients with advanced heart failure (derivation sample). Invasive and noninvasive models (with and without catheterization-derived data) were constructed. Stratum-specific likelihood ratios were used to develop three prognostic-score risk groups. The noninvasive model performed well, and increased performance was not attained by the addition of catheterization-derived variables.

Prognostic-score risk groups derived from the noninvasive model in the derivation sample effectively stratified the risk of an outcome event in both the derivation and validation samples (1-year event-free survival for derivation and validation samples, respectively: low risk [Heart Failure Survival Score or HFSS 8.10–10.47] 93 % and 88 %; medium risk [HFSS 7.20–8.09] 72 % and 60 %; high risk [HFSS 5.51–7.19] 43 % and 35 %). The authors concluded that selection of candidates for cardiac transplantation may be improved by use of this noninvasive risk-stratification model [21]. The beauty of this score does not reside only in its powerful predictive value but also on its easy bedside implementation by the equation:

$$\text{HFSS} = [(0.69 \times \text{CAD}: \text{YES} = 1\ \text{NO} = 0) + (0.022 \times \text{HR}) + (-0.046 \times \text{LVEF}) + (-0.026 \times \text{mBP}) + (0.61 \times \text{IVCD}: \text{YES} = 1\ \text{NO} = 0) + (-0.055 \times \text{VO}_2) + (-0.047 \times \text{Na})]$$

CAD coronary artery disease; HR heart rate; LVEF left ventricular ejection fraction; mBP mean blood pressure; IVCD interventricular conduction delay; VO_2 peak oxygen consumption Na sodium. gathered

Event-free survival rates for the medium- and high-risk strata were much worse than would be expected after cardiac transplantation; the low-risk stratum had an event-free survival rate that was better than would be expected with transplantation. Based on this excellent prognostication tool, patients with HFSS low risk would be considered too well for cardiac transplantation [21]. Risk stratification of hospital-bound cardiac transplantation candidates who are inotrope- or left ventricular assist-device-dependent can be improved by inclusion of further parameters [22].

After the introduction of β-blocker therapy and given the large survival benefit conferred by β-blocker therapy, it was unclear whether the HFSS and pVO_2 were still valid predictors. The fact that β-blockers considerably improved survival while having an inconsistent effect on pVO_2 may explain why pVO_2 did not accurately predict outcomes in patients taking β-blockers. Given the better prognosis for patients with heart failure receiving β-blockade and absence of effect on exercise performance, the clinical guideline value for pVO_2 has probably decreased to the extent that a $pVO_2 \leq 10$ mL/kg/min is a more appropriate target. However, recalibration of the HFSS was not necessary since there were no particular differences in the HFSS pre- or post-β-blocker therapy or its parameters (other than heart rate). The authors conclude that in the β-blocker era, clinicians can continue to rely on the HFSS to accurately predict prognosis in patients with severe heart failure and that pVO_2 may have diminished in value [23].

The predictive accuracy of the HFSS has been noted to be suboptimal in some validation data sets [24]. As a result, the Seattle Heart Failure Model (SHFM) was developed and validated as a multivariate risk model to predict 1-, 2-, and 3-year survival in heart failure patients with the use of easily obtainable characteristics relating to clinical status, therapy (pharmacological as well as devices), and laboratory parameters. The SHFM was derived from a cohort of 1,125 heart failure patients in the Prospective Randomized Amlodipine Survival Evaluation (PRAISE1) with the use of a multivariate Cox model. For medications and devices not available in the derivation database, hazard ratios were estimated from published literature. The model was prospectively validated in five additional cohorts totalling 9,942 heart failure patients. The accuracy of the model was excellent, with predicted versus actual 1-year survival rates of 73.4 % versus 74.3 % in the derivation cohort and

90.5 % versus 88.5 %, 86.5 % versus 86.5 %, 83.8 % versus 83.3 %, 90.9 % versus 91.0 %, and 89.6 % versus 86.7 % in the five validation cohorts. Overall receiver operating characteristic area under the curve was 0.729 (95 % CI, 0.714–0.744). The model also allowed estimation of the benefit of adding medications or devices to an individual patient's therapeutic regimen. The authors concluded that the SHFM provides an accurate estimate of 1-, 2-, and 3-year survival with the use of easily obtained clinical, pharmacological, device, and laboratory characteristics [24].

In a study by Kalogeropoulos and colleagues [25], the SHFM was utilized to predict a composite end point of death, left ventricular assist device (LVAD), and urgent transplantation. However, 98 % of the events in the original SHFM study were death. This fact raises important issues. A higher rate of LVAD implantation and/or urgent transplantation might lead to higher overall event rate. Considering that this patient population was sicker as compared with the original SHFM cohort, it is not surprising that a larger proportion of patients underwent these procedures in their study (16 % vs. 2 %). Thus, miscalibration might not be due to SHFM performance but rather to the SHFM being more accurate for mortality prediction alone rather than a combined outcome. Indeed, when assessing the model performance restricting the outcome to death alone, the model performance improved significantly. Unlike mortality, the timing for urgent transplantation or LVAD implantation can vary between institutions and physicians. With regard to race-based differences, the SHFM needed to be recalibrated by using race-specific coefficients (0.77 for whites and 1.15 for blacks, as estimated in this cohort).

Nonsurgical Management of Heart Failure

Recompensation

The evolution of treatment options for advanced HF patients over the last several decades has been impressive. It includes medical therapies (positive inotropes, vasodilators, angiotensin-converting-enzyme inhibitors and angiotensin-receptor blockers, β-blockade, aldosterone antagonists), defibrillator implantation, resynchronization therapy, heart transplantation, and most recently MCSDs. The comparison of outcomes between different therapies for advanced HF has been challenging. For example, heart transplantation has never been tested in a randomized clinical trial because of the obvious survival advantage in the 1970s in comparison to medical therapy. It is unclear whether this remains true with the recent improvement in HF therapies. Moreover, MCSD is rapidly evolving with advances in technology leading to smaller devices with decreased morbidity. Therefore, the clinical decision-making algorithm is subject to continuing debate and consensus processes, as exemplified by the guideline development initiative of the International Society for Heart and Lung Transplantation [26].

Neurohormonal Blockade

In increasing stages of HF, the adrenergic system, renin-angiotensin-aldosterone system (RAAS), antidiuretic hormone system, and the atrial natriuretic peptide system are chronically activated. These chronic neurohormonal changes lead to compensatory elevation of preload, heart rate, contractility, and cardiac hypertrophy. NYHA class IV is characterized by a flattening and rightward shift of the cardiac function curve to a point where reduced cardiac output does not fulfill the metabolic requirements of the body and capillary wedge pressure reaches a level at which pulmonary edema ensues or both happen [27].

Positive Inotropes/Vasodilators

In the context of refractory acute HF, characterized by peripheral hypoperfusion, renal dysfunction, and marked hypotension present in less than 10 % of acute decompensated HF patients, inotropic agents (classically β-adrenergic agonists and phosphodiesterase inhibitors) have been used as a short-term bridge to cardiac surgery,

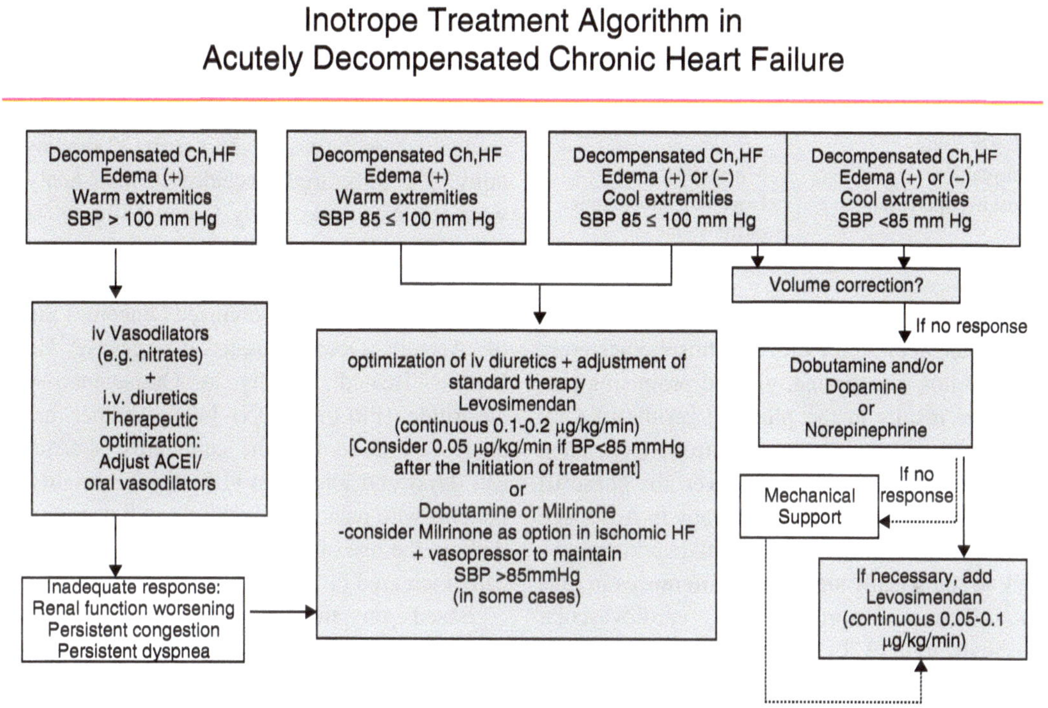

Fig. 2.3 Stepwise approach to use of inotrope therapy

transplantation, or prolonged infusions via improvement of central hemodynamics. The goals outlined for the utilization of inotropes are as follows: (1) provide rapid relief of congestive symptoms and (2) restoration of end-organ perfusion. If the myocardial insult is deemed reversible, inotropic therapy can be transitioned to organ-saving options. However, if end-organ perfusion cannot be achieved, then mechanical circulatory support (e.g., intra-aortic balloon pump) may be required to transition to possible urgent ventricular assist device or heart transplant [28]. A stepwise approach to the use of inotropic therapy is outlined in Fig. 2.3.

Inotropic agents increase myocardial contractility via increase in intracellular cyclic adenylate monophosphate levels (cAMP). This results in an increase in calcium release from the sarcoplasmic reticulum, thereby increasing the contractile force generation. The phosphodiesterase inhibitors such as milrinone and enoximone inhibit phosphodiesterase III, the enzyme that catalyzes the breakdown of cAMP, whereas the β-adrenergic agonists such as dobutamine and dopamine stimulate adenylate cyclase which increases cAMP production. Dopamine has a dose-dependent mechanism of action: ≤2 mcg/kg/min (dopaminergic receptor activity), 2–5 mcg/kg/min (β-adrenergic receptor activity), and ≥5 mcg/kg/min (alpha adrenergic agonist activity). Both milrinone and dobutamine have similar overall hemodynamic effects with key potential distinctions. Milrinone appears to lower filling pressures to a greater extent than dobutamine. It also has a more profound effect of lowering systemic vascular resistance and blood pressure. On the other hand, dobutamine may result in tachycardia with higher heart rates than milrinone [29]. Therefore, the individual clinical setting should dictate which type of inotrope is used (Table 2.1).

Despite short-term hemodynamic and symptomatic improvement, long-term mortality appears to be increased with the use of intravenous and oral inotropes for the treatment of chronic heart failure. Positive inotropes such as vesnarinone [30–34] and vasodilators such as epoprostenol did not demonstrate a survival benefit and, in fact, showed an adverse mortality

Table 2.1 Inotrope selection in various clinical settings

Clinical scenarios	Inotrope
Hypotension	Dobutamine or dopamine
Increased mean pulmonary artery pressure	Milrinone
Tachycardia	Milrinone
Renal hypoperfusion	Dopamine, dobutamine, or milrinone

effect [35]. Over the past years, a large clinical development program with the phosphodiesterase III inhibitor, enoximone, yielded promising preliminary results in the phase II results of Oral Enoximone in Intravenous Inotrope-Dependent Subjects (EMOTE) [36]. However, the phase III studies of Oral Enoximone Therapy in Advanced Heart Failure (ESSENTIAL) trial demonstrated a lack of statistically significant differences in time to all-cause mortality or cardiovascular hospitalization [37].

A novel class of inotropic drugs known as calcium-sensitizing agents, such as levosimendan, had generated excitement due to their ability to induce contractility via enhanced troponin C affinity for calcium and stabilization of the calcium-induced conformation of troponin C. The two phase III trials on levosimendan, "Survival in Patients with Acute Heart Failure in Need of Intravenous Inotropic Support" (SURVIVE) [38] and "Second Randomized Multicenter Evaluation of Intravenous Levosimendan Efficacy Versus Survival in the Short-Term Treatment of Decompensated Heart Failure" (REVIVE-II) [39], demonstrated that levosimendan was superior to dobutamine or placebo, respectively, regarding clinical improvement and neurohormonal modulation but failed to demonstrate superiority with regard to 6-month mortality.

Another potential intravenous therapy which promotes vasodilation, salt and water excretion, and improved diastolic filling properties in order to relieve congestion and reduce cardiac filling pressures is nesiritide, a recombinantly produced intravenous formulation of human B-type natriuretic peptide. Rapid and sustained beneficial hemodynamic effects of nesiritide were demonstrated by Mills et al. [40] in NYHA class II–IV patients over a 24-h infusion period and 4 h post-infusion. Effects on clinical outcomes beyond improvement in symptoms and hemodynamics are not clear. In a meta-analysis [41], Sackner-Bernstein and coworkers expressed the opinion that the use of nesiritide could increase the risk of short-term (30-day) mortality. The three trials included in their analysis were the Nesiritide Study Group Efficacy Trial (NSGET) [42], Vasodilation in the Management of Acute Congestive Heart Failure (VMAC) [43], and the Prospective Randomized Outcomes Study of Acutely Decompensated Congestive Heart Failure Treated Initially as Outpatients with Nesiritide (PROACTION) [44]. Another meta-analysis showed that the cumulative short-term (30 days) and long-term (180 days) mortality in patients who received nesiritide combined with or without the use of inotropes [45] was not statistically increased [46].

Based on this conflicting meta-analysis data, an international, multicenter, randomized, double-blind, placebo-controlled study, the Acute Study of Clinical Effectiveness of Nesiritide in Decompensated Heart Failure Trial (ASCEND-HF), has assessed the safety and efficacy of nesiritide. ASCEND-HF randomized 7,141 patients hospitalized with acute HF within 24 h of hospitalization to receive IV nesiritide or placebo in addition to standard therapy. Although there was a trend toward improvement in dyspnea (measured on the 7-point Likert scale) at 6 and 24 h with nesiritide, the prespecified level for significance was not met. Further, there was no difference between the composite end point of 30-day death and HF hospitalization. It was also shown that nesiritide had no impact on worsening of renal function, which had been a prior concern. The authors concluded that nesiritide cannot be recommended for routine use in patients with acute decompensated HF [47].

Adjunctive intravenous therapy which targets the elevated vasopressin (AVP) levels that activate vasoconstriction and left ventricular hypertrophy/remodeling via V1A/V1B receptors and water retention via V2 receptors have also been studied. Both these mechanisms contribute toward acute decompensation of HF. The utilization of intravenous conivaptan, an AVP-receptor antagonist which binds to both V1A and V2 receptors, has demonstrated favorable changes in hemodynamics, with statistically significant reduction in pulmonary capillary pressure and right atrial pressure, and urine output without affecting blood pressure or heart rate [48]. The Efficacy of Vasopressin Antagonism in Heart Failure Outcome Study with Tolvaptan (EVEREST) trial randomized 4,133 patients hospitalized with HF to oral tolvaptan (selective for V2) or placebo, in addition to standard therapy. Although tolvaptan improved dyspnea, body weight, and edema, there was no significant difference in all-cause mortality or the composite end point of cardiovascular death or HF hospitalization [49]. Thus, vasopressin receptor antagonists may be considered in the management of refractory hyponatremia in HF patients but has no impact on mortality.

RAAS Blockade

Multiple studies have demonstrated the benefit derived from renin-angiotensin system blockade via angiotensin-converting-enzyme inhibitors (ACE-I), including improvements in symptoms, survival, rate of hospitalization, and reverse remodeling. ACE-I decrease the conversion of angiotensin I to angiotensin II, thereby reducing the maladaptive effects of angiotensin II. Furthermore, there is a decrease in the breakdown of bradykinin which promotes vasodilation in the vascular endothelium and promotes natriuresis [7]. At this time, it is unclear if all the different ACE-I demonstrate a similar extent of survival benefit. There is conflicting results from meta-analysis [50], observational studies [51], and comparative trials [52–54]. Moreover, low- versus high-dose enalapril has been studied with no significant differences in survival or clinical and hemodynamic variables [55].

With regard to trial data, the first randomized prospective medical trial demonstrating a survival benefit with ACE-I from a medical treatment in advanced heart failure was the Cooperative North Scandinavian Enalapril Survival Study (CONSENSUS-I) trial [56]. Two hundred fifty-six patients in NYHA class IV heart failure were randomized to enalapril or placebo. This trial demonstrated improved survival in the enalapril cohort. This study is unique in being the first heart failure trial in unselected NYHA class IV patients but also in examining extended survival, with sustained benefit for at least 4 years [57]. The subsequent Studies of Left Ventricular Dysfunction (SOLVD) study in 1991 randomly assigned 2,569 patients with symptomatic NYHA class II to III HF and ejection fraction ≤35 % to either placebo or enalapril, with reduction in all-cause mortality in the enalapril cohort [58].

Despite the inhibition of the angiotensin-converting enzyme with ACE-I, there is evidence of increased plasma levels of aldosterone. Aldosterone has pleiotropic effects, resulting in increased sodium retention, constriction of systemic arterioles, stimulation of cytokine production, inflammatory-cell adhesion, activation of macrophages as well as stimulation of growth of fibroblasts, and the synthesis of type I and III fibrillar collagens involved in scar formation [59]. Mortality reduction was noted with the addition of aldosterone inhibitors, as evidenced by the Randomized Aldactone Evaluation Study (RALES) trial, in which 1,663 NYHA class III–IV HF patients who had severe heart failure and a left ventricular ejection fraction (LVEF) of ≤35 % and who were being treated with an ACE-I, a loop diuretic, and in most cases digoxin were randomly assigned to receive 25 mg of spironolactone daily or placebo. After a mean follow-up period of 24 months, there was a 46 % mortality rate in the placebo group and a 35 % mortality rate in the spironolactone group [60]. The Eplerenone Post-Acute Myocardial Infarction Heart Failure Efficacy and Survival Study (EPHESUS) trial demonstrated that eplerenone also significantly reduces mortality in post-myocardial infarction (MI) patients with HF or diabetes mellitus with LVEF ≤40 % [61]. More recently, the Eplerenone in Mild Patients Hospitalization and Survival Study in Heart Failure (EMPHASIS-HF) trial studied eplerenone in HF patients with LVEF ≤30 % (or 30–35 % if QRS duration ≥130 ms) with milder NYHA class II symptoms. In this population, aldosterone antagonism was also associated with improved survival [62].

Another class of medication utilized in RAAS blockade is angiotensin II type 1 receptor blockers (ARB). In the Valsartan Heart Failure Trial (Val-HeFT) study, valsartan significantly reduced the combined end point of mortality and morbidity and improved clinical signs and symptoms in patients with heart failure compared to placebo. This difference was predominantly driven by a 24 % reduction in the rate of HF hospitalizations, without a clear benefit for survival alone. However, the post hoc observation of an adverse effect on mortality and morbidity in the subgroup receiving combined valsartan, an angiotensin-converting-enzyme (ACE) inhibitor, and a β-blocker raised concern about the potential safety of this specific combination [63].

Candesartan in Heart Failure Assessment of Reduction in Mortality and Morbidity (CHARM) addressed whether the angiotensin-receptor blocker (ARB) candesartan improved outcomes in HF patients in two complementary parallel trials (CHARM-Alternative, for patients who could not tolerate ACE-I, and CHARM-Added, for patients who were receiving ACE-I). NYHA II–IV HF patients with LVEF of ≤V40 % were randomized to candesartan or placebo. The study drug was discontinued in CHARM-Alternative because of adverse effects in 23.1 % of patients in the candesartan group and 18.8 % in the placebo group; the reasons included increased creatinine, hypotension, and hyperkalemia. The authors concluded that candesartan significantly reduces all-cause mortality, cardiovascular death, and heart failure hospitalizations in patients with HF and LVEF ≤F40 % when added to standard therapies including ACE-I, β-blockers, and an aldosterone antagonist. However, routine monitoring of blood pressure, serum creatinine, and serum potassium is warranted [64]. Thus, ARB are a reasonable alternative to ACE inhibitors as first-line agents for HF. ARB or ACE-I are useful to prevent HF in selected stage A and B patients, and candesartan can improve outcomes in patients with impaired cardiac function who are intolerant of ACE-I [64].

Other landmark trials including Evaluation of Losartan in the Elderly (ELITE II) [65], Optimal Trial in Myocardial Infarction with the Angiotensin II Antagonist Losartan (OPTIMAAL) [66], and Valsartan in Acute Myocardial Infarction (VALIANT) [67] that have assessed ARB in comparison to ACE-I for treatment of HF have shown no clear benefit of one pharmacologic agent over the other for mortality in HF-REF patients. Studies that have looked at the addition of ARB to background therapy, including the aforementioned Val-HeFT [63], CHARM-Added [68], and VALIANT [67], that already includes ACE-I have also not shown any clear benefit of ARB in addition to ACE-I in reducing mortality in HF-REF.

β-Adrenergic Blockade

The cornerstone of heart failure treatment is neurohormonal blockade of the RAAS and adrenergic systems. According to the European guidelines, ACE inhibition is the first line of therapy, with the initiation of β-blockers (BB) once the patient is clinically stable and ACE inhibitors have been optimized. This paradigm of treatment has resulted in some degree of controversy, pertaining to whether adrenergic blockade should be the front-runner in medical therapy as opposed to ACE inhibition due to its greater impact on sudden death and its initial presence in the sequence of maladaptive neurohormonal activation [69].

The Carvedilol and ACE-Inhibitor Remodeling Mild Heart Failure Evaluation (CARMEN) and the Cardiac Insufficiency Bisoprolol Study (CIBIS) III studies challenged the concept of ACE inhibitors as first-line treatment in CHF. CARMEN explored the need for combined treatment of ACE-I and β-blocker, as well as the order of introduction of these therapies in HF patients with mild, chronic symptoms. They found that combination therapy is superior to ACE-I alone for left ventricular (LV) remodeling as assessed by LV end-systolic volume index on transthoracic echocardiography. When assessing whether introduction of enalapril or carvedilol first had an impact on outcomes, they found that introduction of carvedilol first had a nonsignificant trend toward benefit. The authors concluded that introduction of beta-blockade should not be delayed [70].

CIBIS III was designed to assess the effectiveness of bisoprolol for 6 months followed by combination therapy with enalapril compared to enalapril for 6 months followed by combination therapy with bisoprolol. HF patients with stable mild to moderate symptoms demonstrated non-inferiority of initial initiation of bisoprolol or enalapril in only the intention-to-treat sample for a combined end point of all-cause mortality or hospitalization. However, there was notably more frequent HF events (defined as requiring hospitalization or occurring in the hospital) observed in the bisoprolol group [71]. As a result, first-line treatment with either ACE inhibitors or BB should be based on personalized medicine.

The Metoprolol CR/XL Randomised Intervention Trial in Congestive Heart Failure (MERIT-HF) study group investigated whether metoprolol succinate controlled release/extended release (CR/XL) once daily, in addition to standard therapy, would lower mortality in patients with decreased ejection fraction (EF) and HF symptoms. The study randomized approximately 2,000 NYHA class II–VI patients with chronic HF and with LVEF ≤40 % to either metoprolol succinate or placebo. All-cause mortality, sudden death, and death from worsening HF were lower in the metoprolol group [72].

The CIBIS study group investigated the efficacy of bisoprolol, a β_1-selective adrenoceptor blocker, in decreasing all-cause mortality in chronic HF. In a multicenter trial in Europe, they randomized 2,647 NYHA III–IV patients with LVEF ≤35 % receiving standard therapy with diuretics and ACE-I to bisoprolol or placebo. CIBIS-II was stopped early because bisoprolol showed a significant mortality benefit. Treatment effects were independent of the severity or cause of heart failure. The authors concluded that β-blocker therapy had benefits for survival in stable heart failure patients [73].

The Carvedilol Prospective Randomized Cumulative Survival (COPERNICUS) trial demonstrated the beneficial effects of carvedilol, a mixed β_1-, β_2-, and α_1-blocker, on mortality in NYHA class IV patients with chronic HF, with reduction in 1-year mortality from 19.6 % to 11 %, when compared to placebo. All subgroups including those with the most advanced HF showed the same beneficial direction of effect [74]. The Carvedilol or Metoprolol European Trial (COMET) reported a significant survival benefit for carvedilol when compared to metoprolol tartrate in patients with mild-to-severe chronic heart failure [75]. However, the implications of COMET are not fully clear, as critics have argued that the target dosing of metoprolol tartrate (50 mg twice daily) and carvedilol (25 mg twice daily) was not equivalent, with the carvedilol dose being substantially higher [76]. Further, others have argued that long-acting metoprolol succinate should have been directly compared to carvedilol rather than the shorter-acting metoprolol tartrate to achieve more steady-state β-blockade over each 24-h period.

Oral Vasodilators

Hydralazine increases intracellular cyclic guanosine monophosphate (cGMP) to promote smooth muscle relaxation, primarily in the arterioles with reduction in afterload. Nitrates act on the nitric oxide pathway to activate guanylate cyclase and increase cGMP, with predominant venodilation at low doses and vasodilation at higher doses. The original Vasodilator-Heart Failure Trial (V-HeFT) study randomized HF-REF patients who were on background digoxin and diuretic to receive additional therapy with placebo, prazosin (α1-blocker), or combination of isosorbide dinitrate-hydralazine (ISDN-HYD). They found that mortality was lower in the ISDN-HYD cohort compared to placebo at 2 years. Prazosin demonstrated no benefit compared to placebo. Thus, it appeared that ISDN-HYD has potential benefit in chronic HF [77]. However, it should be kept in mind that these patients were not on a background therapy of ACE-I and β-blockade. Subsequently, V-HeFT II randomized 804 patients to either ISDN-HYD or enalapril on background therapy of digoxin and diuretics. The study showed that enalapril resulted in significantly improved survival compared to ISDN-HYD in HF patients [78].

However, there appeared to less benefit of ACE-I compared to ISDN-HYD in African

American patients in V-HeFT II. This led to the African American Heart Failure Trial (A-HeFT), which randomized 1,050 NYHA class III–VI HF patients self-described as African American to fixed-dose ISDN-HYD or placebo in addition to standard background therapy that included neurohormonal blockade (including ACE-I, ARB, β-blockers, aldosterone antagonists on the discretion of their regular physicians). The study was terminated early due to significantly improved survival in the ISDN-HYD arm. ISDN-HYD was also associated with improved quality of life. This suggests that there are additional mechanisms of heart failure progression, perhaps decreased NO bioavailability not treated by standard neurohormonal blockade, which are favorably impacted by combined ISDN-HYD [79].

Pulmonary hypertension (PH) is present in 68–78 % of patients with chronic severe LV systolic dysfunction (LVSD) and is commonly associated with right ventricular (RV) dysfunction. Pulmonary vascular resistance (PVR) and RV performance are important determinants of exercise capacity and prognosis in patients with LVSD. The hypothesis that sildenafil, an effective therapy for pulmonary arterial hypertension, would lower PVR and improve exercise capacity in patients with HF complicated by PH was tested in a group of 34 symptomatic HF patients with PH. The patients were randomized to 12 weeks of treatment with sildenafil (25–75 mg orally three times daily) or placebo. Patients underwent cardiopulmonary exercise testing before and after treatment, with greater improvement in pVO_2 for the sildenafil group. Sildenafil reduced PVR and increased cardiac output with exercise without altering pulmonary capillary wedge or mean arterial pressure, heart rate, or systemic vascular resistance. The ability of sildenafil to augment pVO_2 correlated directly with baseline resting PVR and indirectly with baseline resting right ventricular ejection fraction (RVEF). Sildenafil also improved 6-min walk distance and Minnesota Living with Heart Failure score. The sildenafil cohort experienced fewer HF hospitalizations but had a higher incidence of headache without incurring other serious adverse events. Thus, phosphodiesterase 5 inhibition with sildenafil may improve exercise capacity and quality of life in patients with systolic HF with secondary PH [80].

Antiarrhythmic Therapy

Despite a steady decline in the risk of death from pump failure, many patients remain at high risk for sudden cardiac death (SCD). It accounts for one third to one half of the deaths in patients with HF [81]. Severity of HF is associated with higher overall mortality and higher rate of SCD [72]. Patients with HF are at risk of ventricular arrhythmias, ranging from asymptomatic ventricular premature beats to sustained ventricular tachycardia (VT) or ventricular fibrillation (VF), which can develop into malignant form and can lead to SCD. Some studies have shown arrhythmias not to be the only cause of SCD [82]. Regardless, prevention of arrhythmias remains the key strategy for reducing the risk of SCD.

Most clinical trials of implantable cardioverter/defibrillator (ICD) therapy have demonstrated the superiority of ICD to conventional medical therapy in reducing overall mortality. Most of the antiarrhythmic medications, along with their antiarrhythmic effect, are associated with pro-arrhythmic effects limiting their use as an adjunct to the ICD therapy. Currently, the only antiarrhythmics considered safe for use in HF patients with ventricular arrhythmias are amiodarone and dofetilide. Early trials with amiodarone including the Grupo de Estudio de la Sobrevida en la Insuficiencia Cardiaca en Argentina (GESICA) trial [83] found a significant benefit to mortality and SCD, while the Veterans Affairs Congestive HF Survival Trial of Antiarrhythmic Therapy (CHF-STAT) trial [84] found no benefit in terms of mortality or SCD. Thus, amiodarone is not routinely used in the absence of significant arrhythmias. Other studies have demonstrated increased mortality with sotalol [85] and dronedarone [86] in HF-REF. Radiofrequency ablation and surgical options can also be considered in selected patient populations. In patients with prior MI, the border zone of the infarct is frequently the site of the reentrant circuit, and these sites are often amenable to ablation.

Since most HF patients receive β-blocker therapy, some studies have shown that using β-adrenergic blockers in patients with reduced systolic function and HF symptoms leads to significant reductions in overall mortality rates, which is in part related to reduced SCD. The reduced rate of SCD was 3.9 % versus 6.6 % in MERIT-HF [72] and 3.6 % versus 6.3 % in CIBIS-II [73].

Implantable Cardioverter/Defibrillator

Because of the survival benefit of ICDs as compared with medical therapy, ICDs are the treatment of choice for the primary and secondary prevention of malignant arrhythmias which lead to SCD.

Secondary Prevention

Based on the results of three major clinical trials: Cardiac Arrest Study Hamburg (CASH) [87], Canadian Implantable Defibrillator Study (CIDS) [88], and The Antiarrhythmics Versus Implantable Defibrillators (AVID) [89], which compared ICD to pharmacologic therapy in SCD survivors and other high-risk patients with sustained VT, patients who have survived SCD or had sustained VT are recommended to get an ICD because of their high risk for the development of malignant arrhythmia and SCD. Similarly, all patients who have syncope with either spontaneous or induced sustained VT also should get an ICD. It is unclear whether all patients with unexplained syncope should undergo ICD placement. According to the Heart Rhythm Society guidelines, ICD implantation is recommended if there is significant LV dysfunction due to non-ischemic cardiomyopathy in patients with unexplained syncope [90]. On the other hand, patients with ischemic cardiomyopathy and LV dysfunction (LVEF ≤30 %) qualify for an ICD even in the absence of syncope [91].

Primary Prevention

In asymptomatic patients, there is a mortality benefit with prophylactic use of ICD therapy. Multicenter Automatic Defibrillator Implantation Trial (MADIT) I was the first trial to show that an ICD has a role in primary prevention of SCD. However, the trial enrolled a subselective cohort of patients with prior MI, nonsustained VT, LVEF ≤35 %, and inducible sustained monomorphic VT [91]. The Multicenter Unsustained Tachycardia Trial (MUSTT) trial showed that patients with prior MI, asymptomatic nonsustained VT, LVEF ≤40 %, and inducible sustained VT had reduced sudden cardiac death with ICD implantation for primary prevention [92]. MADIT II was subsequently carried out to expand the population compared to earlier studies, enrolling patients with LVEF ≤30 % more than 30 days post-MI. Unlike the earlier studies, electrophysiologic testing and presence of nonsustained VT were not required for enrollment. Patients were randomized to ICD or medical therapy, with the trial terminated early due to significant reduction in all-cause mortality for the ICD cohort, due to reduction in sudden cardiac death [93].

The Sudden Cardiac Death in Heart Failure (SCD-HeFT) trial included all HF patients with LVEF ≤35 % and NYHA class II–III, regardless of ischemic or non-ischemic etiology. Patients were randomized to either ICD implantation, amiodarone, or placebo. At 5 years, mortality was significantly improved with ICD therapy in both ischemic and non-ischemic cardiomyopathy. Amiodarone had no impact on survival [94]. The decision to use ICD therapy in asymptomatic patients with non-ischemic cardiomyopathy can be challenging. Different risk prediction methods (e.g., microvolt T-wave alternans) [95] have been used to predict the risk of arrhythmia, without the identification of any clear risk stratifiers. Some patients might die because of arrhythmia despite ICD therapy, which may be related to heart failure severity or frequency of appropriate and inappropriate shocks received from ICD versus no shocks, as was demonstrated from the SCD-HeFT trial results [96].

The most recent AHA/ACC guidelines [97] for primary prevention with ICD recommend implantation for (1) LVEF ≤35 % due to prior MI, who are at least 40 days post-MI and NYHA class II–III; (2) LVEF ≤35 % in non-ischemic dilated cardiomyopathy who are NYHA class

II–III; (3) LVEF ≤30 % due to prior MI, who are at least 40 days post-MI and NYHA class I; and (4) LVEF ≤40 % due to prior MI, with nonsustained VT and inducible VF or VT at electrophysiological study.

Cardiac Resynchronization Therapy (CRT)

A growing body of evidence suggests that the use of implantable devices to resynchronize ventricular contraction may be a beneficial adjunct in the treatment of chronic heart failure. One third of patients with chronic heart failure have electrocardiographic evidence of a major intraventricular conduction delay, which may worsen left ventricular systolic dysfunction through asynchronous ventricular contraction. Uncontrolled studies suggest that multisite biventricular pacing improves hemodynamics and well-being by reducing ventricular asynchrony.

The Multisite Stimulation in Cardiomyopathies (MUSTIC) trial showed that CRT in NYHA class III HF-REF patients with QRS ≥150 ms resulted in improvement in 6-min walk distance, quality of life, and pVO_2, with reduced hospitalizations [98]. In the Multicenter InSync Randomized Clinical Evaluation (MIRACLE) trial, patients with NYHA class III-IV HF from either ischemic or non-ischemic cardiomyopathy, LVEF ≤35 %, LVEDD ≥55 mm, and QRS duration of ≥130 ms were randomized to CRT or conventional therapy. Patients randomized to CRT had an improvement in 6-min walk distance, quality of life, functional class, time on treadmill during exercise testing, and ejection fraction. Further, CRT reduced hospitalization compared to control [99]. The Comparison of Medical Therapy, Pacing, and Defibrillation in Chronic Heart Failure (COMPANION) trial randomized NYHA class III–IV patients with LVEF ≤35 % and QRS ≥120 ms to receive optimal pharmacologic therapy (diuretics, ACE-I, β-blockers, and spironolactone) alone or in combination with CRT with either a pacemaker or a pacemaker-defibrillator. CRT with either pacemaker or pacemaker-defibrillator resulted in reduction of the primary end point of time to all-cause mortality or hospitalization by 34 % and 40 %, respectively, when compared to pharmacologic-only therapy. The authors concluded that CRT decreases the combined risk of death from any cause or first hospitalization and, when combined with an ICD, significantly reduces mortality [100]. The Cardiac Resynchronization Heart Failure (CARE-HF) study randomized patients with NYHA class III–IV HF, LVEF ≤35 %, and cardiac dyssynchrony to CRT or standard pharmacologic therapy. CRT reduced time to all-cause mortality or cardiovascular hospitalization [37], with reduction in mortality that persisted to an extended follow-up of 38 months [101]. Further, CRT reduced the interventricular mechanical delay, the end-systolic volume index, and the area of the mitral regurgitant jet; increased the LVEF; and improved symptoms and the quality of life. The authors concluded that in patients with heart failure and cardiac dyssynchrony, cardiac resynchronization improves symptoms and the quality of life as well as reducing complications and the risk of death. The beneficial effects of CRT in this group of patients were impressive, considering that these patients were receiving optimal medical therapy with diuretics, β-blockers, spironolactone, ACE-I, or ARB at the time of enrollment. The results showed that for every nine devices implanted, one death and three hospital stays were prevented [37].

Other studies have explored the use of CRT in patients with milder HF symptoms. Resynchronization Reverses Remodeling in Systolic Left Ventricular Dysfunction (REVERSE) demonstrated that in NYHA class I–II symptoms with LVEF ≤40 % and QRS ≥120 ms, CRT resulted in a reduction in HF hospitalization, with improvement of ventricular structure and function. However, the REVERSE study did not examine the impact of CRT on mortality in these patients with milder HF symptoms [102]. The Resynchronization-Defibrillation for Ambulatory Heart Failure Trial (RAFT) randomized patients with NYHA class II–III HF, with LVEF ≤30 %, intrinsic QRS ≥120 ms, or paced QRS ≥200 ms to ICD alone compared to ICD plus CRT. With CRT, there was a reduction in a combined end point all-cause mortality or HF hospitalization. Independently, there was a reduction in mortality alone. However, there was increased rate of device-related complications in the CRT cohort [103]. The recent MADIT-CRT trial explored the use of CRT in patients with NYHA class I–II HF, LVEF ≤30 %, and QRS ≥130 ms, showing a reduction in a composite of all-cause mortality and nonfatal HF event, but was predominantly driven by a 41 % reduction in risk of HF events. There was no difference in risk of death alone [104]. The 2012 AHA/ACC class I recommendation for CRT includes patients with LVEF ≤35 %, sinus rhythm, left bundle branch block (LBBB) morphology with QRS≥150 ms, and NYHA class II–IV symptoms. Class IIa indications include expanded criteria including LBBB with QRS duration of 120–149 ms, non-LBBB with QRS ≥150 ms, and in patients with atrial fibrillation if they require ventricular pacing [105].

After CRT implantation, optimization may be considered. Mullens and colleagues evaluated 75 ambulatory patients with CRT with persistent advanced HF symptoms and/or adverse reverse remodeling referred for CRT optimization. Eighty-eight percent of patients had significantly better echocardiographic indexes of LV filling and LV ejection with optimal setting of their CRT compared with VVI (ventricular pacing, ventricular sensing, inhibition) setting. Most patients had identifiable reasons for suboptimal response, including inadequate device settings (47 %), suboptimal medical treatment (32 %), arrhythmias (32 %), inappropriate lead position (21 %), or lack of baseline dyssynchrony (9 %). Device settings or therapies were modified in 74 % of cases, with a decrease in adverse events [106].

Other studies have sought to determine the effects of CRT on quality of life (QoL). CARE-HF showed that CRT improved QoL (measured with European Quality of Life-5 Dimensions and Minnesota Living with Heart Failure questionnaires) at each timepoint of 3 months, 18 months, and study-end with median follow-up of 29.6 months, mostly due to improved physical functioning. Thus, CRT improves QoL with sustained effects [107].

Further studies have examined the impact of CRT on patients with narrower QRS than the standard criteria. The evaluation of CRT in narrow QRS patients with mechanical dyssynchrony from a multicenter study (ESTEEM-CRT) trial evaluated CRT in patients with QRS ≤120 ms, NYHA class III, LVEF ≤35 %, and mechanical dyssynchrony (standard deviation of time to peak velocity of 12 segments more than 28.7 ms) as a multicenter, nonrandomized, unblinded feasibility trial to determine the effects CRT in this population. Patients with CRT had improvement in QoL and NYHA functional class at 6 months. There was no improvement in pVO_2, LVEF, left ventricular end-systolic volume (LVESV), and left ventricular end-diastolic volume (LVEDV). Mechanical dyssynchrony remained unchanged [108]. One important limitation of this study was the nonblinded single arm design, suggesting that symptom improvement may have been related to a placebo effect.

The Cardiac Resynchronization Therapy in Patients with Heart Failure and Narrow QRS (RethinQ) study sought to determine if CRT benefits individuals with QRS ≤130 ms. They randomized 172 NYHA class III HF patients with LVEF ≤35 %, QRS ≤130 ms, and evidence of mechanical dyssynchrony on echocardiography undergoing ICD to either CRT or no CRT, with a primary end point of increase in pVO_2 of 1.0 cc/kg/min by cardiopulmonary testing at 6 months. They found that there was no difference with CRT in the total cohort. In a subcohort of individuals with QRS ≥120 ms, there was apparent benefit with CRT. CRT does not appear to result in improvement in pVO_2 in HF patients with narrow QRS intervals [109]. It is estimated, however, that approximately 15 % of patients with CHF meet the current indications for CRT. Moreover, clinical trials have demonstrated that approximately 30–40 % of these patients are considered nonresponders clinically or based on echocardiographic remodeling [110]. Therefore, the actual number of patients who benefit from CRT is quite small relative to that of the entire CHF patient population.

ESTEEM-CRT and RethinQ suggest that perhaps echocardiographic tissue Doppler failed to identify patients who would respond to CRT with a narrow QRS and mechanical dyssynchrony or that this patient population does not actually benefit from CRT. Interestingly, when baseline characteristics are compared between the ESTEEM-CRT and RethinQ patient populations, it is evident that the patients in the RethinQ study appeared to be more sick with a lower baseline peak VO_2 and larger LVESV and LVEDV. In addition, there was a higher percentage of non-ischemic patients in the RethinQ patient population as compared with that of the ESTEEM-CRT. Regardless, neither trial identified patients with a narrow QRS and echocardiographic evidence of dyssynchrony who benefited from CRT. In light of these data, the question remains whether or not tissue Doppler is the appropriate diagnostic tool for identifying dyssynchrony in this patient population or whether it is a technology searching for an application. It has been suggested that "Until other technologies for evaluating mechanical dyssynchrony emerge and demonstrate efficacy in large-scale randomized clinical trials, patients with narrow QRS should not receive CRT" [111].

Surgical Management of Heart Failure

Coronary Revascularization Therapy

High-risk revascularization may constitute the treatment of choice in the subgroup of advanced HF patients with ischemic cardiomyopathy, LVEF ≤35 %, viable myocardium, and vessels suitable for grafting. Different trials have suggested the benefit of revascularization in advanced heart failure if angina [112–117] is present. There are several key questions in the management of patients with symptomatic heart failure, left ventricular dysfunction, and coronary artery disease (CAD) amenable to coronary artery bypass grafting (CABG):

- Does surgical coronary revascularization in addition to aggressive medical management confer long-term mortality, morbidity, QoL, or cost benefit beyond aggressive medical management alone?
- Does surgical ventricular shape restoration in combination with CABG improve outcome compared to coronary revascularization alone and medical therapy alone [118]?

To assess the effect of CABG on future risk of death in patients with HF-REF, mortality and modes of death in 5,410 patients with ischemic LV dysfunction from the Studies of Left Ventricular Dysfunction (SOLVD) trials were retrospectively evaluated. Outcomes of patients with and without prior CABG were compared, and stratification by baseline LVEF (≤0.25, 0.25–0.30, and ≥0.30 %) was performed. Prior CABG was associated with a 25 % reduction in risk of death and a 46 % reduction in risk of sudden death independent of LVEF and severity of symptoms [119]. The Veteran Affairs Cooperative Study of Surgery and the Coronary Artery Surgery Study (CASS) confirmed these findings, showing a higher survival rate in HF-REF after CABG compared to medical therapy [120]. The benefits appear to be transient and last shorter than 11 years, with benefit diminished after graft closure. Low-risk patients had no survival benefit with CABG [121].

The Surgical Treatment of Ischemic Heart Failure (STICH) trial was an international randomized controlled clinical trial evaluating the use of CABG on heart failure patients with CAD [122]. In the primary study, 1,212 patients with LVEF ≤35 % were randomized to CABG compared to medical therapy alone. Over a median follow-up of 56 months, there was no significant difference between CABG compared to medical therapy alone for all-cause mortality (HR 0.86, 95 % CI: 0.72–1.04, $p=0.12$). Secondary outcomes appeared to favor CABG compared to medical therapy alone, including cardiovascular mortality. There was significant crossover of the study groups, with 17 % of the medical group receiving CABG and 9 % of patients assigned to CABG not undergoing surgery. An as-treated analysis showed an apparent benefit of CABG compared to medical therapy alone at 1 year ($p \leq 0.001$) [122].

Recent studies have confirmed that CABG on patients with severely depressed LVEF gave a satisfactory survival rate, approaching that of cardiac transplantation. Selection of patients for high-risk myocardial revascularization involves considerations about potential systemic comorbidities like chronic pulmonary disease, renal failure requiring dialysis, cancer, or severe advanced diabetes. Myocardial dysfunction in patients with ischemic cardiomyopathy may be due to impaired blood flow leading to oxygen supply/demand imbalance. This condition can result in myocardial stunning and/or hibernation (which may be reversible after CABG) or scarring. Myocardial stunning follows an acute episode of cardiac ischemia and leads to reversible reduced systolic and diastolic function. Hibernation was described in the late 1980s, and is characterized by decreased myocardial function concomitant with a reduction in blood supply. The identification of viable myocardium usually allows confirmation of contractile reserve, preserved metabolic activity, and myocyte membrane integrity and is associated with convincing improvements in left ventricular function after coronary revascularization. The techniques employed to identify the presence of hibernation include positron emission tomography (PET) with fluorodeoxyglucose (FDG), which is limited by its high costs and availability. Myocardial viability can be demonstrated by dobutamine stress echocardiography and by its predictive biphasic response, characterized by an initial improvement in myocardial contractility at low doses of dobutamine infusion, followed by a decrease at high doses. Nevertheless, the most promising imaging technique seems to be magnetic resonance with gadolinium enhancement because it can reveal scar or viable muscle. Both hibernating and stunned myocardium contribute to progressive systolic dysfunction, remodeling, and the development of HF. Rahimtoola et al. [123] have recently suggested a unifying concept of hibernation and remodeling with emphasis on the importance of early revascularization. In fact, remodeling appears to progress over time, and the ability to reverse the process may be time-sensitive [124].

It has long been suggested that if no viable myocardium is present, the prospect of improvement with revascularization is reduced and, thus, cardiac transplantation should be considered for appropriate candidates [125–128]. Recently, a substudy from the STICH trial assessed the impact of myocardial viability on outcomes after CABG versus medical therapy for ischemic heart disease in 601 HF-REF patients who underwent viability testing with either single photon emission computed tomography (SPECT) or dobutamine echocardiography at the discretion of the recruiting investigators. It demonstrated that viability at baseline did not appear to be associated with all-cause mortality over 5 years and had no interaction with the effectiveness of CABG or medical therapy. The presence of viability did not identify patients with differential survival from CABG compared to medical therapy [129]. The STICH viability substudy must be interpreted with caution due to the loss of true randomization as a subcohort and the fact that the main STICH study had a negative end point, making any further analyses exploratory. Also, the interpretation may either be that viability is not associated with improved survival after CABG but can also be viewed that the lack of viability should not exclude CABG.

Mitral Valve Repair

Severe mitral regurgitation (MR) is a frequent complication of end-stage cardiomyopathy that contributes to HF and predicts a poor survival. A group at University of Michigan, Ann Arbor, studied the intermediate-term outcome of mitral reconstruction in 48 NYHA class III–IV patients with severe 4+ mitral regurgitation (LVEF 16 % ± 3 %) who underwent annuloplasty with improvement to mild MR in 7 and no MR in 41 patients. One- and two-year actuarial survivals were 82 % and 71 %. HF hospitalizations post-MR repair decreased, NYHA functional class improved, and LV volume and sphericity decreased, while LVEF and cardiac output increased [130]. Another group explored the outcomes in a series of 40 patients with LVEF ≤35 % and moderate to severe secondary MR who underwent mitral valve replacement or repair. They found that at mean follow-up of 50 + 34 months, patients had improved NYHA class and improved LVEF, without any difference in survival after mitral valve repair or replacement and with no difference in mortality compared to age- and period-matched controls who underwent cardiac transplantation instead [131].

Ventricular Reconstruction

There has been significant interest in ventricular reconstruction, with the theory that improving LV geometry will theoretically improve function and may translate to better outcomes. Surgical anterior ventricular endocardial restoration (SAVER) involves the exclusion of noncontracting segments in the dilated remodeled LV after anterior myocardial infarction. An international study was performed, with 439 patients undergoing SAVER and followed for 18 months. Concomitant procedures included CABG in 89 %, mitral valve repair in 22 %, and mitral valve replacement in 4 % of patients. After SAVER, there was improvement in LVEF and reduction in LV end-systolic volume index. In-hospital mortality was 6.6 %, with 18-month survival of 84 % in the total cohort [132].

A study at the Cleveland Clinic followed the echocardiographic changes and functional outcome from mitral valve repair combined with partial left ventriculectomy (the Batista procedure) in 57 patients, primarily (95 %) transplant candidates with idiopathic dilated cardiomyopathy. Forty percent of patients were hospitalized on inotropes, with all patients previously NYHA class IV (36.8 % improved to class III by time of surgery). At 3 months, there was improvement in LV end- diastolic diameter (from 8.1 ± 1.0 cm to 6.3 ± 0.9 cm), LVEF (from 13.6 ± 6 % to 23 ± 7.7%), improvement in NYHA functional class, and improved pVO_2. Actuarial survival at 1 year was 82.1 %, and freedom from death, relisting for transplantation, and need for LVAD support was 58 % [133].

The Reconstructive Endoventricular Surgery Returning Torsion Original Radius Elliptical Shape (RESTORE) to the LV study tested how surgical ventricular restoration affects early and late survival in a registry of 1,198 post-anterior infarction HF patients with LVEF ≤35 % between 1998 and 2003. Concomitant procedures included CABG in 95 %, mitral valve repair in 22 %, and mitral valve replacement in 1 %. LVEF improved from 29.6 ± 11.0 % preoperatively to 39.5 ± 12.3 % postoperatively ($p \leq 0.001$), and NYHA functional class also improved in the majority of patients. Overall 30-day survival was 94.7 %, and 5-year survival was 68.6 %. Based on these results, it was felt that surgical ventricular restoration improves LV function [134].

In a substudy of the previously mentioned STICH trial, the use of surgical ventricular reconstruction in addition to CABG compared to CABG alone was examined [135]. They found that patients undergoing CABG with surgical ventricular reconstruction had a reduction in 19 % of end-systolic volume index, while those undergoing CABG alone had a decrease of 6 % in end-systolic volume index ($p < 0.001$). However, there was no significant difference in the primary outcome of all-cause mortality or cardiac hospitalization ($p = 0.90$). Symptoms of patients in each treatment arm were followed, and patients in both groups had improvement of 1.7 CCS angina class ($p = 0.84$) and approximately 1 NYHA HF class ($p = 0.70$). There was also no significant difference in median distance by 6-min walk test ($p = 0.80$). Thus, even though surgical vascular reconstruction appeared to reduce LV volume, this did not translate to clinically meaningful outcomes [135].

Mechanical Circulatory Support Device Implantation

Recompensation after development of advanced HF includes appropriate neurohormonal blockade. Specifically, targets include the adrenergic system, RAAS, antidiuretic hormone system, and the atrial natriuretic peptide system, which are chronically activated in increasing stages of advanced heart failure. If a patient is deemed unsuccessfully recompensated despite maximal tolerated medical therapy, revascularization, and CRT, then one needs to risk stratify the patient for possible urgent heart transplant or MCSD.

Risk stratification of patients with end-stage congestive heart failure is a critical component of the selection process in identifying the best treatment for a given patient. For example, for patients with refractory HF, the choice between optimal medical therapy, heart transplantation, and chronic mechanical circulatory support has to be made. Accurate identification of individuals most likely to survive without a transplant would facilitate more efficient use of scarce donor organs.

Advanced heart failure therapy with MCSD is currently being practiced in approximately 200 selected hospitals out of ≥3,000 in the USA alone. In order to provide equitable and high-quality access to MCSD therapy, a referral network has to be in place. This network requires a structure similar to the referral network for heart transplantation and includes the local general practitioner, internist and cardiologist, the local and regional hospital, and the tertiary care center. The referral is often initiated by the local or regional colleagues who are taking care of a patient at a stage of the advanced heart failure syndrome that is not sufficiently responsive to medical therapy. Upon contacting the tertiary care center, patient history information is shared between the two hospitals. If the patient is deemed to likely benefit from evaluation for mechanical circulatory support, the transfer is initiated.

Advanced Heart Failure Transfer Decision Making

The decision of a local center to ask for transfer of a patient to a center providing MCSD therapy or cardiac transplant is followed by an evaluation and decision of the accepting MCSD/cardiac transplant center. This evaluation is critically important. A transfer is in the interest of a patient who has a higher chance of longevity and good quality of life with more advanced therapies but not for a patient who is either too well or too ill for these potential options.

Tertiary Center Outreach Team

The MCSD/cardiac transplant center may organize an outreach team on call. This team can perform the evaluation in the transfer-requesting hospital. This approach is advantageous for (1) the patient (minimizing unnecessary transfers), (2) the transferring hospital (maximizing educational decision-making experience), and (3) the MCSD/cardiac transplant center (minimizing medically unnecessary resource consumption and maximizing networking in the region).

Decision-Making Algorithm

The decision-making algorithm is initiated when the patient is referred for evaluation into an established MCSD/cardiac transplant center [136–139]. Referral takes place to a designated center when the treating cardiologist or internist has exhausted all lifestyle and medical options without success in the setting of decompensation and progression of advanced heart failure (AHF), a phase known to be associated with a high risk of death. Anytime during management, if a patient is felt to be too end stage to benefit from any of the modern therapies because of multiorgan failure or other comorbidities, there should be ongoing discussions regarding comfort care as a way to facilitate a humane form of death instead of prolongation of suffering [13, 14]. A structured management algorithm should be applied to recompensate the patient and initiate neurohormonal blockade and lifestyle changes, or if recompensation cannot be achieved and the patient is not a suitable candidate for cardiac transplantation, destination MCSD therapy should be considered. In 2005, the International Society Heart Lung Transplantation (ISHLT) organized a consensus conference to provide clinical evidence and expert opinion and experience-based guidelines for consideration of MCSD implantation [26]. More recently in 2013, ISHLT released an executive summary for the use of mechanical circulatory support devices [140]. Care must be taken in MCSD-centers to adhere to evidence-based destination-MCSD-implantation guidelines and not to inadvertently drift to other patient-selection criteria, either patients who are less sick or patients who are sicker than the original Randomized Evaluation of Mechanical Assistance for the Treatment of Congestive Heart Failure (REMATCH) cohort and therefore would have a survival/QoL benefit that would be difficult to predict [6] (see Fig. 2.2).

Patient Selection for MCSD

Despite the potential for explosive growth for MCSD in the future with the aging population, there are no definitive patient-selection criteria for ventricular assist device (VAD) use. Patient selection must take into account the (1) appropriateness for device therapy based on patient condition and (2) risk to the patient.

The landmark REMATCH trial randomized patients with NYHA class IV HF on maximal medical therapy for 90 days, LVEF ≤25 %, and with pVO_2 ≤12 mL/kg/min (later expanded to 14) who were ineligible for cardiac transplantation to a pulsatile, first-generation LVAD compared to optimal medical management. LVAD implantation significantly improved survival compared to medical therapy (relative risk 0.52 with 95 % confidence interval of 0.34–0.78; $p = 0.001$). Quality of life was also improved in the LVAD group [141].

Given this clear benefit in the selective REMATCH cohort, it could be suggested that this population should be eligible for LVAD. However, this excludes a large proportion of patients with advanced HF, including those who are functionally better than NYHA class IV, LVEF better than 25 %, or who are not yet excluded from transplant candidacy. Despite this gap, no consensus guidelines for MCSD or VAD candidacy have been established [142]. Rather, patients continue to be evaluated for VAD implantation across most centers in the USA on a case-by-case basis. Typical inclusion criteria include patients unable to be weaned from inotropic support, who develop intolerance to medical therapies, have poor functional capacity, and cannot be restored to a reasonable NYHA class despite maximal medical therapy.

More recent studies with MCSD have been aimed at newer generations of VAD and development of the total artificial heart (TAH). For example, it was demonstrated that the Heartmate II (Thoratec Corporation, Pleasanton, CA), a second-generation continuous-flow VAD, can be successfully utilized for hemodynamic support as a bridge to cardiac transplantation [143] and that it appears to improve survival free from disabling stroke and reoperation, as well as actuarial survival rates, at 2 years as compared to the first-generation pulsatile devices [144]. It has also been demonstrated that TAH may be a viable alternative to patients as a bridge to transplant in critically ill patients with biventricular failure [145].

The centers for Medicare and Medicaid services (CMS) have requirements in place for reimbursement for MCSD. However, criteria for VAD use in the post-cardiotomy setting or as bridge to cardiac transplantation are not well defined. For destination therapy, current CMS criteria mirror the inclusion criteria from the REMATCH trial [81]. A recent review by Wilson et al. tackles this problem and includes an extensive list of indications, relative contraindications, and absolute contraindications to VAD implantation [142]. The recommendations incorporate a combination of REMATCH inclusion criteria, CMS reimbursement requirements, case series, anecdotal reports, published literature, and experience from general clinical practice.

Heart Transplantation

Based on the initial evaluation and failure of recompensation measures, a patient may be designated as a "potential transplant candidate," who could be placed on a national "potential transplant candidate list." This algorithm combines the psychological benefit for the patient of being accepted by the program with an ongoing openness to a diversity of advanced HF treatment modalities, not committing to transplantation as the only therapeutic option. If the initial evaluation reveals hemodynamic instability and therefore cardiac transplant evaluation and listing is completed, follow-up may still lead to stabilization without transplantation enabling delisting in individual cases.

References

1. Roger VL, Go AS, Lloyd-Jones DM, Benjamin EJ, Berry JD, Borden WB, et al. Heart disease and stroke statistics–2012 update: a report from the American Heart Association. Circulation. 2012;125(1):e2–220.
2. Lloyd-Jones D, Adams R, Carnethon M, De Simone G, Ferguson TB, Flegal K, et al. Heart disease and stroke statistics–2009 update: a report from the American Heart Association Statistics Committee and Stroke Statistics Subcommittee. Circulation. 2009;119(3):480–6.

3. Cappuccio FP. Commentary: epidemiological transition, migration, and cardiovascular disease. Int J Epidemiol. 2004;33(2):387–8.
4. Hunt SA, Abraham WT, Chin MH, Feldman AM, Francis GS, Ganiats TG, et al. ACC/AHA 2005 Guideline update for the diagnosis and management of chronic heart failure in the adult: a report of the American College of Cardiology/American Heart Association Task Force on practice guidelines (writing committee to update the 2001 guidelines for the evaluation and management of heart failure): developed in collaboration with the American College of Chest Physicians and the International Society for Heart and Lung Transplantation: endorsed by the Heart Rhythm Society. Circulation. 2005;112(12):e154–235.
5. Deng MC, Naka Y. Circulatory support in advanced heart failure. Cardiol Rev. 2002;19:28–35.
6. Deng MC. The challenges of generating evidence to guide mechanical circulatory support-based management of advanced heart failure. Eur Heart J. 2005;26(10):953–5.
7. Jessup M, Brozena S. Heart failure. N Engl J Med. 2003;348(20):2007–18.
8. Owan TE, Hodge DO, Herges RM, Jacobsen SJ, Roger VL, Redfield MM. Trends in prevalence and outcome of heart failure with preserved ejection fraction. N Engl J Med. 2006;355(3):251–9.
9. Vasan RS, Larson MG, Benjamin EJ, Evans JC, Reiss CK, Levy D. Congestive heart failure in subjects with normal versus reduced left ventricular ejection fraction: prevalence and mortality in a population-based cohort. J Am Coll Cardiol. 1999;33(7):1948–55.
10. Gottdiener JS, McClelland RL, Marshall R, Shemanski L, Furberg CD, Kitzman DW, et al. Outcome of congestive heart failure in elderly persons: influence of left ventricular systolic function. The cardiovascular health study. Ann Intern Med. 2002;137(8):631–9.
11. Senni M, Tribouilloy CM, Rodeheffer RJ, Jacobsen SJ, Evans JM, Bailey KR, et al. Congestive heart failure in the community: a study of all incident cases in Olmsted County, Minnesota, in 1991. Circulation. 1998;98(21):2282–9.
12. Bhatia RS, Tu JV, Lee DS, Austin PC, Fang J, Haouzi A, et al. Outcome of heart failure with preserved ejection fraction in a population-based study. N Engl J Med. 2006;355(3):260–9.
13. Bramstedt KA, Nash PJ. When death is the outcome of informed refusal: dilemma of rejecting ventricular assist device therapy. J Heart Lung Transplant. 2005;24(2):229–30.
14. Hauptman PJ, Havranek EP. Integrating palliative care into heart failure care. Arch Intern Med. 2005;165(4):374–8.
15. Guyatt GH, Sullivan MJ, Thompson PJ, Fallen EL, Pugsley SO, Taylor DW, et al. The 6-minute walk: a new measure of exercise capacity in patients with chronic heart failure. Can Med Assoc J. 1985;132(8):919–23.
16. Zugck C, Kruger C, Durr S, Gerber SH, Haunstetter A, Hornig K, et al. Is the 6-minute walk test a reliable substitute for peak oxygen uptake in patients with dilated cardiomyopathy? Eur Heart J. 2000;21(7):540–9.
17. Opasich C, Pinna GD, Mazza A, Febo O, Riccardi R, Riccardi PG, et al. Six-minute walking performance in patients with moderate-to-severe heart failure; is it a useful indicator in clinical practice? Eur Heart J. 2001;22(6):488–96.
18. Sharma R, Anker SD. The 6-minute walk test and prognosis in chronic heart failure–the available evidence. Eur Heart J. 2001;22(6):445–8.
19. Mancini DM, Eisen H, Kussmaul W, Mull R, Edmunds Jr LH, Wilson JR. Value of peak exercise oxygen consumption for optimal timing of cardiac transplantation in ambulatory patients with heart failure. Circulation. 1991;83(3):778–86.
20. Stevenson LW, Steimle AE, Fonarow G, Kermani M, Kermani D, Hamilton MA, et al. Improvement in exercise capacity of candidates awaiting heart transplantation. J Am Coll Cardiol. 1995;25(1):163–70.
21. Aaronson KD, Schwartz JS, Chen TM, Wong KL, Goin JE, Mancini DM. Development and prospective validation of a clinical index to predict survival in ambulatory patients referred for cardiac transplant evaluation. Circulation. 1997;95(12):2660–7.
22. Smits JM, Deng MC, Hummel M, De Meester J, Schoendube F, Scheld HH, et al. A prognostic model for predicting waiting-list mortality for a total national cohort of adult heart-transplant candidates. Transplantation. 2003;76(8):1185–9.
23. Lund LH, Aaronson KD, Mancini DM. Predicting survival in ambulatory patients with severe heart failure on beta-blocker therapy. Am J Cardiol. 2003;92(11):1350–4.
24. Levy WC, Mozaffarian D, Linker DT, Sutradhar SC, Anker SD, Cropp AB, et al. The Seattle Heart Failure Model: prediction of survival in heart failure. Circulation. 2006;113(11):1424–33.
25. Kalogeropoulos AP, Georgiopoulou VV, Giamouzis G, Smith AL, Agha SA, Waheed S, et al. Utility of the Seattle Heart Failure Model in patients with advanced heart failure. J Am Coll Cardiol. 2009;53(4):334–42.
26. Mehra MR, Jessup M, Gronda E, Costanzo MR. Rationale and process: International Society for Heart and Lung Transplantation guidelines for the care of cardiac transplant candidates–2006. J Heart Lung Transplant. 2006;25(9):1001–2.
27. Mann D. Heart failure: a companion to Braunwald's heart disease: expert consult. 2nd ed. St. Louis: Saunders; 2010.
28. Petersen JW, Felker GM. Inotropes in the management of acute heart failure. Crit Care Med. 2008;36(1 Suppl):S106–11.
29. Parissis JT, Farmakis D, Nieminen M. Classical inotropes and new cardiac enhancers. Heart Fail Rev. 2007;12(2):149–56.
30. Feldman AM, Bristow MR, Parmley WW, Carson PE, Pepine CJ, Gilbert EM, et al. Effects of vesnarinone on morbidity and mortality in patients with heart failure. Vesnarinone Study Group. N Engl J Med. 1993 ;329(3):149–55.

31. The Xamoterol in Severe Heart Failure Study Group. Xamoterol in severe heart failure. Lancet. 1990;336(8706):1–6.
32. Cohn JN, Goldstein SO, Greenberg BH, Lorell BH, Bourge RC, Jaski BE, et al. A dose-dependent increase in mortality with vesnarinone among patients with severe heart failure. Vesnarinone Trial Investigators. N Engl J Med. 1998;339(25):1810–6.
33. Hampton JR, van Veldhuisen DJ, Kleber FX, Cowley AJ, Ardia A, Block P, et al. Randomised study of effect of ibopamine on survival in patients with advanced severe heart failure. Second Prospective Randomised Study of Ibopamine on Mortality and Efficacy (PRIME II) Investigators. Lancet. 1997; 349(9057):971–7.
34. Packer M, Carver JR, Rodeheffer RJ, Ivanhoe RJ, DiBianco R, Zeldis SM, et al. Effect of oral milrinone on mortality in severe chronic heart failure. The PROMISE Study Research Group. N Engl J Med. 1991;325(21):1468–75.
35. Califf RM, Adams KF, McKenna WJ, Gheorghiade M, Uretsky BF, McNulty SE, et al. A randomized controlled trial of epoprostenol therapy for severe congestive heart failure: the Flolan International Randomized Survival Trial (FIRST). Am Heart J. 1997;134(1):44–54.
36. Feldman AM, Oren RM, Abraham WT, Boehmer JP, Carson PE, Eichhorn E, et al. Low-dose oral enoximone enhances the ability to wean patients with ultra-advanced heart failure from intravenous inotropic support: results of the oral enoximone in intravenous inotrope-dependent subjects trial. Am Heart J. 2007;154(5):861–9.
37. Cleland JG, Daubert JC, Erdmann E, Freemantle N, Gras D, Kappenberger L, et al. The effect of cardiac resynchronization on morbidity and mortality in heart failure. N Engl J Med. 2005;352(15):1539–49.
38. Mebazaa A, Nieminen MS, Packer M, Cohen-Solal A, Kleber FX, Pocock SJ, et al. Levosimendan vs dobutamine for patients with acute decompensated heart failure: the SURVIVE Randomized Trial. JAMA. 2007;297(17):1883–91.
39. Cleland JG, Freemantle N, Coletta AP, Clark AL. Clinical trials update from the American Heart Association: REPAIR-AMI, ASTAMI, JELIS, MEGA, REVIVE-II, SURVIVE, and PROACTIVE. Eur J Heart Fail. 2006;8(1):105–10.
40. Mills RM, LeJemtel TH, Horton DP, Liang C, Lang R, Silver MA, et al. Sustained hemodynamic effects of an infusion of nesiritide (human b-type natriuretic peptide) in heart failure: a randomized, double-blind, placebo-controlled clinical trial. Natrecor Study Group. J Am Coll Cardiol. 1999;34(1):155–62.
41. Sackner-Bernstein JD, Kowalski M, Fox M, Aaronson K. Short-term risk of death after treatment with nesiritide for decompensated heart failure: a pooled analysis of randomized controlled trials. JAMA. 2005;293(15):1900–5.
42. Colucci WS, Elkayam U, Horton DP, Abraham WT, Bourge RC, Johnson AD, et al. Intravenous nesiritide, a natriuretic peptide, in the treatment of decompensated congestive heart failure. Nesiritide Study Group. N Engl J Med. 2000;343(4):246–53.
43. VMAC Investigators. Intravenous nesiritide vs nitroglycerin for treatment of decompensated congestive heart failure: a randomized controlled trial. JAMA. 2002;287(12):1531–40.
44. Peacock WF, Holland R, Gyarmathy R, Dunbar L, Klapholz M, Horton DP, et al. Observation unit treatment of heart failure with nesiritide: results from the proaction trial. J Emerg Med. 2005;29(3):243–52.
45. Dontas ID, Xanthos T, Dontas I, Lelovas P, Papadimitriou L. Impact of nesiritide on renal function and mortality in patients suffering from heart failure. Cardiovasc Drugs Ther. 2009;23(3):221–33.
46. Arora RR, Venkatesh PK, Molnar J. Short and long-term mortality with nesiritide. Am Heart J. 2006;152(6):1084–90.
47. O'Connor CM, Starling RC, Hernandez AF, Armstrong PW, Dickstein K, Hasselblad V, et al. Effect of nesiritide in patients with acute decompensated heart failure. N Engl J Med. 2011;365(1):32–43.
48. Udelson JE, Smith WB, Hendrix GH, Painchaud CA, Ghazzi M, Thomas I, et al. Acute hemodynamic effects of conivaptan, a dual V(1A) and V(2) vasopressin receptor antagonist, in patients with advanced heart failure. Circulation. 2001;104(20):2417–23.
49. Konstam MA, Gheorghiade M, Burnett Jr JC, Grinfeld L, Maggioni AP, Swedberg K, et al. Effects of oral tolvaptan in patients hospitalized for worsening heart failure: the EVEREST Outcome Trial. JAMA. 2007;297(12):1319–31.
50. Garg R, Yusuf S. Overview of randomized trials of angiotensin-converting enzyme inhibitors on mortality and morbidity in patients with heart failure. Collaborative Group on ACE Inhibitor Trials. JAMA. 1995;273(18):1450–6.
51. Wienbergen H, Schiele R, Gitt AK, Juenger C, Heer T, Meisenzahl C, et al. Impact of ramipril versus other angiotensin-converting enzyme inhibitors on outcome of unselected patients with ST-elevation acute myocardial infarction. Am J Cardiol. 2002;90(10):1045–9.
52. Giles TD, Katz R, Sullivan JM, Wolfson P, Haugland M, Kirlin P, et al. Short- and long-acting angiotensin-converting enzyme inhibitors: a randomized trial of lisinopril versus captopril in the treatment of congestive heart failure. The Multicenter Lisinopril-Captopril Congestive Heart Failure Study Group. J Am Coll Cardiol. 1989;13(6):1240–7.
53. Pilote L, Abrahamowicz M, Eisenberg M, Humphries K, Behlouli H, Tu JV. Effect of different angiotensin-converting-enzyme inhibitors on mortality among elderly patients with congestive heart failure. CMAJ. 2008;178(10):1303–11.
54. Vittorio TJ, Ahuja K, Kasper M, Turalic H, Tseng CH, Jorde UP, et al. Comparison of high- versus low-tissue affinity ACE-inhibitor treatment on circulating aldosterone levels in patients with chronic heart failure. J Renin Angiotensin Aldosterone Syst. 2007;8(4):200–4.

55. Nanas JN, Alexopoulos G, Anastasiou-Nana MI, Karidis K, Tirologos A, Zobolos S, et al. Outcome of patients with congestive heart failure treated with standard versus high doses of enalapril: a multicenter study. High Enalapril Dose Study Group. J Am Coll Cardiol. 2000;36(7):2090–5.
56. Swedberg K, Kjekshus J. Effects of enalapril on mortality in severe congestive heart failure: results of the Cooperative North Scandinavian Enalapril Survival Study (CONSENSUS). Am J Cardiol. 1988;62(2):60A–6.
57. Swedberg K, Kjekshus J, Snapinn S. Long-term survival in severe heart failure in patients treated with enalapril. Ten year follow-up of CONSENSUS I. Eur Heart J. 1999;20(2):136–9.
58. The SOLVD Investigators. Effect of enalapril on survival in patients with reduced left ventricular ejection fractions and congestive heart failure. N Engl J Med. 1991;325(5):293–302.
59. Weber KT. Aldosterone in congestive heart failure. N Engl J Med. 2001;345(23):1689–97.
60. Pitt B, Zannad F, Remme WJ, Cody R, Castaigne A, Perez A, et al. The effect of spironolactone on morbidity and mortality in patients with severe heart failure. Randomized Aldactone Evaluation Study Investigators. N Engl J Med. 1999;341(10):709–17.
61. Pitt B, Remme W, Zannad F, Neaton J, Martinez F, Roniker B, et al. Eplerenone, a selective aldosterone blocker, in patients with left ventricular dysfunction after myocardial infarction. N Engl J Med. 2003;348(14):1309–21.
62. Zannad F, McMurray JJ, Krum H, van Veldhuisen DJ, Swedberg K, Shi H, et al. Eplerenone in patients with systolic heart failure and mild symptoms. N Engl J Med. 2011;364(1):11–21.
63. Cohn JN, Tognoni G. A randomized trial of the angiotensin-receptor blocker valsartan in chronic heart failure. N Engl J Med. 2001;345(23):1667–75.
64. Young JB, Dunlap ME, Pfeffer MA, Probstfield JL, Cohen-Solal A, Dietz R, et al. Mortality and morbidity reduction with Candesartan in patients with chronic heart failure and left ventricular systolic dysfunction: results of the CHARM low-left ventricular ejection fraction trials. Circulation. 2004;110(17):2618–26.
65. Pitt B, Poole-Wilson PA, Segal R, Martinez FA, Dickstein K, Camm AJ, et al. Effect of losartan compared with captopril on mortality in patients with symptomatic heart failure: randomised trial–the Losartan Heart Failure Survival Study ELITE II. Lancet. 2000;355(9215):1582–7.
66. Dickstein K, Kjekshus J. Effects of losartan and captopril on mortality and morbidity in high-risk patients after acute myocardial infarction: the OPTIMAAL randomised trial. Optimal Trial in Myocardial Infarction with Angiotensin II Antagonist Losartan. Lancet. 2002;360(9335):752–60.
67. Pfeffer MA, McMurray JJ, Velazquez EJ, Rouleau JL, Kober L, Maggioni AP, et al. Valsartan, captopril, or both in myocardial infarction complicated by heart failure, left ventricular dysfunction, or both. N Engl J Med. 2003;349(20):1893–906.
68. McMurray JJ, Ostergren J, Swedberg K, Granger CB, Held P, Michelson EL, et al. Effects of candesartan in patients with chronic heart failure and reduced left-ventricular systolic function taking angiotensin-converting-enzyme inhibitors: the CHARM-Added trial. Lancet. 2003;362(9386):767–71.
69. Dobre D, van Veldhuisen DJ, Goulder MA, Krum H, Willenheimer R. Clinical effects of initial 6 months monotherapy with bisoprolol versus enalapril in the treatment of patients with mild to moderate chronic heart failure. Data from the CIBIS III Trial. Cardiovasc Drugs Ther. 2008;22(5):399–405.
70. Remme WJ, Riegger G, Hildebrandt P, Komajda M, Jaarsma W, Bobbio M, et al. The benefits of early combination treatment of carvedilol and an ACE-inhibitor in mild heart failure and left ventricular systolic dysfunction. The carvedilol and ACE-inhibitor remodelling mild heart failure evaluation trial (CARMEN). Cardiovasc Drugs Ther. 2004;18(1):57–66.
71. Willenheimer R, van Veldhuisen DJ, Silke B, Erdmann E, Follath F, Krum H, et al. Effect on survival and hospitalization of initiating treatment for chronic heart failure with bisoprolol followed by enalapril, as compared with the opposite sequence: results of the randomized Cardiac Insufficiency Bisoprolol Study (CIBIS) III. Circulation. 2005;112(16):2426–35.
72. Metoprolol CR/XL Randomised Intervention Trial in Congestive Heart Failure (MERIT-HF). Effect of metoprolol CR/XL in chronic heart failure. Lancet. 1999;353(9169):2001–7.
73. The Cardiac Insufficiency Bisoprolol Study II (CIBIS-II). A randomised trial. Lancet. 1999; 353(9146):9–13.
74. Packer M, Coats AJ, Fowler MB, Katus HA, Krum H, Mohacsi P, et al. Effect of carvedilol on survival in severe chronic heart failure. N Engl J Med. 2001;344(22):1651–8.
75. Poole-Wilson PA, Swedberg K, Cleland JG, Di Lenarda A, Hanrath P, Komajda M, et al. Comparison of carvedilol and metoprolol on clinical outcomes in patients with chronic heart failure in the Carvedilol Or Metoprolol European Trial (COMET): randomised controlled trial. Lancet. 2003;362(9377):7–13.
76. Hjalmarson A, Waagstein F. COMET: a proposed mechanism of action to explain the results and concerns about dose. Lancet. 2003;362(9389):1077. author reply -8.
77. Cohn JN, Archibald DG, Ziesche S, Franciosa JA, Harston WE, Tristani FE, et al. Effect of vasodilator therapy on mortality in chronic congestive heart failure. Results of a Veterans Administration Cooperative Study. N Engl J Med. 1986;314(24):1547–52.
78. Cohn JN, Johnson G, Ziesche S, Cobb F, Francis G, Tristani F, et al. A comparison of enalapril with hydralazine-isosorbide dinitrate in the treatment of chronic congestive heart failure. N Engl J Med. 1991;325(5):303–10.

79. Taylor AL, Ziesche S, Yancy C, Carson P, D'Agostino Jr R, Ferdinand K, et al. Combination of isosorbide dinitrate and hydralazine in blacks with heart failure. N Engl J Med. 2004;351(20):2049–57.
80. Lewis GD, Shah R, Shahzad K, Camuso JM, Pappagianopoulos PP, Hung J, et al. Sildenafil improves exercise capacity and quality of life in patients with systolic heart failure and secondary pulmonary hypertension. Circulation. 2007;116(14):1555–62.
81. Narang R, Cleland JG, Erhardt L, Ball SG, Coats AJ, Cowley AJ, et al. Mode of death in chronic heart failure. A request and proposition for more accurate classification. Eur Heart J. 1996;17(9):1390–403.
82. Cleland JG, Erhardt L, Murray G, Hall AS, Ball SG. Effect of ramipril on morbidity and mode of death among survivors of acute myocardial infarction with clinical evidence of heart failure. A report from the AIRE Study Investigators. Eur Heart J. 1997;18(1):41–51.
83. Doval HC, Nul DR, Grancelli HO, Perrone SV, Bortman GR, Curiel R. Randomised trial of low-dose amiodarone in severe congestive heart failure. Grupo de Estudio de la Sobrevida en la Insuficiencia Cardiaca en Argentina (GESICA). Lancet. 1994;344(8921):493–8.
84. Singh SN, Fletcher RD, Fisher SG, Singh BN, Lewis HD, Deedwania PC, et al. Amiodarone in patients with congestive heart failure and asymptomatic ventricular arrhythmia. Survival Trial of Antiarrhythmic Therapy in Congestive Heart Failure. N Engl J Med. 1995;333(2):77–82.
85. Waldo AL, Camm AJ, deRuyter H, Friedman PL, MacNeil DJ, Pauls JF, et al. Effect of d-sotalol on mortality in patients with left ventricular dysfunction after recent and remote myocardial infarction. The SWORD Investigators. Survival With Oral d-Sotalol. Lancet. 1996;348(9019):7–12.
86. Kober L, Torp-Pedersen C, McMurray JJ, Gotzsche O, Levy S, Crijns H, et al. Increased mortality after dronedarone therapy for severe heart failure. N Engl J Med. 2008;358(25):2678–87.
87. Kuck KH, Cappato R, Siebels J, Ruppel R. Randomized comparison of antiarrhythmic drug therapy with implantable defibrillators in patients resuscitated from cardiac arrest: the Cardiac Arrest Study Hamburg (CASH). Circulation. 2000;102(7):748–54.
88. Connolly SJ, Gent M, Roberts RS, Dorian P, Roy D, Sheldon RS, et al. Canadian implantable defibrillator study (CIDS): a randomized trial of the implantable cardioverter defibrillator against amiodarone. Circulation. 2000;101(11):1297–302.
89. The Antiarrhythmics versus Implantable Defibrillators (AVID) Investigators. A comparison of antiarrhythmic-drug therapy with implantable defibrillators in patients resuscitated from near-fatal ventricular arrhythmias. N Engl J Med. 1997;337(22):1576–83.
90. Epstein AE, DiMarco JP, Ellenbogen KA, Estes 3rd NA, Freedman RA, Gettes LS, et al. ACC/AHA/HRS 2008 Guidelines for device-based therapy of cardiac rhythm abnormalities: a report of the American College of Cardiology/American Heart Association Task Force on practice guidelines (writing committee to revise the ACC/AHA/NASPE 2002 Guideline update for implantation of cardiac pacemakers and antiarrhythmia devices) developed in collaboration with the American Association for Thoracic Surgery and Society of Thoracic Surgeons. J Am Coll Cardiol. 2008;51(21):e1–62.
91. Moss AJ, Hall WJ, Cannom DS, Daubert JP, Higgins SL, Klein H, et al. Improved survival with an implanted defibrillator in patients with coronary disease at high risk for ventricular arrhythmia. Multicenter Automatic Defibrillator Implantation Trial Investigators. N Engl J Med. 1996;335(26):1933–40.
92. Buxton AE, Lee KL, Fisher JD, Josephson ME, Prystowsky EN, Hafley G. A randomized study of the prevention of sudden death in patients with coronary artery disease. Multicenter Unsustained Tachycardia Trial Investigators. N Engl J Med. 1999 ;341(25):1882–90.
93. Moss AJ, Zareba W, Hall WJ, Klein H, Wilber DJ, Cannom DS, et al. Prophylactic implantation of a defibrillator in patients with myocardial infarction and reduced ejection fraction. N Engl J Med. 2002;346(12):877–83.
94. Bardy GH, Lee KL, Mark DB, Poole JE, Packer DL, Boineau R, et al. Amiodarone or an implantable cardioverter-defibrillator for congestive heart failure. N Engl J Med. 2005;352(3):225–37.
95. Grimm W, Christ M, Bach J, Muller HH, Maisch B. Noninvasive arrhythmia risk stratification in idiopathic dilated cardiomyopathy: results of the Marburg Cardiomyopathy Study. Circulation. 2003;108(23):2883–91.
96. Poole JE, Johnson GW, Hellkamp AS, Anderson J, Callans DJ, Raitt MH, et al. Prognostic importance of defibrillator shocks in patients with heart failure. N Engl J Med. 2008;359(10):1009–17.
97. Epstein AE, DiMarco JP, Ellenbogen KA, Estes 3rd NA, Freedman RA, Gettes LS, et al. ACC/AHA/HRS 2008 Guidelines for device-based therapy of cardiac rhythm abnormalities: a report of the American College of Cardiology/American Heart Association Task Force on practice guidelines (writing committee to revise the ACC/AHA/NASPE 2002 Guideline update for implantation of cardiac pacemakers and antiarrhythmia devices): developed in collaboration with the American Association for Thoracic Surgery and Society of Thoracic Surgeons. Circulation. 2008;117(21):e350–408.
98. Cazeau S, Leclercq C, Lavergne T, Walker S, Varma C, Linde C, et al. Effects of multisite biventricular pacing in patients with heart failure and intraventricular conduction delay. N Engl J Med. 2001;344(12):873–80.
99. Abraham WT, Fisher WG, Smith AL, Delurgio DB, Leon AR, Loh E, et al. Cardiac resynchronization in chronic heart failure. N Engl J Med. 2002; 346(24):1845–53.

100. Bristow MR, Saxon LA, Boehmer J, Krueger S, Kass DA, De Marco T, et al. Cardiac-resynchronization therapy with or without an implantable defibrillator in advanced chronic heart failure. N Engl J Med. 2004;350(21):2140–50.
101. Cleland JG, Daubert JC, Erdmann E, Freemantle N, Gras D, Kappenberger L, et al. Longer-term effects of cardiac resynchronization therapy on mortality in heart failure [the CArdiac REsynchronization-Heart Failure (CARE-HF) trial extension phase]. Eur Heart J. 2006;27(16):1928–32.
102. Linde C, Abraham WT, Gold MR, St John Sutton M, Ghio S, Daubert C. Randomized trial of cardiac resynchronization in mildly symptomatic heart failure patients and in asymptomatic patients with left ventricular dysfunction and previous heart failure symptoms. J Am Coll Cardiol. 2008;52(23):1834–43.
103. Tang AS, Wells GA, Talajic M, Arnold MO, Sheldon R, Connolly S, et al. Cardiac-resynchronization therapy for mild-to-moderate heart failure. N Engl J Med. 2010;363(25):2385–95.
104. Moss AJ, Hall WJ, Cannom DS, Klein H, Brown MW, Daubert JP, et al. Cardiac-resynchronization therapy for the prevention of heart-failure events. N Engl J Med. 2009;361(14):1329–38.
105. Tracy CM, Epstein AE, Darbar D, Dimarco JP, Dunbar SB, Estes 3rd NA, et al. 2012 ACCF/AHA/HRS Focused update of the 2008 guidelines for device-based therapy of cardiac rhythm abnormalities: a report of the American College of Cardiology Foundation/American Heart Association Task Force on practice guidelines. Circulation. 2012;126(14):1784–800.
106. Mullens W, Grimm RA, Verga T, Dresing T, Starling RC, Wilkoff BL, et al. Insights from a cardiac resynchronization optimization clinic as part of a heart failure disease management program. J Am Coll Cardiol. 2009;53(9):765–73.
107. Cleland JG, Calvert MJ, Verboven Y, Freemantle N. Effects of cardiac resynchronization therapy on long-term quality of life: an analysis from the CArdiac Resynchronisation-Heart Failure (CARE-HF) study. Am Heart J. 2009;157(3):457–66.
108. Donahue T, Niazi I, Leon A, Stucky M, Herrmann K. Acute and chronic response to CRT in narrow QRS patients. J Cardiovasc Transl Res. 2012;5(2):232–41.
109. Beshai JF, Grimm RA, Nagueh SF, Baker 2nd JH, Beau SL, Greenberg SM, et al. Cardiac-resynchronization therapy in heart failure with narrow QRS complexes. N Engl J Med. 2007;357(24):2461–71.
110. Yu CM, Wing-Hong Fung J, Zhang Q, Sanderson JE. Understanding nonresponders of cardiac resynchronization therapy–current and future perspectives. J Cardiovasc Electrophysiol. 2005;16(10):1117–24.
111. Beshai JF, Khunnawat C, Lin AC. Mechanical dyssynchrony from the perspective of a cardiac electrophysiologist. Curr Opin Cardiol. 2008;23(5):447–51.
112. Winkel E, Piccione W. Coronary artery bypass surgery in patients with left ventricular dysfunction: candidate selection and perioperative care. J Heart Lung Transplant. 1997;16(6):S19–24.
113. Di Carli MF, Asgarzadie F, Schelbert HR, Brunken RC, Laks H, Phelps ME, et al. Quantitative relation between myocardial viability and improvement in heart failure symptoms after revascularization in patients with ischemic cardiomyopathy. Circulation. 1995;92(12):3436–44.
114. Hausmann H, Topp H, Siniawski H, Holz S, Hetzer R. Decision-making in end-stage coronary artery disease: revascularization or heart transplantation? Ann Thorac Surg. 1997;64(5):1296–301. discussion 302.
115. Elefteriades JA, Tolis Jr G, Levi E, Mills LK, Zaret BL. Coronary artery bypass grafting in severe left ventricular dysfunction: excellent survival with improved ejection fraction and functional state. J Am Coll Cardiol. 1993;22(5):1411–7.
116. Olsen PS, Kassis E, Niebuhr-Jorgensen U. Coronary artery bypass surgery in patients with severe left-ventricular dysfunction. Thorac Cardiovasc Surg. 1993;41(2):118–20.
117. Mickleborough LL, Maruyama H, Takagi Y, Mohamed S, Sun Z, Ebisuzaki L. Results of revascularization in patients with severe left ventricular dysfunction. Circulation. 1995;92(9 Suppl):II73–9.
118. Joyce D, Loebe M, Noon GP, McRee S, Southard R, Thompson L, et al. Revascularization and ventricular restoration in patients with ischemic heart failure: the STICH trial. Curr Opin Cardiol. 2003;18(6):454–7.
119. Veenhuyzen GD, Singh SN, McAreavey D, Shelton BJ, Exner DV. Prior coronary artery bypass surgery and risk of death among patients with ischemic left ventricular dysfunction. Circulation. 2001;104(13):1489–93.
120. Alderman EL, Bourassa MG, Cohen LS, Davis KB, Kaiser GG, Killip T, et al. Ten-year follow-up of survival and myocardial infarction in the randomized Coronary Artery Surgery Study. Circulation. 1990;82(5):1629–46.
121. The VA Coronary Artery Bypass Surgery Cooperative Study Group. Eighteen-year follow-up in the Veterans Affairs Cooperative Study of Coronary Artery Bypass Surgery for stable angina. Circulation. 1992;86(1):121–30.
122. Velazquez EJ, Lee KL, Deja MA, Jain A, Sopko G, Marchenko A, et al. Coronary-artery bypass surgery in patients with left ventricular dysfunction. N Engl J Med. 2011;364(17):1607–16.
123. Rahimtoola SH. Concept and evaluation of hibernating myocardium. Annu Rev Med. 1999;50:75–86.
124. Nicolini F, Gherli T. Alternatives to transplantation in the surgical therapy for heart failure. Eur J Cardiothorac Surg. 2009;35(2):214–28.
125. Dreyfus G, Duboc D, Blasco A, Dubois C, Brodaty D, Chatel D, et al. Coronary surgery can be an alternative to heart transplantation in selected patients with end-stage ischemic heart disease. Eur J Cardiothorac Surg. 1993;7(9):482–7. discussion 8.
126. Kron IL. When does one replace the heart in ischemic cardiomyopathy? Ann Thorac Surg. 1993;55(3):581.

127. Lansman SL, Ergin MA, Griepp RB. The history of heart and heart-lung transplantation. Cardiovasc Clin. 1990;20(2):3–19.
128. Tjan TD, Kondruweit M, Scheld HH, Roeder N, Borggrefe M, Schmidt C, et al. The bad ventricle–revascularization versus transplantation. Thorac Cardiovasc Surg. 2000;48(1):9–14.
129. Bonow RO, Maurer G, Lee KL, Holly TA, Binkley PF, Desvigne-Nickens P, et al. Myocardial viability and survival in ischemic left ventricular dysfunction. N Engl J Med. 2011;364(17):1617–25.
130. Bolling SF, Pagani FD, Deeb GM, Bach DS. Intermediate-term outcome of mitral reconstruction in cardiomyopathy. J Thorac Cardiovasc Surg. 1998;115(2):381–6. discussion 7-8.
131. Rukosujew A, Klotz S, Welp H, Bruch C, Ghezelbash F, Schmidt C, et al. Surgery of secondary mitral insufficiency in patients with impaired left ventricular function. J Cardiothorac Surg. 2009;4:36.
132. Athanasuleas CL, Stanley Jr AW, Buckberg GD, Dor V, DiDonato M, Blackstone EH. Surgical anterior ventricular endocardial restoration (SAVER) in the dilated remodeled ventricle after anterior myocardial infarction. RESTORE group. Reconstructive Endoventricular Surgery, returning Torsion Original Radius Elliptical Shape to the LV. J Am Coll Cardiol. 2001;37(5):1199–209.
133. McCarthy JF, McCarthy PM, Starling RC, Smedira NG, Scalia GM, Wong J, et al. Partial left ventriculectomy and mitral valve repair for end-stage congestive heart failure. Eur J Cardiothorac Surg. 1998;13(4):337–43.
134. Athanasuleas CL, Buckberg GD, Stanley AW, Siler W, Dor V, Di Donato M, et al. Surgical ventricular restoration in the treatment of congestive heart failure due to post-infarction ventricular dilation. J Am Coll Cardiol. 2004;44(7):1439–45.
135. Jones RH, Velazquez EJ, Michler RE, Sopko G, Oh JK, O'Connor CM, et al. Coronary bypass surgery with or without surgical ventricular reconstruction. N Engl J Med. 2009;360(17):1705–17.
136. Allen LA, Stevenson LW, Grady KL, Goldstein NE, Matlock DD, Arnold RM, et al. Decision making in advanced heart failure: a scientific statement from the American Heart Association. Circulation. 2012;125(15):1928–52.
137. Crespo-Leiro MG, Barge-Caballero E, Marzoa-Rivas R, Paniagua-Martin MJ. Heart transplantation. Curr Opin Organ Transplant. 2010;15(5):633–8.
138. McMurray JJ, Pfeffer MA. Heart failure. Lancet. 2005;365(9474):1877–89.
139. Nieminen MS, Bohm M, Cowie MR, Drexler H, Filippatos GS, Jondeau G, et al. Executive summary of the guidelines on the diagnosis and treatment of acute heart failure: the Task Force on Acute Heart Failure of the European Society of Cardiology. Eur Heart J. 2005;26(4):384–416.
140. Feldman D, Pamboukian SV, Teuteberg JJ, Birks E, Lietz K, Moore SA, et al. The 2013 International Society for Heart and Lung Transplantation Guidelines for mechanical circulatory support: executive summary. J Heart Lung Transplant. 2013:32(2):157–87.
141. Rose EA, Gelijns AC, Moskowitz AJ, Heitjan DF, Stevenson LW, Dembitsky W, et al. Long-term use of a left ventricular assist device for end-stage heart failure. N Engl J Med. 2001;345(20):1435–43.
142. Wilson SR, Mudge Jr GH, Stewart GC, Givertz MM. Evaluation for a ventricular assist device: selecting the appropriate candidate. Circulation. 2009;119(16):2225–32.
143. Miller LW, Pagani FD, Russell SD, John R, Boyle AJ, Aaronson KD, et al. Use of a continuous-flow device in patients awaiting heart transplantation. N Engl J Med. 2007;357(9):885–96.
144. Slaughter MS, Rogers JG, Milano CA, Russell SD, Conte JV, Feldman D, et al. Advanced heart failure treated with continuous-flow left ventricular assist device. N Engl J Med. 2009;361(23):2241–51.
145. Copeland JG, Smith RG, Arabia FA, Nolan PE, Sethi GK, Tsau PH, et al. Cardiac replacement with a total artificial heart as a bridge to transplantation. N Engl J Med. 2004;351(9):859–67.

3 Surgical Coronary Artery Revascularization in Patients with Advanced Ischemic Cardiomyopathy

Benjamin C. Sun

Introduction

Coronary artery disease (CAD) is becoming the dominant cause of heart failure [1]. Coronary artery bypass grafting (CABG) has only recently been more broadly utilized to address this population. There are only two studies comparing medical therapy to CABG in patients with ischemic cardiomyopathy, the Coronary Artery Surgery Study (CASS) [2] and the Surgical Treatment of Congestive Heart Failure (STICH) trial Hypothesis I [3]. In the CASS study, only patients with three-vessel disease benefited CABG over medical therapy demonstrated at 7 years of follow-up. This is a study performed in the 1980s with limited practical relevance today. The recently published STICH Hypothesis I data showed there was no significant difference between medical therapy alone and medical therapy plus CABG with respect to the primary end point of death from any cause. However, patients assigned to CABG, as compared with those assigned to medical therapy alone, had lower rates of death from cardiovascular causes and of death from any cause or hospitalization for cardiovascular causes [3].

B.C. Sun, M.D., FACS (✉)
Department of Cardiothoracic Surgery,
Minneapolis Heart Institute, Allina Health System,
920 E. 28th St.–Suite 400, Minneapolis, MN 55407, USA
e-mail: benjamin.sun@allina.com

Other smaller series and single center studies add to the increasing evidence supporting this therapeutic option as beneficial to our patients both for survival benefit and symptom relief for those having chronic CAD and left ventricular (LV) dysfunction with viable myocardium [4]. The surgical techniques whether performed off pump, pump assisted, or with the heart cross clamped can all be performed successfully without clear benefit from one technique over another. Several important patient and anatomic factors must be assessed prior to determining the appropriateness of an individual for this therapy.

"Stunned" Versus "Hibernating" Myocardium

"Stunned" myocardium occurs as a sequela to an acute ischemic insult and the associated regional dysfunction from inflammation despite adequate perfusion (can be remote myocardium) or as part of reperfusion. This is largely a reversible process as the inflammatory process abates and is associated with adequate perfusion leading to a perfusion-contraction mismatch [5]. Revascularization, if needed, can be performed safely with "stunned" myocardium, though patients may benefit from an interval recovery phase prior to surgery pending the size of the infarct [6]. Short-term mechanical circulatory support may be required in some of these patients to maintain end-organ function as well as facilitate some myocardial recovery with ventricular unloading prior to revascularization.

J.A. Morgan and Y. Naka (eds.), *Surgical Treatment for Advanced Heart Failure*,
DOI 10.1007/978-1-4614-6919-3_3, © Springer Science+Business Media New York 2013

"Hibernating" myocardium is a decrease of myocardial contractility and metabolism due to sustained hypoperfusion of the myocyte. Hibernating myocardium requires the restoration of a normal blood supply for an improvement in contractile function; global increases in left ventricular ejection fraction (LVEF) following CABG may be seen in as many as 40 % of patients with ischemic cardiomyopathy [7]. Chronic hypoperfusion may convert hibernating myocardium into dedifferentiated myocytes as well as fibrosis. Revascularization can be beneficial during the window where myocardial function may be restored. Identifying this window can be problematic. The information below draws largely on the growing body of nonrandomized studies evaluating efficacy of various techniques to quantify myocardial viability pre- and post-revascularization to help develop a strategy for patient selection and treatment.

Anatomic

Determining myocardial viability and functional myocardial recovery corresponding to coronary anatomy that is amenable to revascularization is the key to patient selection. Though conceptually obvious, the tools for this execution have variable sensitivity and specificity with no consensus. A feature of viable myocardium is the presence of inotropic reserve, which may be elicited by catecholamine stimulation. Hence dobutamine or adenosine is used, and many of the subsequently described imaging techniques employ this response to help differentiate attenuated regions from scar [8].

Echocardiography

Stress echocardiography is widely used as the yard stick to determine the potential for myocardial recovery after revascularization. The thickness of the myocardial wall corresponding to anatomic targets is the first-pass assessment of viability. Incremental diastolic wall thickness changes >0.8 cm with dobutamine infusion may improve the sensitivity, though decrease the specificity of this technique in akinetic regions [9].

Scintigraphy

Single-photon emission computed tomography perfusion scintigraphy, whether using thallium-201, Tc-99m sestamibi, or Tc-99m tetrofosmin, in stress and/or rest protocols, has consistently been shown to be an effective modality for identifying myocardial viability and guiding appropriate management. Metabolic imaging with positron emission tomography (PET) radiotracers frequently adds additional information and is a powerful tool for predicting which patients will have an improved outcome from revascularization [10].

The number of viable segments per patient may be related to the improvement in LVEF after revascularization. In a recent study using TC-99m sestamibi, patients with more than four viable segments representing 24 % of the left ventricle yielded a sensitivity of 83 % and specificity of 79 %, respectively, for predicting improvement in LVEF. Furthermore, the presence of four or more viable segments predicted improvement in heart failure symptoms and quality of life after surgical revascularization [11].

PET using rubidium 82 (Rb 82) or ammonia N-13 can be used in lieu of a single-photon emission computer tomography (SPECT) scan or when a SPECT scan is inconclusive [12].

Cardiac Magnetic Resonance

This noninvasive diagnostic tool is evolving into a one-stop shop for evaluation of myocardial dysfunction. Myocardial wall thickness can be accurately measured as can regional wall motion abnormalities. In addition, delayed contrast enhancement after the intravenous (IV) administration of gadolinium-based contrast material is a very reliable indicator of acute myocardial infarction.

Hyperenhancement is not seen in areas of ischemia whether by stunning or hibernation. In addition, the degree of hyperenhancement can correlate with transmural versus subendocardial infarction and may predict improvements in myocardial function after revascularization [13].

Cardiac CT

In ischemic cardiomyopathy, there is limited added benefit with a cardiac computed tomography (CT). Its role in cardiovascular imaging is important in anatomic variants of the coronary anatomy. However its use in determining ischemia or viability as a stand-alone diagnostic modality is very limited. The use of PET with cardiac CT may make this a useful tool for ischemic myopathy.

Results

The recently published STICH trial Hypothesis I is a prospective multicenter, nonblinded, randomized study at 99 clinical sites in 22 countries trial comparing a strategy of medical therapy alone versus medical therapy and surgical revascularization for qualified patients with depressed ejection fractions. There were 1,212 patients randomly assigned to receive medical therapy alone (602 patients) or medical therapy plus CABG (610 patients). There was no significant difference between the two study groups with respect to the primary end point of the rate of death from any cause. The rates of death from cardiovascular causes and of death from any cause or hospitalization for cardiac causes were lower among patients assigned to CABG than among those assigned to medical therapy [3]. This landmark study is clearly important in comparing these two strategies; however, it did not have the fidelity to correlate ischemic regions with coronary targets.

Several nonrandomized studies have retrospectively assessed outcomes in patients with CAD and low left ventricular function. Nardi et al. published a series of 302 consecutive patients with ejection fraction (EF) <35 % who underwent CABG with 298 patients 292 patients receiving complete revascularization subsequently resulting in a 5 % operative mortality and an 87 % freedom from myocardial infarction at 10 years [14]. Shapira et al. published a series of 115 consecutive patients with EF<30 % operative mortality was a very low 2.6 %. Three- and five-year survival rates were 91±3 % and 76±6 %, respectively, for this group of patients [15]. Filsoufi et al. also published his series of 2,725 consecutive patients undergoing isolated CABG, of whom 495 patients had EF<30 %. Postoperative mortality was higher in the low ejection fraction group (3.6 % vs. 1.4 %). Long-term survival was significantly decreased in patients with EF of 0.30 or less: 1-year and 5-year survival 88±1.5 % and 75±2.2 % versus 96±0.4 % and 81±1.2 %, respectively ($p=0.001$) [16].

Successful coronary revascularization can be successfully performed in patients with low ejection fractions and ischemic cardiomyopathies. Long-term survival is worse in this subpopulation than patients with more normal cardiac function. Nevertheless, long-term survival appears to be robust. There are many different imaging modalities that can be utilized to identify viable myocardium. The STICH trial Hypothesis I is the only contemporary randomized prospective study comparing surgical revascularization to medical therapy in a group of patients with low ejection fraction and CAD. Though the primary end point of all cause mortality did not demonstrate a benefit from the surgical arm, death from cardiovascular causes was lower in the group treated with CABG.

Correlating the quality and the size of the coronary targets to these viable myocardial segments has not been well studied. One would intuitively believe that a complete revascularization would address this limitation. Nevertheless, we currently do not have the tools to accurately answer the question most commonly posed to us from this patient group, "How much better will my heart be when you are finished with the surgery?"

References

1. Gheorghiade M, Sopko G, De Luca L, Velazquez EJ, Parker JD, Binkley PF, et al. Navigating the crossroads of coronary artery disease and heart failure. Circulation. 2006;114:1202–13.
2. Passamani E, Davis K, Gillespie M, Killip T. and the CASS Principal Investigators and their associates. A randomized trial of coronary artery bypass surgery. Survival in patients with low ejection fraction. N Engl J Med. 1985;312:1665–71.
3. Velazquez E, Lee K, Deja M, Jain A, Sopko G, Marchenko A, et al. Coronary-artery bypass surgery in patients with left ventricular dysfunction. N Engl J Med. 2011;364:1607–16.
4. Allman KC, Shaw LJ, Hachamovitch R, Udelson JE. Myocardial viability testing and impact of revascularization on prognosis in patients with coronary artery disease and left ventricular dysfunction: a meta-analysis. J Am Coll Cardiol. 2002;39(7):1151–8.
5. Ross Jr J. Myocardial perfusion–contraction matching. Implications for coronary heart disease and hibernation. Circulation. 1991;83(3):1076–83.
6. Antman EM, Anbe DT, Armstrong PW, Bates ER, Green LA, Hand M, et al. ACC/AHA guidelines for the management of patients with ST-elevation myocardial infarction: a report of the American College of Cardiology/American Heart Association Task Force on Practice Guidelines (Committee to Revise the 1999 Guidelines for the Management of patients with acute myocardial infarction). J Am Coll Cardiol. 2004;44:E1–211.
7. Bonow RO. The hibernating myocardium: implications for management of congestive heart failure. Am J Cardiol. 1995;75(3):17A–25.
8. Bax JJ, Poldermans D, Elhendy A, Cornel JH, Boersma E, Rambaldi R, et al. Improvement of left ventricular ejection fraction, heart failure symptoms and prognosis after revascularization in patients with chronic coronary artery disease and viable myocardium detected by dobutamine stress echocardiography. J Am Coll Cardiol. 1999;34(1):163–9.
9. Zaglavara T, Pillay T, Karvounis H, Haaverstad R, Parharidis G, Louridas G, et al. Detection of myocardial viability by dobutamine stress echocardiography: incremental value of diastolic wall thickness measurement. Heart. 2005;91(5):613–7.
10. Travin MI, Bergmann SR. Assessment of myocardial viability. Semin Nucl Med. 2005;35(1):2–16.
11. Peovska I, Maksimovic J, Vavlukis M, Gorceva DP, Majstorov V. Functional outcome and quality of life after coronary artery bypass surgery in patients with severe heart failure and hibernated myocardium. Nucl Med Commun. 2008;29(3):215–21.
12. Lalonde L, Ziadi MC, Beanlands R. Cardiac positron emission tomography: current clinical practice. Cardiol Clin. 2009;27(2):237–55.
13. Weinsaft JW, Klem I, Judd RM. MRI for the assessment of myocardial viability. Cardiol Clin. 2007;25(1):35–56.
14. Nardi P, Pellegrino A, Scafuri A, Colella D, Bassano C, Polisca P, et al. Long-term outcome of coronary artery bypass grafting in patients with left ventricular dysfunction. Ann Thorac Surg. 2009;87(5):1401–7.
15. Shapira OM, Hunter CT, Anter E, Bao Y, DeAndrade K, Lazar HL, et al. Coronary artery bypass grafting in patients with severe left ventricular dysfunction–early and mid-term outcomes. J Card Surg. 2006;21(3):225–32.
16. Filsoufi F, Rahmanian PB, Castillo JG, Chikwe J, Kini AS, Adams DH. Results and predictors of early and late outcome of coronary artery bypass grafting in patients with severely depressed left ventricular function. Ann Thorac Surg. 2007;84(3):808–16.

Mitral Valve Repair for Ischemic Mitral Regurgitation with Advanced Cardiomyopathy

4

Leora B. Balsam, Eugene A. Grossi, and Aubrey Galloway

Introduction

Functional ischemic mitral regurgitation (FIMR) is a frequent end-stage complication of coronary artery disease which results from the process of negative left ventricular remodeling. Chronic myocardial ischemia and infarction effect an increase in left ventricular size secondary to myocyte loss and lengthening. As left ventricular size increases, the mitral annulus dilates and papillary muscle displacement tethers the mitral valve leaflets, causing FIMR. FIMR causes further impairment of ventricular function through volume overload, leading to the cycle of progressive left ventricular dilatation and worsening mitral regurgitation (MR) known as negative left ventricular remodeling [1–4]. With viable ischemic myocardium, revascularization of significant coronary artery disease may prevent further damage, relieve the contributing ischemia, and stop or reverse the remodeling process. However, the effect of correcting the ischemia alone on valve function has been unpredictable and often transient, leaving the majority of patients with residual, recurrent, or progressive MR [5]. Significant mitral regurgitation is treated by either valve repair or replacement. Mitral repair, while in the distant past was performed by suture annuloplasty, is now primarily performed by reduction annuloplasty (RA) with placement of an undersized annuloplasty device. This strategy increases the coaptive leaflet margin and reduces or eliminates the regurgitation [6]. Current surgical techniques for FIMR have significant procedural risk, and the late survival remains poor [7]. Due to the risk associated with current surgical therapies, the vast majority of patients with FIMR are treated medically [8]. In this chapter we will review current clinical and experimental data on the mechanisms and treatment of FIMR.

Clinical Scope and Consequences of Functional Ischemic MR

Heart failure affects over five million patients in the United States, with nearly 500,000 new cases diagnosed each year [9]. Coronary artery disease is a leading cause of systolic heart failure, affecting 40–60 % of heart failure patients [10]. In these patients, mitral regurgitation frequently coexists with systolic heart failure due to regional and global left ventricular remodeling. This mitral regurgitation, known as FIMR, is distinguished from other organic causes of mitral regurgitation, such as leaflet prolapse due to myxomatous change, leaflet flail secondary to chordal rupture, or leaflet perforation from endocarditis.

Functional ischemic MR can occur with preserved global left ventricular (LV) function

L.B. Balsam, M.D. (✉) • E.A. Grossi, M.D.
A. Galloway, M.D.
Department of Cardiothoracic Surgery,
New York University Langone Medical Center,
530 First Avenue, Suite 9V, New York, NY 10016, USA
e-mail: leora.balsam@nyumc.org;
eugene.grossi@nyumc.org; Aubrey.Galloway@nyumc.org

J.A. Morgan and Y. Naka (eds.), *Surgical Treatment for Advanced Heart Failure*,
DOI 10.1007/978-1-4614-6919-3_4, © Springer Science+Business Media New York 2013

(left ventricular ejection fraction [LVEF] > 30 %) or with severe LV dysfunction (LVEF < =30 %). In the former case, regional tethering and restriction of the posterior mitral valve leaflet result in FIMR, while in the latter case, increased LV dimensions and sphericity result in FIMR. Following myocardial infarction, there is a graded independent association between the severity of FIMR and the late development of heart failure. Aronson et al. prospectively studied 1,190 patients with acute myocardial infarction (MI) for the late development of congestive heart failure (CHF) [11]. In this cohort, FIMR, which was quantified echocardiographically during the hospitalization for acute MI, was mild in 39.7 % and moderate or severe in 6.3 %. All grades of FIMR (mild through severe) were associated with a significantly increased risk of CHF and death. Another large cohort study reported a similar relationship between moderate or severe FIMR and the late risk of CHF or death; importantly, this relationship was independent of left ventricular ejection fraction [12]. FIMR occurs in the majority of patients with ischemic cardiomyopathy, and their survival correlates with the degree of FIMR. In a recent observational study, Trichon et al. found an incidence of FIMR of 59 % in a cohort of 1,214 ischemic cardiomyopathy patients at a single center undergoing diagnostic work-up for heart failure (New York Heart Association [NYHA] class 2–4) [13]. The FIMR was mild (grade 1+ or 2+) in 38 % of the patients and moderate or severe (grade 3+ or 4+) in 17 %. Survival rates at 1, 3, and 5 years were significantly lower in patients with moderate to severe MR versus those with mild or no MR, and the degree of mitral regurgitation was an independent predictor of mortality by multivariable analysis.

Grigioni et al. also published their data on long-term outcomes in patients with chronic FIMR. In their series of 303 patients with previous transmural MI, 64 % developed chronic FIMR [14]. Patients with FIMR experienced worse survival rates than those without MR (38 ± 5 % vs. 61 ± 6 % at 5 years). Survival was also affected by FIMR grade (61 ± 6 % at 5 years for no MR; 47 ± 8 % at 5 years for effective regurgitant orifice (ERO) <20 mm^2; 29 ± 9 % at 5 years for ERO ≥ 20 mm^2).

Because FIMR has been associated with excess cardiac mortality, there has been considerable interest in the impact of its surgical correction on long-term outcomes. It is hypothesized that FIMR itself is an important contributor to the process of negative left ventricular remodeling, and elimination of FIMR, in combination with revascularization and/or medical therapy, may allow for normalization of left ventricular geometry. While FIMR can be reduced or eliminated with valve replacement or repair techniques, there has not been a direct correlation between elimination of FIMR and long-term reverse left ventricular remodeling. Moreover, valve repair techniques may have limited durability in certain clinical circumstances, leading to recurrent FIMR. As a consequence, long-term results of mitral surgery for FIMR have been inconsistent.

Experimental Studies of Functional Ischemic MR: Animal Models

The varied clinical presentation of patients makes it extremely difficult to analyze outcomes of FIMR treatment. Patients have varying amounts of ischemia, infarct, and subvalvular distortion which are both difficult to quantify and impossible to stratify for in the analysis of clinical trials. Fortunately, various animal models have been developed which, despite their limitations, offer insight into this complex disease and its treatment.

The Gorman research group at the University of Pennsylvania has performed a series of ovine myocardial infarct experiments which investigate the complex relationship of ischemic myocardial injury, LV remodeling, and functional mitral regurgitation. Their initial experimental series demonstrated that after a severe ischemic injury, ongoing negative LV remodeling will continue to occur even if the FIMR is "pretreated" or prevented by restrictive annuloplasty performed at the time of ischemic insult [15]. Lateral wall infarcts were induced in two groups of sheep; one group was pretreated with reduction annuloplasty (RA), while the other group was given a sham intervention (control). After 8 weeks, the RA group had successful prevention of FIMR, yet both groups had equal increases in left ventricular end-diastolic dimension (LVEDD; 68 ± 23 % for RA and 89 ± 16 % for control; p = NS) and equal decreases in ejection fraction (36.7 ± 3.7 % to 25.3 ± 2.9 % for RA and 42.4 ± 2.6 % to 32.4 ± 2.0 % for control; p = NS). In a more recent experimental report, restrictive mitral annuloplasty performed 8 weeks after large ischemic injury and myocardial infarction did not alter the ongoing process of LV dilation and negative remodeling, despite "successful" elimination of FIMR. In this model, after a severe infarction, negative remodeling progressed over a period of 6 months (twofold increase in end-diastolic volume and threefold increase in end-systolic volume) and was unaffected by eliminating the volume overload associated with the FIMR. Nevertheless, elimination of FIMR with reduction annuloplasty did significantly reduce pulmonary artery hypertension and was associated with greater forward cardiac output in the treated animals.

These experimental results are in marked opposition to ovine infarct experiments from Levine's group at Massachusetts General Hospital. In his series [16], all sheep had anteroapical infarcts, and two-thirds were also given controlled MR via a left ventricular to left atrial shunt (creating a 30 % regurgitant fraction). At one month postinfarction, half of the sheep had their shunts closed. The negative remodeling in this "MR-treated" group reversed, such that at 3 months, LV end-diastolic dimensions were the same as infarct alone and significantly better than infarct plus untreated MR. The authors concluded that repair of moderate MR substantially reverses the otherwise progressive remodeling process, with reduced left ventricular volumes, relatively maintained contractility, persistently activated intracellular signals promoting hypertrophy and opposing apoptosis, and reduced matrix proteolytic activity.

These seemingly contradictory results lead us to question the driving mechanisms for ongoing cardiac remodeling in ventricles with large infarcts zones and functional MR. Autopsy series [17] suggest that the remodeling pathway is related to the degree of myocardial mass lost and the amount of scarring, both of which lead to an increase in LV dimension that triggers cardiac myocyte apoptosis in border zones and to a lesser extent in remote regions of the ventricle. Also, there is strong laboratory evidence that mechanical tension (stress/strain) is responsible for activating the apoptotic pathway [18]. Another driving force in cardiac remodeling is the increase in cardiac myocyte length and decrease in end-diastolic wall thickness via chronic volume overload, as well the activation of neurohumoral systems including activation of adrenergic pathways, activation of the renin-angiotensin-aldosterone system, and release of atrial natriuretic peptide. We are left with the unanswered question as to which of the above mechanisms predominates in the remodeling response in these animal models.

Clinical data does provide insight into the ventricular response to the elimination of FIMR in the setting of preexisting damage. Dion demonstrated that when LV end-diastolic dimension is less than 6.5 cm, restrictive annuloplasty can reliably eliminate MR and is associated with sustained reverse ventricular remodeling [19]. This size stratification method may make it possible to identify ventricles in which the activation of cardiac myocyte apoptosis is not overwhelming and in which elimination of FIMR would allow for reversal of the cardiac myocyte lengthening due to chronic volume overload. Similarly, Alfieri reported two different patient responses to reduction annuloplasty for FIMR [20]. In his series, those patients who responded with reverse remodeling had long-term elimination of FIMR, and those who had ongoing negative remodeling had recurrence of their mitral insufficiency. In these patients, the degree of ventricular end-diastolic enlargement had a borderline significance in predicting ongoing negative remodeling.

It is possible to argue that the Gorman laboratory model is congruous with the "nonresponders" and does not reflect the group of patients who are capable of the reverse remodeling response (as demonstrated in the Levine model). Further laboratory work will be necessary to elucidate the above listed factors which control the ultimate fate of the ventricle. With an understanding of this, we will not only be able to clearly identify "responders" to reduction annuloplasty but also be able to develop other strategies to deal with the evolving pattern of ventricular remodeling.

Surgical Techniques for the Treatment of Functional Ischemic MR

While either mitral repair or replacement is acceptable for treating functional mitral regurgitation (FMR), there are two well-known confounding factors which impact the utilization of these therapies. The first factor is that the degree of functional mitral regurgitation is often downgraded during intraoperative transesophageal echocardiography (TEE) evaluation; as a result FMR tends to go untreated. Aklog et al. demonstrated in a population of patients with 3+ FMR documented preoperatively on transthoracic echocardiogram that only 10 % of the patients have 3+ MR on intraoperative TEE [5]. Unfortunately, their postoperative transthoracic echocardiogram reveals that 89 % still have 2+ or worse FMR. The second confounding factor is the misperception that CABG alone will improve MR of ischemic etiology. In patients with preoperative baseline MR of 3+ who underwent CABG alone, 40 % of these patients had no improvement in MR postoperatively, with 86 % having 2+ or worse FMR [5].

Having acknowledged some uncertainty in patient selection, the primary surgical intervention for functional ischemic mitral insufficiency is reduction annuloplasty or mitral valve replacement. While there are multiple factors which influence the decision whether to replace or repair FIMR valves, first we shall review the comparative outcomes. Gillinov et al. presented the Cleveland Clinic series of 397 mitral valve repairs and 85 mitral valve replacements analyzed by propensity case matching [21]. They demonstrated improved survival with valve repair versus valve replacement in "better risk patients." However, the 5-year survival was 56 % for repair and 36 % for replacement even in these patients. No survival benefit was demonstrated for repair over replacement in NYHA class 4 patients or in patients greater than 70 years of age. At the same time, we reported the experience at New York University. It was clear in our series that there was a significant difference in preoperative risk between those patients who received mitral repair and those that received mitral valve replacement for FIMR. The patients in our series who underwent replacement were more likely to be intubated, have preoperative shock, or have preoperative intra-aortic balloon pump placement. Our repair strategy was downsizing annuloplasty to treat the annular dilation and/or moderate to severe leaflet tethering. Our multivariable analysis demonstrated that hospital death was predicted by NYHA class 4 and a lack of angina. Analysis of death or complication via multiple logistic regression revealed that repair had half the risk compared to replacement. Indeed, when we analyzed the different preoperative risk subgroups, the hazard ratio for death or death and complication was always less than 1. This indicated that there was always a benefit to repair over replacement; the only subgroup in which this was not true was those patients who had previous surgery. Our 5-year complication-free survival was 63 % in our repair patients as compared to 30 % in the replacement patients. While late death was predicted by NYHA class 4 and the presence of prior cardiac surgery, complication-free survival was favored (odds ratio = 0.29) by mitral valve repair.

The above-mentioned datasets have therefore been used to support a preference for repair versus replacement. However, there are some patients in whom mitral repair may not have durability; this is discussed later in this chapter in the "Clinical Results" section.

In addition to the standard procedure of reduction annuloplasty, multiple alternative techniques have been advocated to treat FMR. These include the cutting of secondary chordae [22], posterior papillary muscle relocation [23, 24], anterior leaflet augmentation [25], and posterior leaflet patching. Division of secondary chordae releases the downward tented leaflet of the anterior mitral valve and decreases mitral leaflet tenting area. However, it is also argued that this effectively removes support from the papillary muscles, increases the sphericity of the ventricle, and worsens left ventricular performance [26].

The leaflet augmentation strategies with patching have demonstrated success in small series with limited follow-up. Of interest are the papillary muscle relocation procedures. Kron's group has limited data showing outcomes of placement of a traction suture placed into the posterior papillary muscle which shortens the distance to the right fibrous trigone [22]. Recently, the follow-up results of the "papillary muscle sling" technique have been published. A 4 mm graft is used to bring the papillary muscles together to reduce ventricle distortion. In a patient population at high risk for recurrence of MR (larger LV dimension), 4-year follow-up has been accrued. These results demonstrated good freedom from recurrent MR and improvements in ventricular diameter, volume, ejection fraction, and sphericity index [24].

Clinical Results of Surgical Treatment of Functional Ischemic MR

The strategy for surgical intervention in FIMR is based on four observations. First is the theoretical argument that FIMR imposes an important secondary remodeling stimulus on a ventricle that has already sustained a severe primary injury. Second, there is strong evidence that even mild MR is a poor prognostic sign in acute patients and those who have suffered an MI [14]. Third, there is a dramatic beneficial effect reported with valve repair for structural mitral valve disease. And fourth, there are limited alternative surgical options for FIMR patients with end-stage CHF. Clearly, from retrospective studies, there is little data at this time to support the concept that repairing these valves increases long-term survival [27, 28]. In rough summation, these clinical series show 50–60 % 5-year survival in patients undergoing treatment for their FIMR. This contrasts to Ellis et al.'s follow-up of patients undergoing percutaneous coronary intervention: those with either grade 3 or 4 MR at the time of intervention had only a 50 % survival at 36 months [29].

There is data, however, demonstrating that intervention on moderate or worse mitral insufficiency provides symptomatic benefits in those with patients with heart failure [27]. This has been excellently demonstrated by Dion in a subset of patients [19]. Specifically, in those patients with FIMR and LVEDD <6.5 cm, the 5-year survival for CABG and mitral repair was 80 %. These patients had an improvement in NYHA class from 2.9 to 1.6. Moreover, there was negligible recurrence of MR: mean follow-up MR grade was 0.8 (scale of 0–4), and 85 % of patients had less than grade 2. In contrast, patients with preoperative LVEDD greater than 6.5 cm had a 5-year survival of only 49 %, and there was little evidence of reverse remodeling. The authors concluded that for patients with an end-diastolic dimension of 6.5 cm or less, restrictive annuloplasty with revascularization provides a "cure" for ischemic MR and heart failure. While this may be an optimistic evaluation, their work does demonstrate the dramatic clinical benefit of surgical treatment of FIMR in appropriately selected patients.

Although valve repair is generally believed to be superior over replacement, there are several important technical considerations. First, most authors agree that either a rigid or semirigid remodeling device should be used and aggressive downsizing should be performed. Mitral insufficiency recurs at unacceptable rates when either flexible devices, tissue reinforcement, or suture-only techniques are used [7, 30, 31]. Secondly, multiple authors have noted that in patients with excessive distortion of the subvalvular apparatus, recurrent MR after reduction annuloplasty is not infrequent. Calafiore et al. noted that when the tenting distance was greater than 1 cm, the return of MR was "inevitable" [30]. Similarly, Duran noted that the degree of papillary displacement with respect to depth and angle correlated with return of MR [32].

Therefore, for treatment of FIMR, we do not recommend attempting a repair with reduction annuloplasty alone when the LVEDD is greater than 6.5 cm or the depth of leaflet coaptation is greater than 1 cm. Their results can be unpredictable and disappointing; patients with these dimensions are best served by chordal-sparing tissue valve replacement which reliably provides symptomatic relief.

Acker and colleagues published outcomes of the CorCap study in which patients underwent mitral valve surgery alone as a control arm of a Food and Drug Administration (FDA)-monitored investigational device study [33]. These medically optimized patients with significant functional MR, myopathic hearts, and symptomatic CHF underwent mitral valve surgery alone as control therapy. The patients were NYHA class 3 or 4, had EF < 35 % (mean EF 23 ± 9 %), and had dilated left ventricles (mean LVEDV 270.1 ± 100.3 mL). These patients had a remarkable 1.6 % 30-day mortality and significant improvements in quality of life, exercise performance, and NYHA functional class over the 2-year follow-up. Equally as important, mitral valve operations led to improvements in LV volumes (mean decrease of 45 mL), mass, and shape, all consistent with reverse remodeling. Finally, unlike other reported experiences in the literature, the operations were durable, as recurrence of clinically significant MR was uncommon in this patient cohort. The authors' concluded that "the improvement in LV structure and clinical function along with a very low mortality rate justifies strong consideration to offering mitral valve (MV) surgery to heart failure patients who are on an optimal medical regimen." The outcomes do support the hypothesis that these patients with cardiomyopathy benefit from the surgical correction of the functional mitral insufficiency. The results of this study add to a growing experience of clinical improvement with mitral valve repair. There is a significant caveat to this dataset however; 90 % of these FMR patients had a nonischemic etiology. How generalizable this is to the ischemic functional MR population is yet to be determined.

The New York University Experience

Our institutional experience with MV repair in the setting of impaired left ventricular function, including long-term echocardiographic and clinical outcomes, was recently presented at the annual meeting of the American College of Cardiology. Over 14 years, 193 patients with severe mitral regurgitation and EF < 50 % underwent mitral repair alone (reduction annuloplasty) without CABG. Sternotomy was utilized in 56 patients, and a mini-thoracotomy approach was used in 137 patients. Mean age was 63.7 years (range 24–90). Preoperative NYHA class was 2.8 (54.4 % were 3 or 4), and 41 (21.2 %) patients had previous cardiac surgery. Preoperative EF distribution was 40–49 % in 52 patients (26.9 %), 30–39 % in 81(42.0 %), 20–29 % in 37(19.2 %), and <20 % in 23(11.9 %).

Hospital mortality was 5.7 % overall and 3.6 % for mini-thoracotomy. Propensity-adjusted multivariate predictors (odds ratio; *p*-value) of hospital mortality were ischemic etiology (22.7; $p = 0.03$), age ($p = 0.04$), and chronic obstructive pulmonary disease or COPD (6.5; 0.03). The sternotomy approach (4.8; $p = 0$ .10) and peripheral vascular disease (5.8; $p = 0.10$) were weakly associated with hospital mortality. Freedom from all cause death was 74 % at 5 years (84 % for nonischemic patients and 51 % for ischemic patients; $p < 0.001$). Predictors of decreased survival were age ($p < 0.001$), severely impaired ejection fraction ($p = 0.01$), ischemic etiology ($p < 0.04$), and cerebrovascular disease ($p = 0.06$). NYHA class improved 0.9 grades ($p = 0.01$). At 5 years, freedom from valve reoperation was 92 %; freedom from valve reoperation or severe recurrent mitral insufficiency was 88 %. We concluded that reduction annuloplasty in FMR patients with decreased EF improves late NYHA functional status and is associated with good late survival. Significantly, the predictors of poor survival were age, lower EF, ischemic etiology, and cerebrovascular disease.

We recently published standard outcomes of CABG and reduction annuloplasty for FIMR in a controlled, prospective multicenter series [34]. Seventy patients with coronary artery disease requiring revascularization, severe or symptomatic moderate FIMR, ejection fraction ≥25 %, LVEDD ≤7.0 cm, and >30 days since acute myocardial infarction were treated with CABG and device reduction annuloplasty. Two patients underwent immediate intraoperative conversion to

Table 4.1 Structural and functional changes in patients treated with CABG and reduction annuloplasty

	Baseline	1 year	1.5 years	2 years
MR grade	2.54±0.81 (*N*=70)	0.52±0.66* (*N*=46)	0.35±0.63* (*N*=33)	0.48±0.62* (*N*=26)
LV EF	37.9±11.7 (*N*=67)	47.0±12.5** (*N*=46)	46.5±11.8** (*N*=33)	47.0±12.9*** (*N*=25)
LVEDD (cm)	5.83±0.68 (*N*=60)	5.34±0.86** (*N*=38)	5.55±0.80 (*N*=26)	5.16±0.75*** (*N*=17)
LVESD (cm)	4.66±0.89 (*N*=57)	3.94±1.08** (*N*=35)	4.26±1.03 (*N*=23)	3.96±0.95*** (*N*=17)

*$p<0.001$; **$p=0.001$; ***$p=0.01$

Mixed model, pairwise comparison versus baseline, adjusted for multiple comparisons

Reprinted from the Journal of Thoracic Cardiovascular Surgery, Vol. 141, Grossi EA, Woo YJ, Patel N, et al., Outcomes of coronary artery bypass grafting and reduction annuloplasty for functional ischemic mitral regurgitation: a prospective multicenter study (Randomized Evaluation of a Surgical Treatment for Off-Pump Repair of the Mitral Valve), pp. 91–97, copyright 2011, with permission from Elsevier

a valve replacement due to inability of reduction annuloplasty to correct MR. The as-treated results included a 30-day mortality of 4.1 %, with the patients receiving an average of 2.8 bypass grafts. Mean follow-up was 24.6 months. MR severity was significantly reduced from 2.54±0.80 at baseline to 0.52±0.66 and 0.35±0.63 at 1 and 2 years, respectively (MR scale was 0=none, 1=mild, 2=moderate, 3=moderate-severe, 4=severe). Freedom from death or valve reoperation was 78±5 % at 2 years. Ejection fraction significantly improved from 38 % to 47 % at 2 years. Reverse remodeling was evident with significant decreases in end-diastolic and end-systolic dimensions (Table 4.1). NYHA class was improved one or greater grades in 65.9 % at 1 year and 72.0 % at 2 years. Cox regression analyses suggested that increasing age ($p=0.001$; hazard ratio (HR) 1.16/year, 95 % CI 1.06–1.26) and renal disease ($p=0.018$; HR=3.48; 95 % CI 1.25–9.72) were associated with decreased survival.

From these data, we can conclude that CABG with reduction annuloplasty for FIMR predictably reduces MR and relieves symptoms in patients without excessive preexisting ventricular distortion. This operative strategy for the treatment of moderate to severe MR is associated with improved indices of ventricular geometry, improved NYHA functional class, and excellent freedom from recurrent mitral insufficiency. While long-term prognosis and outcomes remain uncertain, this dataset delineates the midterm benefits of such an approach.

Future Approaches in the Treatment of Functional Ischemic MR

Novel Clinical Research

One characteristic of functional MR is the presence of "normal" leaflet structure in the setting of ventricular remodeling which distorts the subvalvular apparatus and impairs valve function. A novel approach to treating this FMR is offered by the Coapsys device (Myocor, Inc., Maple Grove, MI), a ventricular shape change device that can be placed without the need for cardiopulmonary bypass to reduce FMR. This device consists of two pads which are connected by a transventricular "chordal" suture. After echocardiographically assisted placement across the left ventricle, the device is tightened to compress the mitral annulus, thereby reducing FMR and positively reshaping the ventricle [35]. An FDA-monitored investigational device trial was conducted in patients requiring CABG who had severe MR or symptomatic moderate MR, ejection fractions >=25 %, and LVEDD<=7.0 cm. The hypotheses tested were that investigative "off-pump" treatment would have non-inferior efficacy (as measured by MR degree) and superior safety efficacy as compared to standard mitral repair [36]. The trial was terminated prematurely when the recent financial collapse resulted in the bankruptcy of the trial sponsor (Myocor Inc.).

Recruitment had accrued 165 patients, the prespecified value for the "first-look" data analysis. The Coapsys device was associated with greater

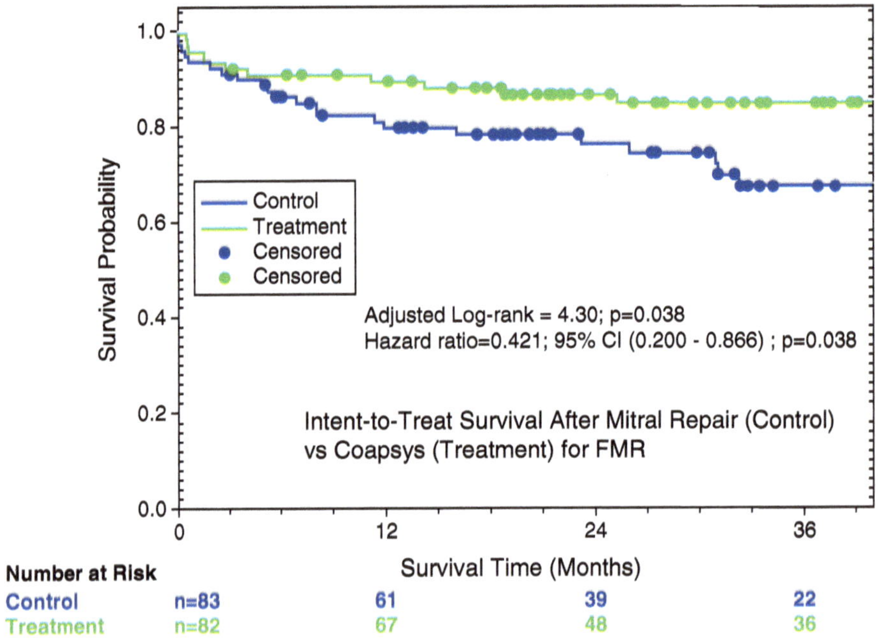

Fig. 4.1 Randomized Coapsys trial demonstrating late superior survival from all cause death for the Coapsys+CABG patients as compared to the control mitral repair+CABG patients (Reprinted from the Journal of the American College of Cardiology, Vol. 56, Grossi EA, Patel N, Woo YJ, et al., Outcomes of the RESTOR-MV Trial (Randomized Evaluation of a Surgical Treatment for Off-Pump Repair of the Mitral Valve), pp. 1984–1993, copyright 2010, with permission from Elsevier)

long-term positive ventricular reshaping, with the LVEDD decreasing from 6.0±0.8 to 5.4±0.8 cm as compared to 5.9±0.7 to 5.6±0.9 cm for the control MV repair (effect of time $p<0.001$, repeated measures analysis of variance [ANOVA]; effect of treatment $p=0.02$). However, the MR treatment efficacy was not as effective with the Coapsys treatment: the standard mitral repair technique reduced MR (0=none, 1=mild, 2=moderate, 3=moderate-severe, 4=severe scale) from 2.54±0.80 to 0.35±0.63 at 24 months, while Coapsys reduced MR from 2.40±0.87 to 1.24±0.97 (both effect of time and treatment $p=0.0001$, repeated measures ANOVA). What was totally unanticipated was that the trial discerned a significant survival benefit to the Coapsys treatment; at 24 months, there was nearly half the incidence of death with the Coapsys device as compared to standard mitral repair (Fig. 4.1). Twenty-four-month survival from all cause death was 89 % in the Coapsys randomized group as compared to 78 % in the standard treatment group (adjusted log-rank 4.30; $p=0.038$; intent-to-treat analysis); a more powerful benefit to the Coapsys treatment was noted in the as-treated analysis ($p=0.020$).

These findings are very provocative: patients with FIMR requiring revascularization treated with ventricular reshaping rather than standard mitral repair surgery had improved survival and significant reduction of major adverse outcomes. This unique dataset should guide further research in this area towards “ventricular solutions.”

Current Clinical Trials

Currently two topical clinical trials regarding the outcomes of ischemic mitral regurgitation are being conducted by the National Heart, Lung, and Blood Institute (NHLBI)-sponsored Cardiothoracic Surgical Trials Network. The first trial is entitled “Evaluation of Outcomes Following Mitral Valve Repair or Replacement in Severe Chronic Ischemic Mitral Regurgitation.” In this study, patients with severe FIMR will be randomized to either mitral repair or replacement; concomitant CABG will be performed if indicated. Pre- and postoperative evaluation will include cardiopulmonary exercise evaluation. The patients will be followed for 24 months. Interestingly, no restrictions are being applied as to the mitral valve repair technique employed by an individual surgeon.

The second trial is entitled "Surgical Interventions for Moderate Ischemic Mitral Regurgitation." The purpose of this trial is to determine whether repairing moderate mitral insufficiency at the time of planned CABG will have beneficial effects. Again, cardiopulmonary exercise testing, neurocognitive tests, and quality of life surveys will be conducted over a 2-year period. Unfortunately, patient recruitment has been an issue for both trials. It has been speculated that there is a lack of clinical equipoise when treating "stentable" coronary artery disease in the presence of moderate MR which has limited patient referral. The NHLBI has announced a request for additional investigative sites to correct this issue.

Summary

FIMR is a common end-stage complication of coronary artery disease that develops from myocardial injury and subsequent negative LV remodeling. While various animal models have been developed to offer insight into this complex pathologic process, data inferred from them is conflicting. More sensitive and specific models are warranted to gain insight into patient-specific disease status and treatment outcomes.

FIMR can be eliminated with valve replacement or repair techniques, and this provides documented relief of heart failure symptoms. Notably, in patients with smaller ventricles, a majority will have positive LV remodeling. Mitral repair appears to have benefit over replacement for the majority of patients. However, in those patients who are NYHA class 4 or greater than 70 years of age, there is no advantage to repair over replacement. Extensive valvular distortion is probably best treated with mitral replacement. Novel techniques are being developed not only to treat the valve but also to treat the underlying ventricular disease. The combined approaches of annular repair and ventricular reshaping may offer the best therapy for this very sick patient cohort in the future.

References

1. Hendren WG, Nemec JJ, Lytle BW, Loop FD, Taylor PC, Stewart RW, et al. Mitral valve repair for ischemic mitral insufficiency. Ann Thorac Surg. 1991;52(6):1246–51.
2. Sabbah HN, Rosman H, Kono T, Alam M, Khaja F, Goldstein S. On the mechanism of functional mitral regurgitation. Am J Cardiol. 1993;72(14):1074–6.
3. Komeda M, Glasson JR, Bolger AF, Daughters GT, 2nd, MacIsaac A, Oesterle SN, et al. Geometric determinants of ischemic mitral regurgitation. Circulation. 1997;96(9 Suppl):II-128–33.
4. Trichon BH, Glower DD, Shaw LK, Cabell CH, Anstrom KJ, Felker GM, et al. Survival after coronary revascularization, with and without mitral valve surgery, in patients with ischemic mitral regurgitation. Circulation. 2003;108 Suppl 1:II103–10.
5. Aklog L, Filsoufi F, Flores KQ, Chen RH, Cohn LH, Nathan NS, et al. Does coronary artery bypass grafting alone correct moderate ischemic mitral regurgitation? Circulation. 2001;104(12 Suppl 1):I68–75.
6. Bax JJ, Braun J, Somer ST, Klautz R, Holman ER, Versteegh MI, et al. Restrictive annuloplasty and coronary revascularization in ischemic mitral regurgitation results in reverse left ventricular remodeling. Circulation. 2004;110(11 Suppl 1):II103–8.
7. Grossi EA, Bizekis CS, LaPietra A, Derivaux CC, Galloway AC, Ribakove GH, et al. Late results of isolated mitral annuloplasty for "functional" ischemic mitral insufficiency. J Card Surg. 2001;16(4):328–32.
8. Mirabel M, Iung B, Baron G, Messika-Zeitoun D, Detaint D, Vanoverschelde JL, et al. What are the characteristics of patients with severe, symptomatic, mitral regurgitation who are denied surgery? Eur Heart J. 2007;28(11):1358–65.
9. Jessup M, Brozena S. Heart failure. N Engl J Med. 2003;348(20):2007–18.
10. He J, Ogden LG, Bazzano LA, Vupputuri S, Loria C, Whelton PK. Risk factors for congestive heart failure in US men and women: NHANES I epidemiologic follow-up study. Arch Intern Med. 2001;161(7):996–1002.
11. Aronson D, Goldsher N, Zukermann R, Kapeliovich M, Lessick J, Mutlak D, et al. Ischemic mitral regurgitation and risk of heart failure after myocardial infarction. Arch Intern Med. 2006;166(21):2362–8.
12. Bursi F, Enriquez-Sarano M, Nkomo VT, Jacobsen SJ, Weston SA, Meverden RA, et al. Heart failure and death aftery myocardial infarction in the community: the emerging role of mitral regurgitation. Circulation. 2005;111(3):295–301.

13. Trichon BH, Felker GM, Shaw LK, Cabell CH, O'Connor CM. Relation of frequency and severity of mitral regurgitation to survival among patients with left ventricular systolic dysfunction and heart failure. Am J Cardiol. 2003;91(5):538–43.
14. Grigioni F, Enriquez-Sarano M, Zehr KJ, Bailey KR, Tajik AJ. Ischemic mitral regurgitation: long-term outcome and prognostic implications with quantitative Doppler assessment. Circulation. 2001;103(13):1759–64.
15. Guy TSt, Moainie SL, Gorman JH, 3rd, Jackson BM, Plappert T, Enomoto Y, et al. Prevention of ischemic mitral regurgitation does not influence the outcome of remodeling after posterolateral myocardial infarction. J Am Coll Cardiol. 2004;43(3):377–83.
16. Beeri R, Yosefy C, Guerrero JL, Abedat S, Handschumacher MD, Stroud RE, et al. Early repair of moderate ischemic mitral regurgitation reverses left ventricular remodeling: a functional and molecular study. Circulation. 2007;116(11 Suppl):I288–93.
17. Abbate A, Biondi-Zoccai GG, Bussani R, Dobrina A, Camilot D, Feroce F, et al. Increased myocardial apoptosis in patients with unfavorable left ventricular remodeling and early symptomatic post-infarction heart failure. J Am Coll Cardiol. 2003;41(5): 753–60.
18. Pimentel DR, Amin JK, Xiao L, Miller T, Viereck J, Oliver-Krasinski J, et al. Reactive oxygen species mediate amplitude-dependent hypertrophic and apoptotic responses to mechanical stretch in cardiac myocytes. Circ Res. 2001;89(5):453–60.
19. Braun J, van de Veire NR, Klautz RJ, Versteegh MI, Holman ER, Westenberg JJ, et al. Restrictive mitral annuloplasty cures ischemic mitral regurgitation and heart failure. Ann Thorac Surg. 2008;85(2):430–6.
20. De Bonis M, Lapenna E, Verzini A, La Canna G, Grimaldi A, Torracca L, et al. Recurrence of mitral regurgitation parallels the absence of left ventricular reverse remodeling after mitral repair in advanced dilated cardiomyopathy. Ann Thorac Surg. 2008;85(3): 932–9.
21. Gillinov AM, Wierup PN, Blackstone EH, Bishay ES, Cosgrove DM, White J, et al. Is repair preferable to replacement for ischemic mitral regurgitation? J Thorac Cardiovasc Surg. 2001;122(6):1125–41.
22. Komeda M, Shimamoto T. Cutting secondary chordae and placing dual taut stitches between the anterior mitral fibrous annulus and the heads of each papillary muscle to treat ischemic mitral regurgitation without deteriorating left ventricular function. J Thorac Cardiovasc Surg. 2008;135(1):226–7.
23. Kron IL, Green GR, Cope JT. Surgical relocation of the posterior papillary muscle in chronic ischemic mitral regurgitation. Ann Thorac Surg. 2002;74(2): 600–1.
24. Hvass U, Joudinaud T. The papillary muscle sling for ischemic mitral regurgitation. J Thorac Cardiovasc Surg. 2010;139(2):418–23.
25. Kincaid EH, Riley RD, Hines MH, Hammon JW, Kon ND. Anterior leaflet augmentation for ischemic mitral regurgitation. Ann Thorac Surg. 2004;78(2): 564–8.
26. Rodriguez F, Langer F, Harrington KB, Tibayan FA, Zasio MK, Liang D, et al. Cutting second-order chords does not prevent acute ischemic mitral regurgitation. Circulation. 2004;110(11 Suppl 1):II91–7.
27. Harris KM, Sundt TM, 3rd, Aeppli D, Sharma R, Barzilai B. Can late survival of patients with moderate ischemic mitral regurgitation be impacted by intervention on the valve? Ann Thorac Surg. 2002;74(5): 1468–75.
28. Diodato MD, Moon MR, Pasque MK, Barner HB, Moazami N, Lawton JS, et al. Repair of ischemic mitral regurgitation does not increase mortality or improve long-term survival in patients undergoing coronary artery revascularization: a propensity analysis. Ann Thorac Surg. 2004;78(3):794–9.
29. Ellis SG, Whitlow PL, Raymond RE, Schneider JP. Impact of mitral regurgitation on long-term survival after percutaneous coronary intervention. Am J Cardiol. 2002;89(3):315–8.
30. Calafiore AM, Gallina S, Di Mauro M, Gaeta F, Iaco AL, D'Alessandro S, et al. Mitral valve procedure in dilated cardiomyopathy: repair or replacement? Ann Thorac Surg. 2001;71(4):1146–52.
31. McGee EC, Gillinov AM, Blackstone EH, Rajeswaran J, Cohen G, Najam F, et al. Recurrent mitral regurgitation after annuloplasty for functional ischemic mitral regurgitation. J Thorac Cardiovasc Surg. 2004;128(6): 916–24.
32. Matsunaga A, Tahta SA, Duran CM. Failure of reduction annuloplasty for functional ischemic mitral regurgitation. J Heart Valve Dis. 2004;13(3):390–7. discussion 397–8.
33. Acker MA, Bolling S, Shemin R, Kirklin J, Oh JK, Mann DL, et al. Mitral valve surgery in heart failure: insights from the Acorn Clinical Trial. J Thorac Cardiovasc Surg. 2006;132(3):568–77.
34. Grossi EA, Woo YJ, Patel N, Goldberg JD, Schwartz CF, Subramanian VA, et al. Outcomes of coronary artery bypass grafting and reduction annuloplasty for functional ischemic mitral regurgitation: a prospective multicenter study (Randomized evaluation of a surgical treatment for off-pump repair of the mitral valve). J Thorac Cardiovasc Surg. 2011;141(1):91–7.
35. Grossi EA, Woo YJ, Schwartz CF, Gangahar DM, Subramanian VA, Patel N, et al. Comparison of Coapsys annuloplasty and internal reduction mitral annuloplasty in the randomized treatment of functional ischemic mitral regurgitation: impact on the left ventricle. J Thorac Cardiovasc Surg. 2006;131(5):1095–8.
36. Grossi EA, Patel N, Woo YJ, Goldberg JD, Schwartz CF, Subramanian V, et al. Outcomes of the RESTOR-MV Trial (Randomized evaluation of a surgical treatment for off-pump repair of the mitral valve). J Am Coll Cardiol. 2010;56(24):1984–93.

5 Aortic Valve Replacement for Severe Aortic Stenosis or Aortic Insufficiency with Advanced Left Ventricular Dysfunction

S. Chris Malaisrie and Patrick M. McCarthy

Introduction

Surgery for aortic valvular lesions, in particular severe symptomatic aortic stenosis (AS), can result in excellent relief of symptoms and prolongation of survival. Similarly, successful surgical correction of aortic insufficiency (AI) can result in resolution of left ventricular dilatation and subsequent improvement in ejection fraction. Heart failure (HF) is the eventual endpoint of aortic valvular lesions if the diagnosis or treatment is delayed. Aortic valvular disease with advanced heart failure can result from either disregarded aortic valvular disease or, uncommonly, from concomitant aortic valvular disease in the setting of a preexisting cardiomyopathy. In the latter case, surgical therapy carries an increased risk of operative mortality; however, patients may benefit from surgical intervention as continued medical therapy is associated with a dismal prognosis.

This chapter will review the two aortic valvular lesions of AS and AI in the setting of advanced heart failure. The utilization of surgical treatment will be addressed with a focus on improved contemporary surgical results and possible future therapy aimed at high-risk patients as an alternative to traditional open heart surgery.

S.C. Malaisrie, M.D. (✉) • P.M. McCarthy, M.D.
Division of Cardiac Surgery,
Northwestern Memorial Hospital, 201 East Huron St., Suite 11-140, Chicago, IL 60611, USA
e-mail: cmalaisr@nmh.org; pmccart@nmh.org

Aortic Insufficiency and Heart Failure

The causes of AI are multiple, but the most frequent are annuloaortic ectasia from thoracic aortic aneurysmal disease and bicuspid aortic valve. The role of echocardiography is to determine the presence and severity of AI, the mechanism of AI, the degree of left ventricular (LV) dysfunction and dilatation, and the presence of associated aortic root and ascending aortic aneurysms (Fig. 5.1). Cardiac magnetic resonance angiography (MRA) or computed tomographic angiography (CTA) may be helpful in cases where the mechanism of AI or the degree of aortic dilatation is unclear by echocardiography (Fig. 5.2). We perform MRA or CTA in all patients with bicuspid aortic valves (BAV) who are to undergo surgery to determine the presence of an ascending aortic aneurysm.

When symptoms from severe AI are mild, LV dilatation can become severe with left ventricular end-diastolic diameter (LVEDD) >70 mm and left ventricular end-systolic diameter (LVESD) >50 mm due to chronic volume overload of the LV (Fig. 5.3). Severe LV dysfunction, particularly with ejection fraction (EF) less than 25 %, may be irreversible. Whereas patients that undergo aortic valve replacement (AVR) before the development of advanced heart failure can expect a reduction in LV dimensions in the first several months after surgery and subsequent long-term improvement in EF [1], patients with advanced heart failure may not realize such improvement even after successful correction of the AI with AVR [2].

J.A. Morgan and Y. Naka (eds.), *Surgical Treatment for Advanced Heart Failure*,
DOI 10.1007/978-1-4614-6919-3_5, © Springer Science+Business Media New York 2013

Prognosis of Aortic Insufficiency with Heart Failure

Patients who develop acute, severe AI, most commonly from an acute type A aortic dissection or infective endocarditis, have a life-threatening condition as the LV cannot compensate for the abrupt onset of volume overload. Because patients with acute severe AI often present with LV deterioration, manifested by pulmonary edema and

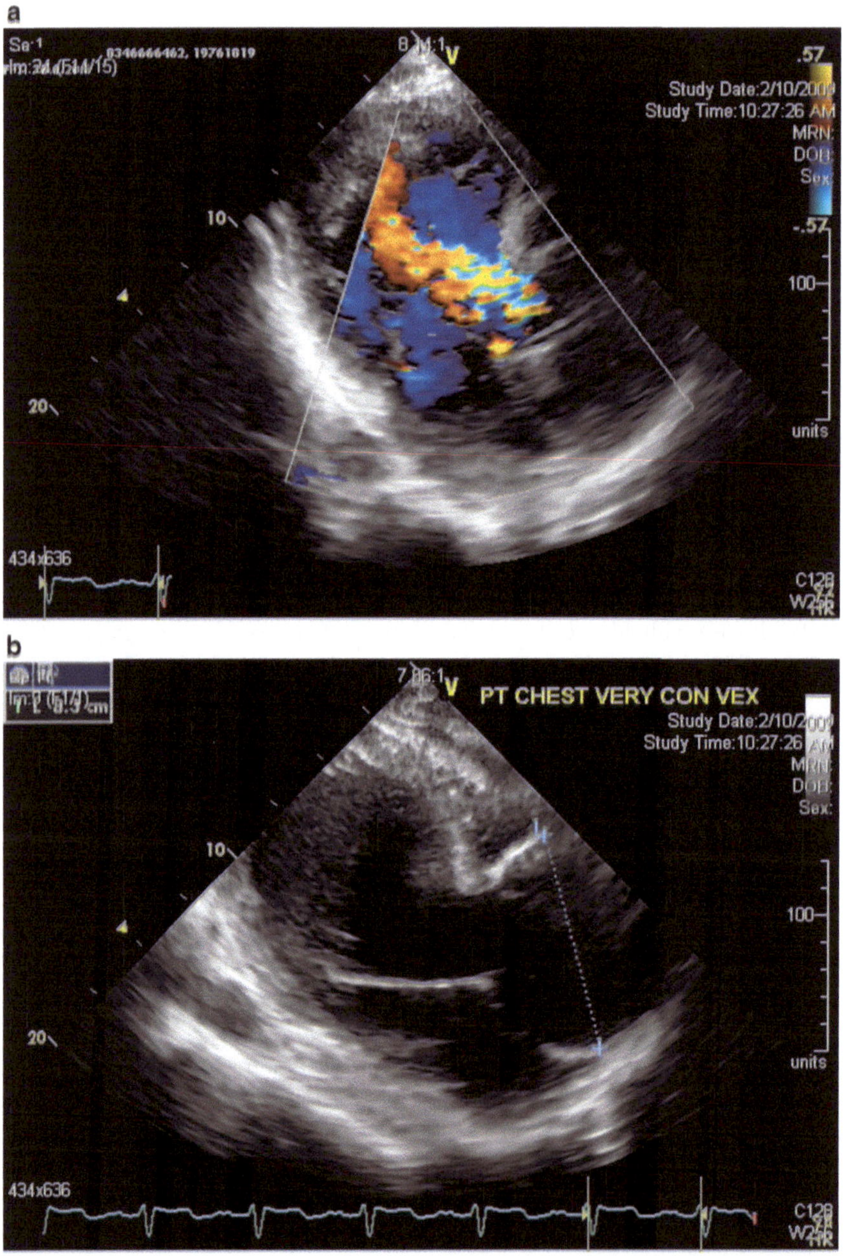

Fig. 5.1 (**a**) Parasternal long-axis view with color flow imaging by transthoracic echocardiography shows severe aortic insufficiency. (**b**) Parasternal long-axis view shows severe annuloaortic ectasia causing poor coaptation of the aortic valve leaflets. (**c**) Parasternal long-axis view shows severe left ventricular dilatation and poor ejection fraction resulting from long-standing severe aortic insufficiency

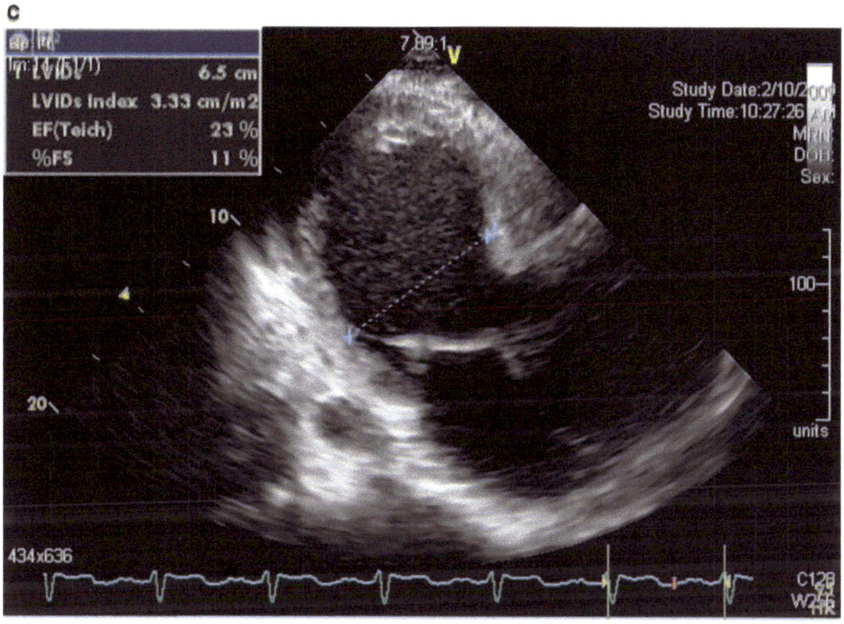

Fig. 5.1 (continued)

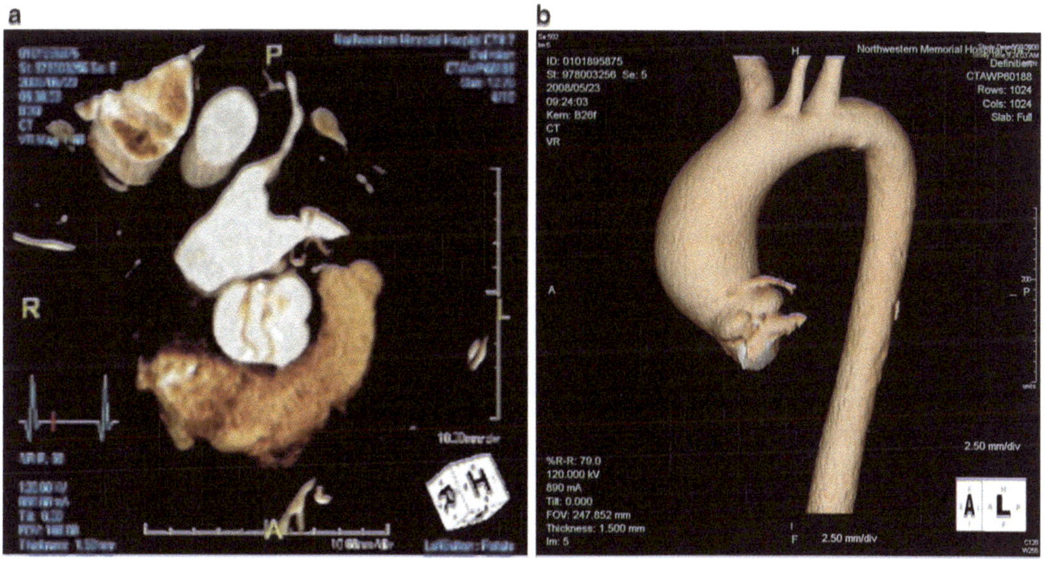

Fig. 5.2 (**a**) Echocardiogram (ECG)-gated dual-source computer tomography with 3-dimensional reconstruction shows an aortic valve with bicuspid morphology. (**b**) ECG-gated dual-source computer tomography with 3-dimensional reconstruction shows an associated ascending aortic aneurysm

cardiogenic shock, urgent treatment is necessary. Intensive vasodilator therapy is beneficial when feasible, but urgent surgical intervention is required.

Patients with chronic AI, however, can tolerate the gradual onset of volume overload with compensatory eccentric hypertrophy of the LV. Asymptomatic patients with severe AI and

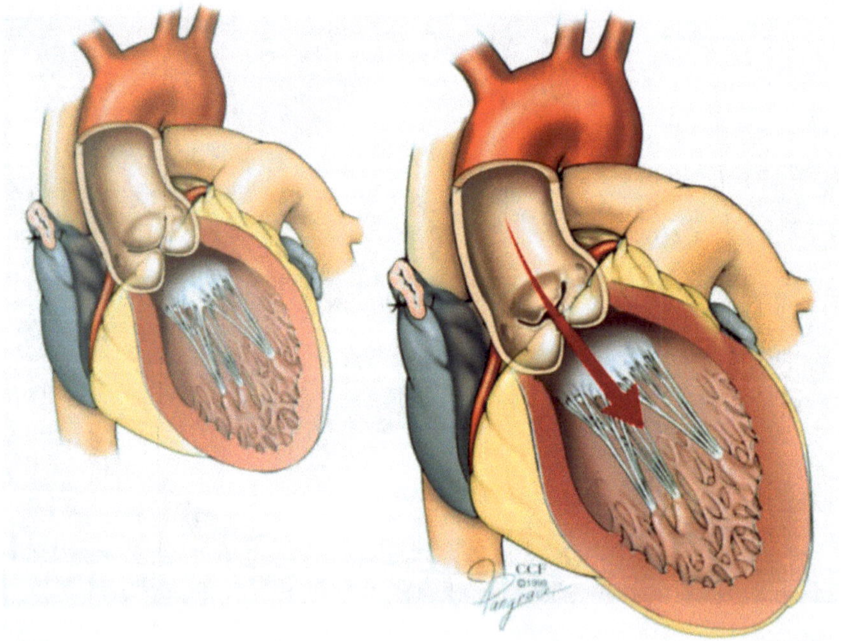

Fig. 5.3 Left ventricular dilatation resulting from chronic aortic insufficiency (Reprinted with permission, Cleveland Clinic Center for Medical Art & Photography © 1999–2013)

normal LV function have a risk of sudden death of less that 0.2 % per year. However, the natural history of symptomatic patients with severe AI is poor with a risk of death greater than 10 % per year for patients with angina pectoris and greater than 20 % per year for patients with heart failure [3–5]. Studies in animals shows that long-standing chronic AI results in myocardial fibrosis with increased deposition of extracellular matrix [6]. The resulting myocardial fibrosis may be the pathologic basis of irreversible LV dysfunction and end-stage heart failure for patients with severe AI.

Historical Results of Aortic Valve Replacement for Aortic Insufficiency

AVR for patients with AI and advanced heart failure (EF <25 %) can be associated with an operative mortality of up to 10 % and poor long-term survival [7]. Because of such poor outcomes, consideration of heart transplantation for these patients has been recommended in the past. However, results of AVR for AI with advanced heart failure (EF <30 %) have improved dramatically over time with operative mortality of 17 % before 1985 compared to 0 % after 1985 in a large surgical series (Fig. 5.4) [8]. Moreover, patients with advanced heart failure undergoing AVR after 1985 can have a long-term survival similar to patients without advanced heart failure (Fig. 5.5).

Current Recommendation for AVR for AI and HF

Recommendation from the 2008 American Heart Association/American College of Cardiology (AHA/ACC) and 2007 European Society of Cardiology (ESC) guidelines for chronic AI are similar [7, 9]. Class I indications for surgery for patients with severe AI include the presence of symptoms, LV dysfunction with EF <50 %. Class IIa indications include LV dilatation with LVESD >55 mm or LVEDD >75 mm and concomitant cardiac

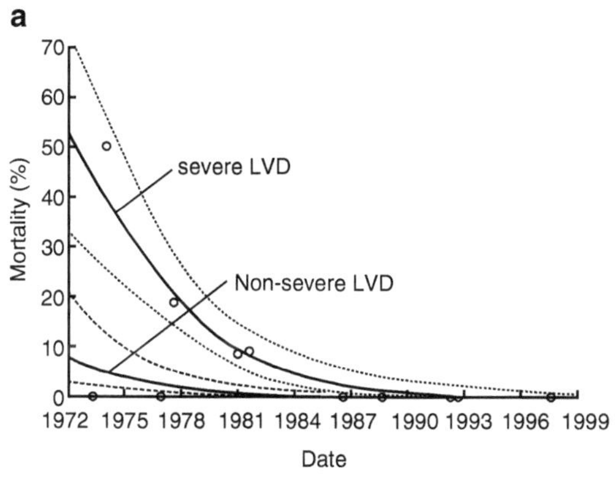

Fig. 5.4 Improved operative mortality after aortic valve replacement for patients with chronic aortic insufficiency and advanced heart failure over time (Reprinted from Journal of the American College of Cardiology, Vol. 49, Bhudia SK, McCarthy PM, Kumpati GS, Helou J, Hoercher KJ, Rajeswaran J, Blackstone EH, Improved outcomes after aortic valve surgery for chronic aortic regurgitation with severe left ventricular dysfunction, pages 1465–1471, copyright 2007, with permission from Elsevier)

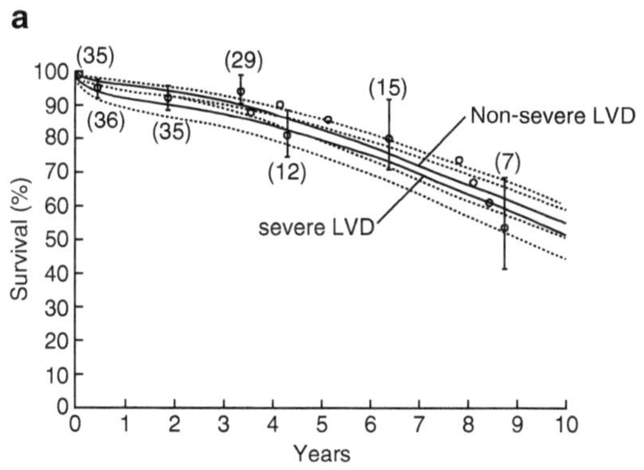

Fig. 5.5 Long-term survival of patients undergoing aortic valve replacement after 1985 for patients with ejection fraction <30 % is similar to that for patients with ejection fraction >30 % (Reprinted from Journal of the American College of Cardiology, Vol. 49, Bhudia SK, McCarthy PM, Kumpati GS, Helou J, Hoercher KJ, Rajeswaran J, Blackstone EH, Improved outcomes after aortic valve surgery for chronic aortic regurgitation with severe left ventricular dysfunction, pages 1465–1471, copyright 2007, with permission from Elsevier)

surgery including coronary artery bypass graft (CABG), other valvular surgery, or aortic aneurysm repair. Class IIb indications include LV dilatation with LVESD >50 mm or LVEDD >70 mm. No particular recommendations are made by either set of guidelines regarding patients with advanced heart failure. Although patients with recent onset of symptoms and patients that improve with intensive medical therapy including intensive vasodilators, diuretics, or inotropic support may demonstrate LV recovery after AVR, exactly which patients will demonstrate an improvement in LV function after a successful AVR is unknown. AVR is, nevertheless, a better alternative than the higher risk of long-term medical management alone for severe AI with advanced heart failure [10]. Therefore, it is reasonable to proceed with AVR in patients with severe AI and advanced heart failure in order to stop further decompensation and facilitate the chronic medical management of the patient's heart failure, especially the use of beta-blockers which is contraindicated in patients with AI. If possible, the use of blood transfusion should be avoided in patients with advanced heart disease in case further deterioration occurs, resulting in candidacy for heart transplantation.

Aortic Stenosis and Heart Failure

Aortic stenosis can be caused by senile, calcific aortic stenosis, which is the most common cause for patients older the 75 years; bicuspid aortic valve, which commonly manifest in younger patients between 65 and 75 years; or, less frequently, rheumatic heart disease. The diagnosis of severe aortic stenosis is made with echocardiography based on a combination of parameters. Peak jet velocity and mean pressure gradients can be reliably measured but are flow dependent and therefore affected by the left ventricular stroke volume and cardiac output. Aortic valve area, calculated using the continuity equation, is less dependent on stroke volume and cardiac output and most reliably identifies patients with severe AS in advanced heart failure. When peak jet velocity >4.0 m/s, mean valvular gradient >40 mmHg, or aortic valve area <1.0 cm^2, the AS is considered severe [7].

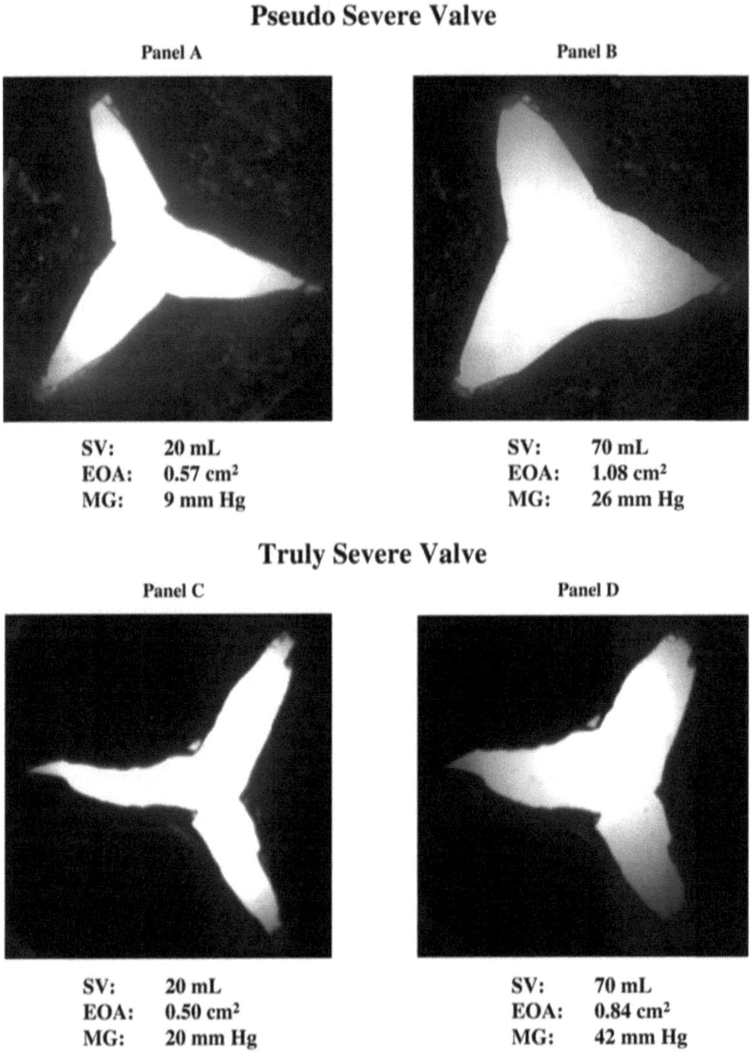

Fig. 5.6 In vitro comparison of fixed severe aortic stenosis with pseudo-severe aortic stenosis. (Reprinted with permission from Blais C, Burwash IG, Mundigler G, Dumesnil JG, Loho N, Rader F, Baumgartner H, Beanlands RS, Chayer B, Kadem L, Garcia D, Durand L-G, Pibarot P. Projected valve area at normal flow rate improves the assessment of stenosis severity in patients with low-flow, low-gradient aortic stenosis: the multicenter TOPAS (Truly or Pseudo-Severe Aortic Stenosis) study. Circulation. 2006;113(5):711–721)

In advanced heart failure, the left ventricle is unable to generate either a significant peak jet velocity or mean pressure gradient despite an aortic valve area that is diagnostic for severe aortic stenosis. This condition, termed low-gradient aortic stenosis (LGAS), can present a diagnostic challenge for clinicians because patients with LGAS can have either truly severe aortic stenosis with resulting poor ejection fraction or primary cardiomyopathy with only moderate aortic stenosis. The latter condition, termed pseudo-severe AS, occurs because the calculated aortic valve area may not be a reliable measurement of the severity of AS. In advanced heart failure, the aortic valve may fail to open completely not as a result of a fixed stenosis but as a result of low stroke volume (Fig. 5.6). Patients with pseudo-severe AS, therefore, have

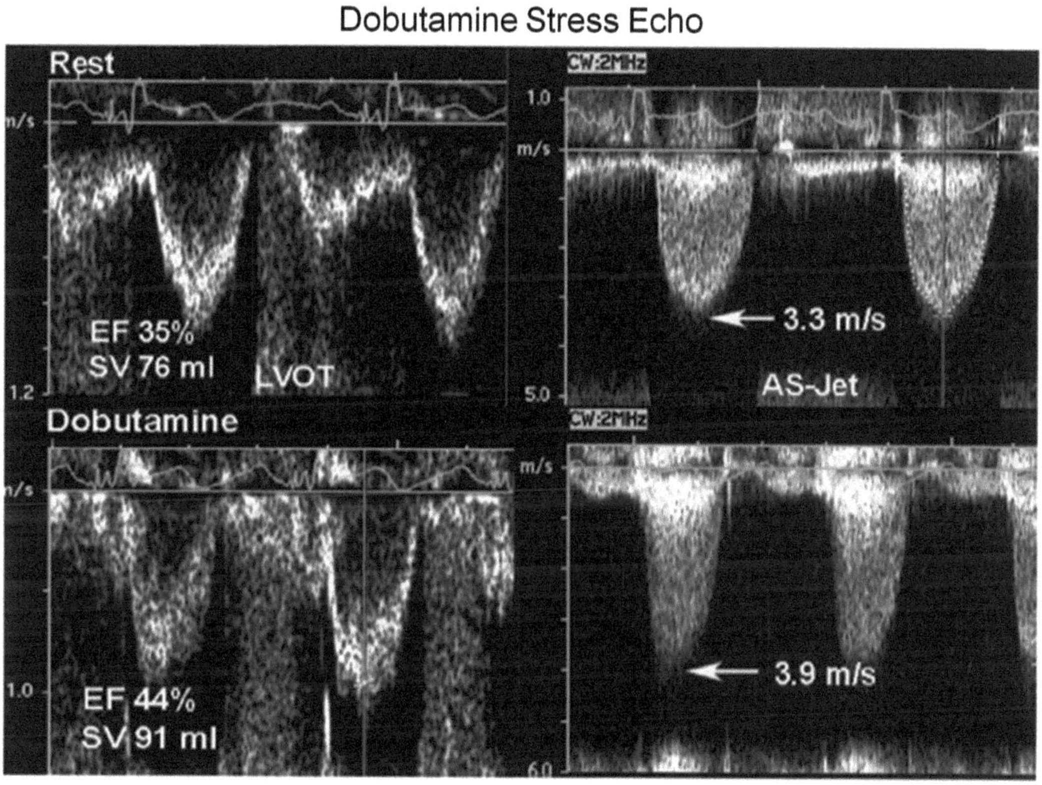

Fig. 5.7 Dobutamine stress echocardiography demonstrates the difference in response in patients with fixed aortic stenosis and pseudo-severe aortic stenosis (Reprinted from Journal of the American College of Cardiology, Vol. 47, Otto CM, Valvular aortic stenosis: disease severity and timing of intervention, pages 2141–2151, copyright 2006, with permission from Elsevier)

a calculated aortic valve area which is falsely reduced.

In order to distinguish between fixed severe AS and pseudo-severe AS, a dobutamine stress study either with echocardiography (Fig. 5.7) or direct pressure measurements during cardiac catheterization (Fig. 5.8) can be performed in patients with LGAS. Doses of up to 20 mcg/kg/min of dobutamine are infused under physician surveillance, while the peak jet velocity, mean pressure gradient, and aortic valve area are measured. In patients with fixed aortic stenosis, the peak jet velocity and mean pressure gradient will increase while the valve area remains unchanged as stroke volume and ejection fraction increases. In patients with pseudo-severe AS, on the other hand, the valve area increases while the peak jet velocity and mean pressure gradient remain unchanged [11, 12].

Prognosis of Aortic Stenosis with Heart Failure

The natural history of asymptomatic AS is indolent with a risk of sudden death without preceding symptoms of approximately 1 % per year [7]. The prognosis of severe AS when patients are symptomatic, however, is poor. The average life expectancy is approximately 2 years after the onset of symptoms and less after the onset of heart failure (Fig. 5.9). As the left ventricle responds to the pressure overload with concentric hypertrophy caused by chronic outflow obstruction, patients

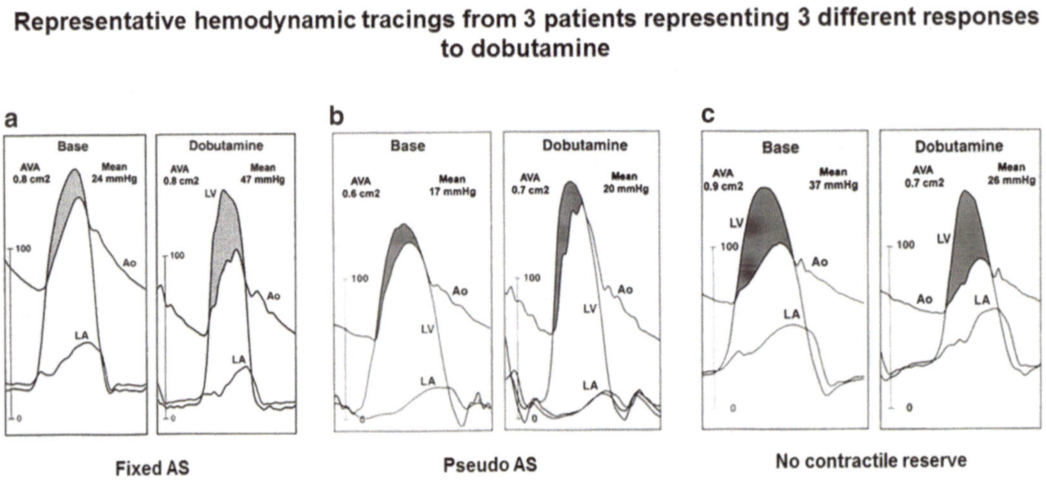

Fig. 5.8 Response to dobutamine during cardiac catheterization demonstrates the hemodynamic changes in patients with fixed aortic stenosis, pseudo-severe aortic stenosis, and no contractile reserve (Reprinted with permission from Nishimura RA, Grantham JA, Connolly HM, Schaff HV, Higano ST, Holmes DR Jr. Low-output, low-gradient aortic stenosis in patients with depressed left ventricular systolic function: the clinical utility of the dobutamine challenge in the catheterization laboratory. Circulation. 2002;106(7):809–813)

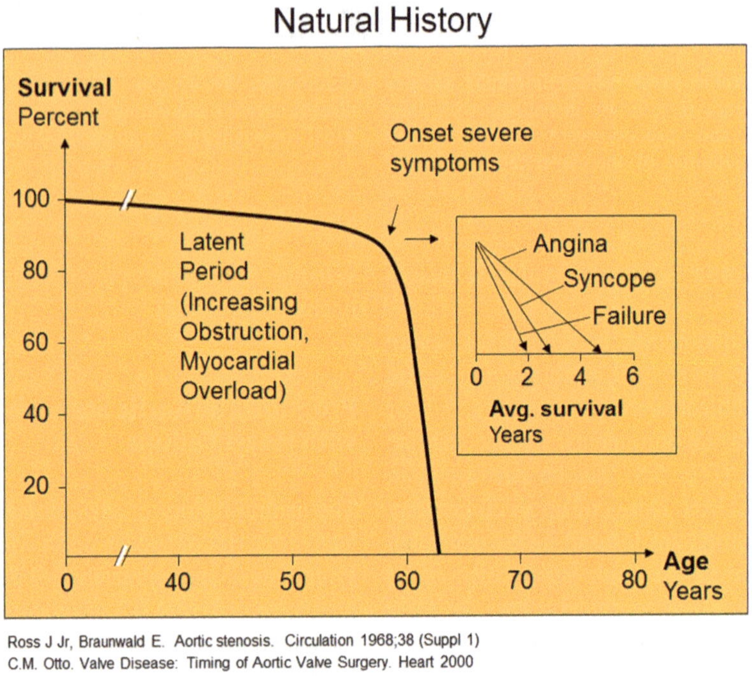

Fig. 5.9 Natural history of aortic stenosis is indolent until the onset of symptoms (Reprinted with permission from Ross J Jr, Braunwald E. Aortic stenosis. Circulation 1968;38(1S5):61–67)

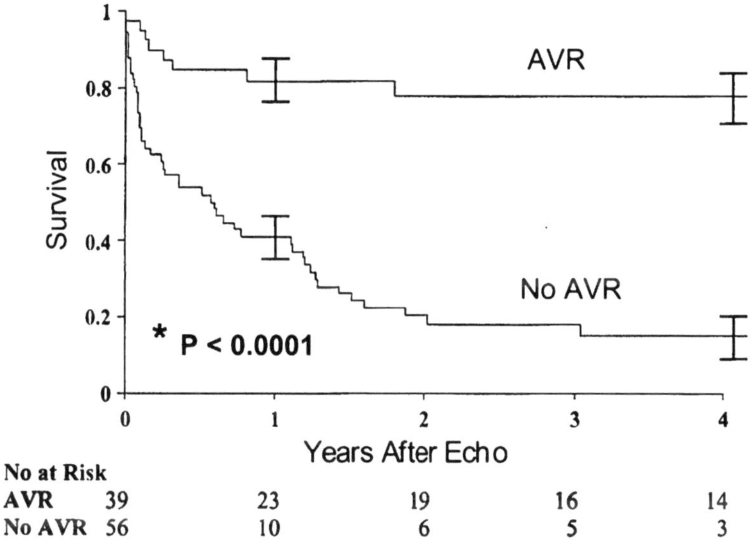

Fig. 5.10 Long-term survival after aortic valve replacement for patients with low-gradient aortic stenosis is superior to medical therapy (Reprinted from Journal of the American College of Cardiology, Vol. 39, Pereira JJ, Lauer MS, Bashir M, Afridi I, Blackstone EH, Stewart WJ, McCarthy PM, Thomas JD, Asher CR, Survival after aortic valve replacement for severe aortic stenosis with low transvalvular gradients and severe left ventricular dysfunction, pages 1356–1363, copyright 2002, with permission from Elsevier)

experience progressive dyspnea on exertion, angina, and syncope. In advanced heart failure secondary to untreated AS, patient survival with medical therapy is less than 50 % at 1 year [13].

Historical Results of Aortic Valve Replacement for Aortic Stenosis

AVR for patients with LGAS was previously associated with poor operative outcomes with mortality as high as 21 % [14]. Improved surgical outcomes have led to a reexamination of AVR for patients with AS and advanced heart failure. Reduced operative mortality and increased long-term survival can be achieved as compared to dismal outcomes associated with medical therapy (Fig. 5.10). In an effort to identify which patients with LGAS would benefit from AVR, a multicenter study in Europe studied patients with and without contractile reserve of the left ventricle as measured by dobutamine stress echocardiography [15]. In patients whose left ventricular stroke volume was augmented with dobutamine infusion, operative mortality was as low as 5 %. In contrast, patients without contractile reserve whose stroke volume were unable to be augmented with dobutamine infusion had a poor operative mortality of up to 31 %. Despite this poor operative mortality, patients with LGAS and no contractile reserve that survived surgery demonstrated recovery of LV function similar to patients with contractile reserve [16].

Current Recommendation for AVR for AS and HF

No particular recommendation are made in the AHA/ACC guidelines in regards to patients with AS and advanced heart failure [7]. The European guidelines state that patients with LGAS with contractile reserve have a class IIa indication and patients with LGAS without contractile reserve have a class IIb indication for surgery [9]. Prognosis for patients with AS and advanced heart failure managed medically is dismal, and although AVR is associated with an elevated operative mortality, long-term survival after a successful operation to relieve AS is superior even in patients without contractile.

Operative Concerns for AVR and HF

Current excellent outcomes after AVR can be attributed to improved preoperative medical optimization, operative technique, and postoperative care. Medical management with current regimens including angiotensin-converting enzyme inhibitors and beta-blockers has improved substantially over time. In the operating room over the past two decades, refinement in cardioplegia has permitted safer myocardial protection, and intraoperative echocardiography has permitted a reduction in complications. Optimization of inotropic management with agents such as phosphodiesterase inhibitors and the use of antiarrhythmic agents such as amiodarone have reduced deaths. Postoperatively, devices such as biventricular synchronous pacemakers and implantable cardioverter-defibrillators may also be used to improve midterm survival.

Concerns related to an AVR with advanced heart failure can be addressed with minimal alteration in surgical technique. Although minimally invasive approach is possible in the majority of patient, this approach is avoided in patients with advanced heart failure to allow complete decompression of the left ventricle. Myocardial protection must be meticulous particularly for those patients with extensive left ventricular hypertrophy. In these cases, antegrade cardioplegia is the preferred technique in order to minimize the possibility of subendocardial ischemia from inadequate distribution of cardioplegia. Although mechanical circulatory support such as intra-aortic balloon pulsation (IABP) may become necessary for postoperative low-cardiac output syndrome, we do not use it prophylactically due to known IABP complications.

Finally, newer-generation heart valves both mechanical and bioprosthetic have lower pressure gradients, reducing the incidence of patient-prosthesis mismatch (PPM) [17]. Two studies have examined the role of PPM in perioperative mortality in patients with LGAS and have not found a statistically significant difference in survival between patients with PPM (defined as an indexed effective orifice area (EOA) ≤ 0.85 cm^2/m^2) as compared to those without PPM, although data from one study suggested a trend in worse 10-year survival [18, 19]. This same study demonstrated an increased rate of congestive heart failure and impaired LV mass regression in patients with PPM [19]. It is unclear, however, that extensive surgical procedures such as aortic annular enlargement or aortic root replacement with either stentless xenografts or human allografts justify the increased operative risk to avoid PPM.

Future of Aortic Valve Surgery in Heart Failure

Resurgence of Aortic Balloon Valvuloplasty

Aortic balloon valvuloplasty (ABV) is not an acceptable alternative to AVR; however, it can be used as a staging procedure prior to AVR in patients with hemodynamic instability or as a purely palliative procedure for inoperable patients [7]. Increased interest in wider application of ABV for patients with heart failure has resulted as a result of patient referrals for transcatheter aortic valve implantation (TAVI). In current trials, patients with EF <20 % are not eligible for enrollment due to advanced heart failure. A strategy being used by many centers is to perform an ABV as a potential bridge to enrollment in ongoing trials. This strategy aims to relieve afterload to determine the response in LV function. If LV function improves, further definitive intervention whether standard AVR or TAVI becomes a viable option. Without a response in LV function, it becomes unlikely that definitive surgery will be beneficial.

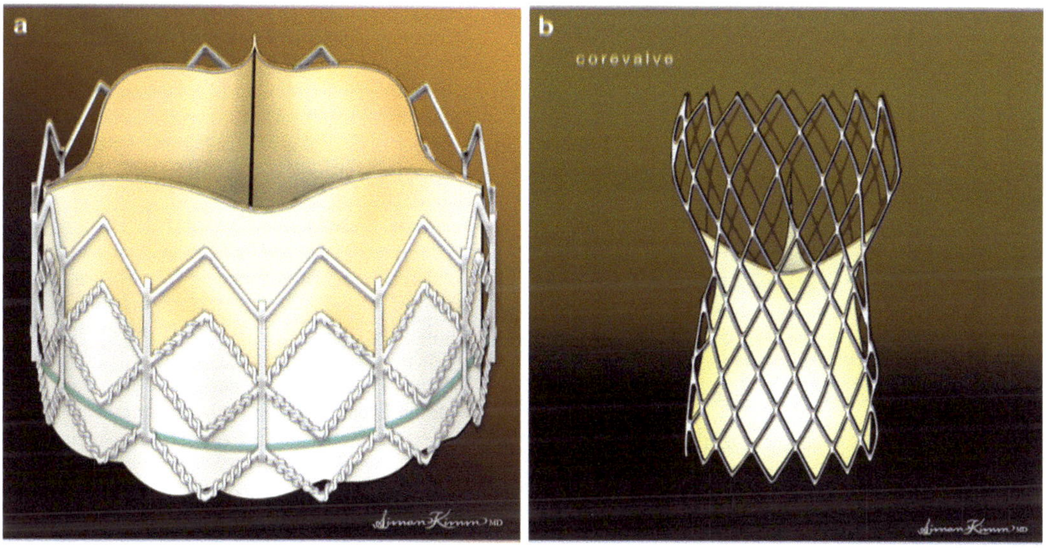

Fig. 5.11 (**a**) Edwards Lifesciences, Sapien valve (Irvine, CA). A bovine pericardial valve is attached to a balloon-expandable stainless-steel stent. (**b**) CoreValve Revalving System (Medtronic, Minneapolis, MN). A porcine pericardial valve is attached to a self-expandable nitinol stent

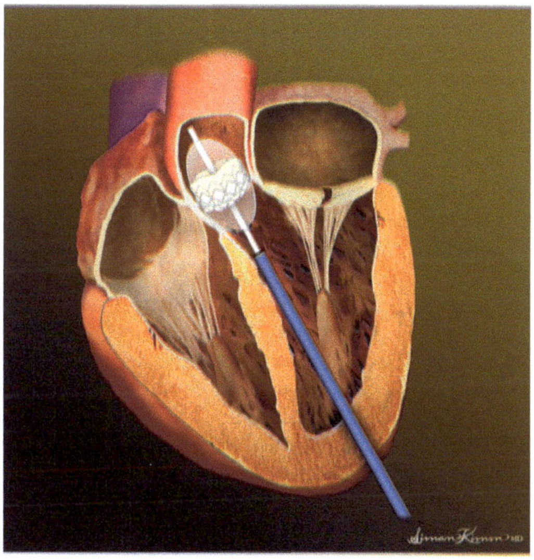

Fig. 5.12 Transapical approach for aortic valve implantation. A stent valve is introduced through the apex of the left ventricle. The stent valve is mounted on a delivery catheter which deploys the stent valve using balloon expansion

Transcatheter Aortic Valve Implantation

Catheter-based therapy for AS (but not AI) is currently being investigated for patients considered high risk for traditional AVR [20]. Current experimental devices (Fig. 5.11) are mounted on a catheter which can be delivered either by a retrograde arterial approach via the femoral artery or by an antegrade approach via the left ventricular apex (Fig. 5.12). Many comorbidities can contribute to the risk profile for these patients, but heart failure is a powerful predictor of operative mortality. Patients with low-gradient AS without contractile reserve determined by dobutamine stress testing may be a subset of patients with AS and advanced heart failure that are particularly suited for TAVI. The reduced invasiveness of TAVI as compared to AVR may result in improved operative mortality and morbidity. If the durability of these catheter-based valves is proven, patients with AS and advanced heart failure may also enjoy improved long-term survival (Fig. 5.13) [21].

Conclusions

The treatment of aortic valvular disease in advanced heart failure must be individualized. Recovery of LV function after successful surgical correction of the aortic valvular pathology is

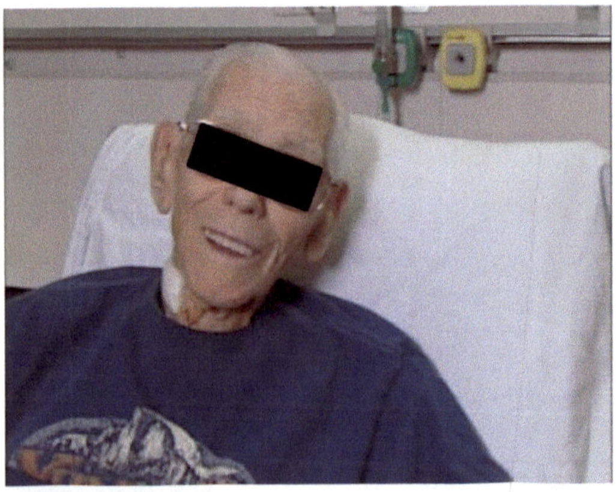

Fig. 5.13 Successful transapical aortic valve implantation for aortic stenosis in a patient at high risk for surgical aortic valve implantation due to advanced heart failure

typical but may not be reliably determined before surgery. Dobutamine stress echocardiography and ABV may be used to stratify patients with AS, but no modality exists to stratify patients with AI. Nevertheless, operative mortality has decreased significantly over the years, and AVR is a better option than continued medical therapy of heart transplantation for patients and can result in improvement of LV function. Moreover, the correction of the aortic valvular pathology can significantly facilitate subsequent medical management of chronic heart failure in patients with irreversible myocardial damage secondary to their aortic valvular disease.

References

1. Bonow RO, Dodd JT, Maron BJ, O'Gara PT, White GG, McIntosh CL, et al. Long-term serial changes in left ventricular function and reversal of ventricular dilatation after valve replacement for chronic aortic regurgitation. Circulation. 1988;78(5 Pt 1):1108–20.
2. Bonow RO, Picone AL, McIntosh CL, Jones M, Rosing DR, Maron BJ, et al. Survival and functional results after valve replacement for aortic regurgitation from 1976 to 1983: impact of preoperative left ventricular function. Circulation. 1985;72(6):1244–56.
3. Hegglin R, Scheu H, Rothlin M. Aortic insufficiency. Circulation. 1968;38(1 Suppl):77–92.
4. Rapaport E. Natural history of aortic and mitral valve disease. Am J Cardiol. 1975;35(2):221–7.
5. Spagnuolo M, Kloth H, Taranta A, Doyle E, Pasternack B. Natural history of rheumatic aortic regurgitation. Criteria predictive of death, congestive heart failure, and angina in young patients. Circulation. 1971;44(3):368–80.
6. Borer JS, Truter S, Herrold EM, Falcone DJ, Pena M, Carter JN, et al. Myocardial fibrosis in chronic aortic regurgitation: molecular and cellular responses to volume overload. Circulation. 2002;105(15):1837–42.
7. Bonow RO, Carabello BA, Kanu C, de Leon Jr AC, Faxon DP, Freed MD, et al. ACC/AHA 2006 guidelines for the management of patients with valvular heart disease: a report of the American College of Cardiology/American Heart Association Task Force on Practice Guidelines (writing committee to revise the 1998 Guidelines for the Management of Patients With Valvular Heart Disease): developed in collaboration with the Society of Cardiovascular Anesthesiologists: endorsed by the Society for Cardiovascular Angiography and Interventions and the Society of Thoracic Surgeons. Circulation. 2006;114(5):e84–231.
8. Bhudia SK, McCarthy PM, Kumpati GS, Helou J, Hoercher KJ, Rajeswaran J, et al. Improved outcomes after aortic valve surgery for chronic aortic regurgitation with severe left ventricular dysfunction. J Am Coll Cardiol. 2007;49(13):1465–71.
9. Vahanian A, Baumgartner H, Bax J, Butchart E, Dion R, Filippatos G, et al. Guidelines on the management of valvular heart disease: The Task Force on the Management of Valvular Heart Disease of the European Society of Cardiology. Eur Heart J. 2007;28(2):230–68.
10. Bonow RO, Nikas D, Elefteriades JA. Valve replacement for regurgitant lesions of the aortic or mitral valve in advanced left ventricular dysfunction. Cardiol Clin. 1995;13(1):73–83, 85.
11. Nishimura RA, Grantham JA, Connolly HM, Schaff HV, Higano ST, Holmes Jr DR. Low-output, low-gradient aortic stenosis in patients with depressed left ventricular systolic function: the clinical utility of the dobutamine challenge in the catheterization laboratory. Circulation. 2002;106(7):809–13.
12. Otto CM. Valvular aortic stenosis: disease severity and timing of intervention. J Am Coll Cardiol. 2006;47(11):2141–51.
13. Pereira JJ, Lauer MS, Bashir M, Afridi I, Blackstone EH, Stewart WJ, et al. Survival after aortic valve replacement for severe aortic stenosis with low transvalvular gradients and severe left ventricular dysfunction. J Am Coll Cardiol. 2002;39(8):1356–63.
14. Carabello BA, Green LH, Grossman W, Cohn LH, Koster JK, Collins Jr JJ. Hemodynamic determinants of prognosis of aortic valve replacement in critical aortic stenosis and advanced congestive heart failure. Circulation. 1980;62(1):42–8.
15. Monin JL, Quere JP, Monchi M, Petit H, Baleynaud S, Chauvel C, et al. Low-gradient aortic stenosis: operative risk stratification and predictors for long-term outcome: a multicenter study using dobutamine stress hemodynamics. Circulation. 2003;108(3):319–24.
16. Quere JP, Monin JL, Levy F, Petit H, Baleynaud S, Chauvel C, et al. Influence of preoperative left ventricular contractile reserve on postoperative ejection

fraction in low-gradient aortic stenosis. Circulation. 2006;113(14):1738–44.
17. Pibarot P, Dumesnil JG. Prosthetic heart valves: selection of the optimal prosthesis and long-term management. Circulation. 2009;119(7):1034–48.
18. Monin JL, Monchi M, Kirsch ME, Petit-Eisenmann H, Baleynaud S, Chauvel C, et al. Low-gradient aortic stenosis: impact of prosthesis-patient mismatch on survival. Eur Heart J. 2007;28(21):2620–6.
19. Kulik A, Burwash IG, Kapila V, Mesana TG, Ruel M. Long-term outcomes after valve replacement for low-gradient aortic stenosis: impact of prosthesis-patient mismatch. Circulation. 2006;114(1 Suppl):I553–8.
20. Vahanian A, Alfieri OR, Al-Attar N, Antunes MJ, Bax J, Cormier B, et al. Transcatheter valve implantation for patients with aortic stenosis: a position statement from the European Association of Cardio-Thoracic Surgery (EACTS) and the European Society of Cardiology (ESC), in collaboration with the European Association of Percutaneous Cardiovascular Interventions (EAPCI). Eur J Cardiothorac Surg. 2008;34(1):1–8.

Ventricular Remodeling for Ischemic Cardiomyopathy and Ventricular Asynergy Post Myocardial Infarction

6

John V. Conte

Introduction

Following myocardial infarction the ventricle undergoes a process of pathological and physiological adaptation which has come to be known as ventricular remodeling. Unchecked, the process can result in a ventricle that is enlarged, spherical and exhibits diminished ventricular function in the area of the infarction as well as in viable areas remote from the infarct and mitral regurgitation [1, 2]. Electrical and mechanical dyssynchrony can develop following infarction due to ventricular remodeling and further impairing the postinfarction ventricular dysfunction [3].

The ultimate impact of postinfarction remodeling is congestive heart failure (CHF) and death. Ischemic cardiomyopathy is the leading cause of heart failure in this country and in the Western world [4]. Mortality in CHF patients has been shown to be related to ventricular size and residual left ventricular function [2, 5–8]. Survival in patients with CHF due to ischemic cardiomyopathy is, in addition, impacted by revascularization of viable, even if nonfunctional myocardium [8] and preservation of left ventricular geometry [9].

Surgical ventricular restoration (SVR) is a term which has come to be applied to a group of related surgical procedures designed to counteract the effects of postinfarction ventricular remodeling. All of the procedures are intended to reduce the size and sphericity of the left ventricle by excluding akinetic and dyskinetic areas in conjunction with complete revascularization and repair of any valvular defects. The goal is to revascularize ischemic myocardium, reduce end-diastolic pressure and ventricular dyssynchrony resulting in an improvement in ventricular function, including the remote areas. This chapter will describe the surgical techniques used to achieve these goals.

Patient Selection

Patients who are candidates for SVR have many different clinical and morphological characteristics. Most commonly, patients are considered candidates if they have had a remote anterior or anteroseptal myocardial infarction, significant ventricular enlargement with a large area of akinesis or dyskinesis, and a clinical picture consistent with CHF. They should have retained function of the basilar and lateral portions of the heart and have good right ventricular function. They should also be candidates for revascularization and valve repair if indicated. Indications and contraindications to SVR are shown in Table 6.1. The only truly absolute contraindications to SVR are viability of anterior wall and documented ischemia of other ventricular walls with coronary artery disease not amenable to revascularization.

J.V. Conte, M.D. (✉)
Division of Cardiac Surgery, Zayad Tower, Suite 7107, Johns Hopkins Hospital, 1800 Orleans Street, Baltimore, MD 21287-4618, USA
e-mail: jconte@jhmi.edu

J.A. Morgan and Y. Naka (eds.), *Surgical Treatment for Advanced Heart Failure*,
DOI 10.1007/978-1-4614-6919-3_6,

Table 6.1 Indications for surgical ventricular restoration

Indications
• Anteroseptal myocardial infarction
• Congestive heart failure
• Depressed ejection fraction %
• Large area of akinesis/dyskinesis
– Asynergy of >30 % of LV surface
• Enlarged ventricle
– End-diastolic volume index >120 cc/m^2
– End-systolic volume index >60 cc/m^2
• Retained basilar heart function
• Candidate for revascularization
• Candidate for valve repair/replacement
• Good right ventricular function
Relative contraindications
• Multiple areas of infarction
• Loss of basilar myocardial function
• Pulmonary hypertension and right ventricular dysfunction
• Unreconstructable coronary artery disease
Absolute contraindications
• Viable myocardium anterior wall
• Active ischemia with unreconstructable coronary artery disease

Surgical Procedures

There is no one SVR operation. Although all of the different procedures generally referred to as SVR have the same surgical goals and achieve the same or similar morphological results, they do so via different techniques.

All require median sternotomy and cardiopulmonary bypass. Bicaval cannulation is preferred when there is a possibility of valve intervention. It is a good idea to place a femoral arterial line in the event that an intra-aortic balloon pump is necessary. Concomitant coronary artery bypass grafting (CABG) is usually performed; the standard approach for CABG at that institution is utilized, including myocardial protection.

The sequence of procedures performed is a matter of personal preference. We generally use a variation of the Dor technique of endoventricular circular patch plasty but have used most of the major described techniques [10, 11]. Our approach is to perform the CABG first, followed by the mitral repair and the SVR last. The mitral valve repair can be performed in a standard trans-atrial fashion or via a left ventricular approach [12]. Our preference is to perform the entire procedure under full cardioplegic arrest. If the cardiac function is poor, we will complete the proximal anastomoses, remove the cross clamp, and perform the SVR after the heart has been reperfused and in extreme cases have done the entire operation beating.

What follows is a description of the primary SVR procedures.

Dor Procedure

This procedure was named after Dr Vincent Dor who first described it as endoventricular circular patch plasty. This procedure is what people generally are referring to when they use the terms SVR, remodeling, or reconstruction or the surgical anterior ventricular endocardial reconstruction (SAVER) procedure. The technique was introduced to improve geometric reconstruction compared to standard linear repair of left ventricle (LV) aneurysms [10]. Subsequently, Dor and colleagues showed that it was applicable not only to classic aneurysms but also to large akinetic ventricles. Results with the Dor procedure have changed the approach to patients with CHF. SVR has become a standard part of the heart failure surgical armamentarium in patients with advanced heart failure and dilated and dysfunctional ventricles [13, 14].

The procedure begins with CABG and valve repair if indicated, on an arrested heart. The heart is vented through the aortic root which results in a collapsed left ventricle in patients with the classic thinned-out anterior wall (Fig. 6.1a). In patients without full-thickness infarction and thinned-out walls, collapse may not occur. A ventriculotomy is then made in the anterior wall parallel to the left anterior descending coronary artery through the center of the scarred tissue (Fig. 6.1b). It is extended proximally and distally as necessary. Retraction sutures are then placed to aid in exposure.

The LV is assessed by visualization and palpation to identify the presence or absence of ventricular thrombus, the extent of septal anterior, lateral, and inferior wall infarction, papillary muscle infarction and the interpapillary muscle distance.

An encircling stitch is then placed which outlines the margins of the reconstructed anterior wall

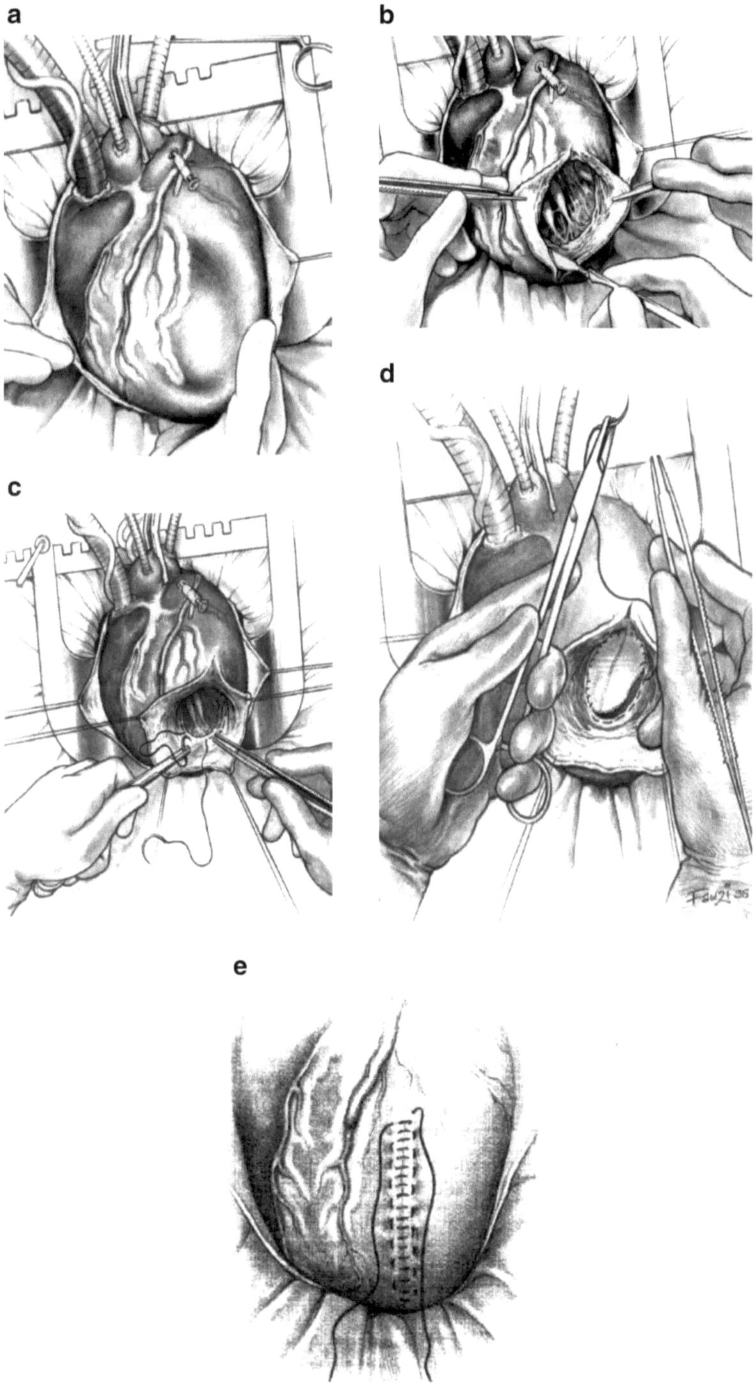

Fig. 6.1 (**a**) Anterior wall of infarcted left ventricle with sunken appearance while on suction. (**b**) Ventriculotomy parallel and lateral to left anterior descending coronary artery through scar tissue on anterior wall exposing left ventricular chamber. (**c**) Circumferential purse string ("Fontan stitch") outlining border of new anterior wall and apex of left ventricle. (**d**) Patch closure of anterior left ventricular opening. (**e**) Final two-layered closure of residual scar over patch. (Reprinted from Operative Techniques in Cardiac & Thoracic Surgery, Vol. 2, Dor V, Surgical management of left ventricular aneurysms by the endoventricular circular patch plasty technique, pages 139–150, copyright 1997, with permission from Elsevier)

(Fig. 6.1c). It runs from the point selected as the new apex cephalad along the septum and then crosses over the most superior margin of the anterior ventriculotomy and down the anterolateral wall back to the new apex. This is commonly referred to as the "Fontan stitch" after Dr Francis Fontan [15]. I routinely use two stitches. Many select the location of this stitch at the visual border of the infarcted and normal tissue; some will perform the ventricular reconstruction on a beating heart and will use the border of the beating and non beating myocardium or between the palpably thinned-out and normal tissue as a guide. Many others will use homemade or commercially available sizing devices. The concept of ventricular sizing was introduced by Dr Dor who used an inflated balloon to size the ventricles. I routinely use a device inflated to a volume of 50–60 cc/m^2 body surface area to estimate the patients' own end-diastolic volume. As a general rule of thumb the height of the septum is not reduced greater than 50 % regardless of the extent of septal infarction.

The encircling stitch is tied to reduce the size of the opening. If the residual opening is greater than 3 cm, a patch is used to close the opening (Fig. 6.1d). If smaller, a linear closure is then performed (Fig. 6.1e). If the quality of the remaining tissue is suboptimal, the linear closure is reinforced with wither bovine pericardium or felt strips.

Modified Linear Closure Technique with Septoplasty

This technique is very similar to a standard linear closure technique for ventricular aneurysms. In this technique, the anterior wall is opened as described above. Once the margins of reconstruction of the anterior wall are identified, horizontal mattress sutures are placed externally through the anterior wall down through the scarred septum medially and continued laterally up through the endocardial scar of the anterolateral wall . These sutures are generally reinforced externally with felt or pericardial strips (Fig. 6.2a, b). A standard linear ventricular closure is performed in layers.

What makes this technique unique is when a septoplasty is added in patients with large septal infarctions to reduce the volume of the septum. Dr Linda Mickleborough of Toronto has popularized this technique [16, 17]. A curvilinear patch of Dacron or pericardium is sewn along the margins of the septal wall along three sides (Fig. 6.2c). The anterior linear closure sutures are then placed in such a fashion to sandwich the remaining side of the patch between the medial and lateral walls creating a new septum and anterior wall (Fig. 6.2d). This can be seen diagrammatically in Fig. 6.2e.

Jatene Modified Septoplasty Technique

The technique introduced and popularized by Dr Adib Jatene [18]. This technique is similar to the Dor technique in that it utilizes a concentric purse string to demarcate the border of the new anterior wall and can be performed with or without a patch.

It is rendered a unique technique by the addition of a septoplasty to reduce the volume in the septum. The septoplasty is accomplished by imbricating the septum with several horizontal mattress sutures which are placed along the septum taking multiple bites of scar tissue beginning near the apex of the heart and running towards the base of the heart until normal tissue is encountered. Sutures are placed in the full height of the infarcted septal tissue and when tied reduce the length of the septum. The encircling stitch is then placed, and the remainder of the reconstruction and closure of the ventricle can proceed in a fashion with or without a patch analogous to the Dor procedure [19].

Septal Exclusion Technique

This technique was described by the French surgeon Guillmet in 1984 to treat aneurysms which primarily involved the septum [20]. This technique is quite unique in that it employs interrupted U-shaped stitches to reapproximate the anterior wall to the septum directly from within the ventricle. The procedure begins like any of the SVR procedures with an anterior ventriculotomy (Fig. 6.3a). A series of interrupted horizontal mattress or U-shaped sutures are placed from the most lateral portion of the anterior wall and anchored on the septal scar (Fig. 6.3b). The sutures are placed from the base towards the apex,

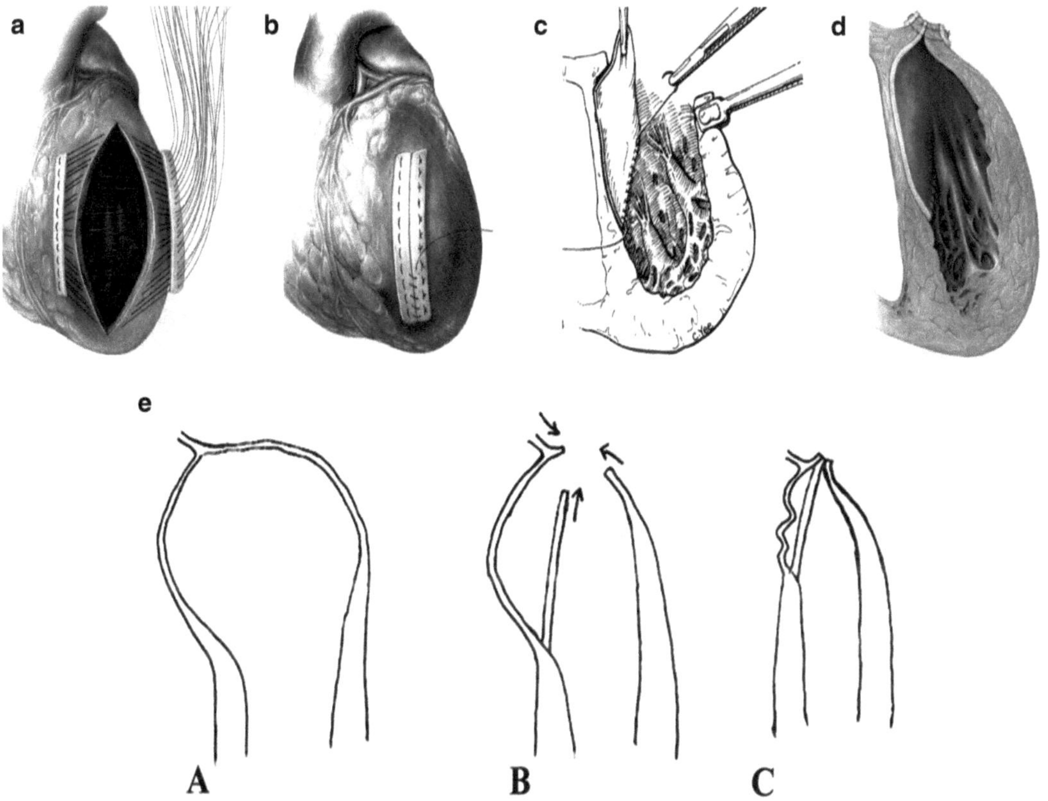

Fig. 6.2 (**a**) Reinforced linear closure of left ventricle. (**b**) Final reinforced linear closure of left ventricle. (**c**) Septal patch over infarcted septal scar. (**d**) Final view of reinforced linear closure with septal patch. (Fig. 6.2**a–d** reprinted from Operative Techniques Cardiac & Thoracic Surgery, Vol. 2, Mickleborough LL, Left ventricular aneurysm: modified linear closure technique, pages 118–131, copyright 1997, with permission from Elsevier.) (**e**) Longitudinal view of linear closure with septal patch. (Reprinted from The Journal of Thoracic and Cardiovascular Surgery, Vol. 128, Mickleborough LL, Merchant N, Ivanov J, Rao V, Carson S, Left ventricular reconstruction: early and late results, pages 27–37, copyright 2004, with permission from Elsevier)

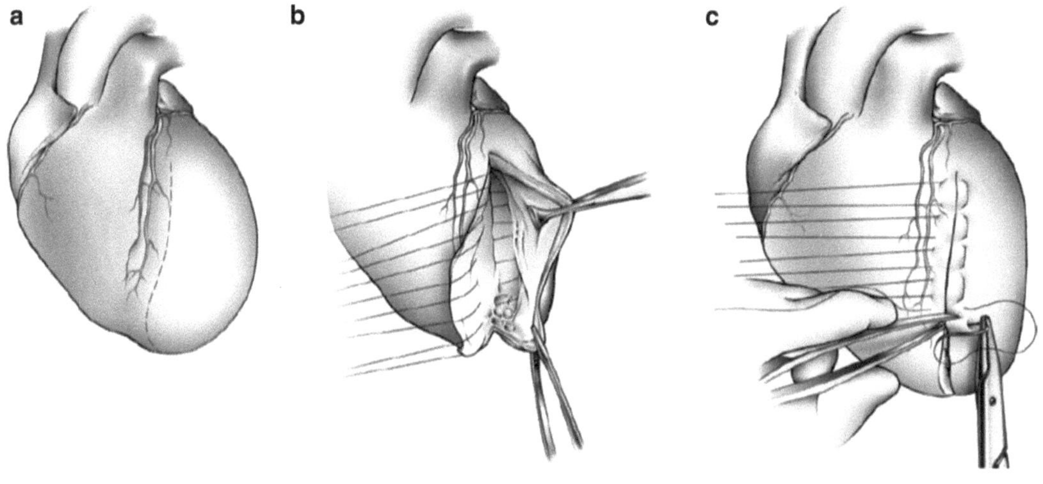

Fig. 6.3 (**a**) Line of ventricular incision lateral to left anterior descending coronary artery. (**b**) Primary septal lateral left ventricular ("Guillmet") repair. (**c**) Final closure of anterior left ventricle. (Reprinted with permission from Calafiore AM, Gallina S, Di Mauro M, Pano M, Teodori G, Di Giammarco G, et al. Left ventricular aneurysmectomy: endoventricular circular patch plasty or septoexclusion. J Card Surg. 2003 Mar–Apr; 18(2):93–100)

and after all the sutures are placed, they are tied in the same sequence. The remaining tissue is reapproximated providing a hemostatic closure in a standard fashion (Fig. 6.3c) [21].

Cerclage Technique

Another modification of the Dor procedure is the concentric purse string or cerclage technique described by Caldeira and McCarthy in 2001 [22]. This technique utilizes multiple concentric purse strings to reapproximate the septal and lateral wall scar tissue in sequential steps until the residual anterior ventriculotomy is small enough that the opening can be closed in a standard linear fashion. This technique uses multiple purse strings with each successive purse string placed approximately 0.5 cm apart.

Other Issues

Mitral regurgitation (MR) is a frequent finding in dilated ischemic ventricles. The mechanism of mitral regurgitation is restriction of the subvalvar apparatus in addition to annular dilation. In patients with significant mitral regurgitation and an increased interpapillary muscle distance, the degree of MR can be reduced by reducing the papillary muscle tethering by reducing the interpapillary muscle distance and displacing the base of the papillary muscles up towards the mitral annulus. In patients with a distance greater than 2.5–3 cm, this can be done by placing mattress sutures between the two papillary muscles or by running an imbricating suture from the base of the papillary muscles up towards the mitral annulus [23] (Fig. 6.4).

Outcomes

The literature is replete with studies documenting the morphological, physiological, and functional improvements seen following SVR in properly selected patients who undergo successful operations. It has been shown to improve ventricular size, morphology, EF %, stroke volume index, endocrine markers of CHF, ventricular energetics, ventricular synchrony, and mechanical efficiency (Table 6.2). Clinically it results in an improved

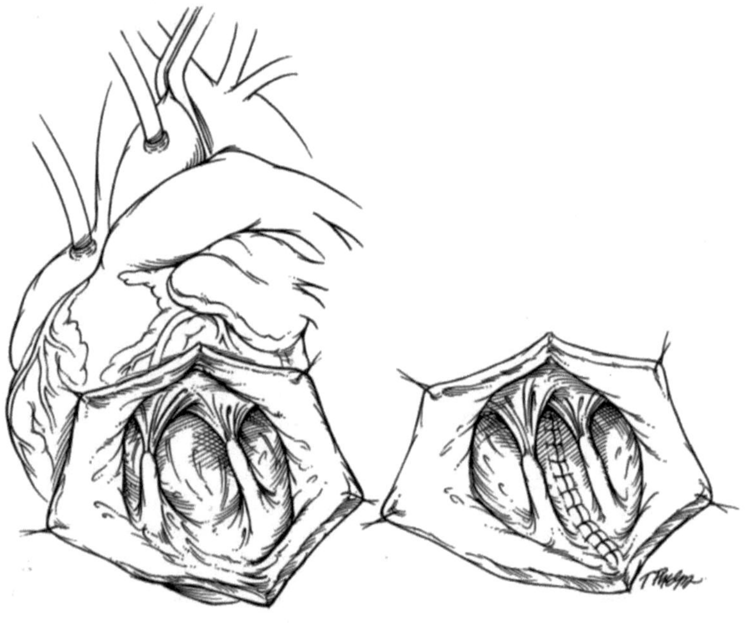

Fig. 6.4 Ventriculoplasty suture line to reapproximate papillary muscles. (Reprinted from The Journal of Thoracic and Cardiovascular Surgery, Vol. 130, Patel ND, Williams JA, Barreiro CJ, Bonde PN, Waldron MM, Chang DC, Bluemke DA, Conte JV, Surgical ventricular remodeling for multi-territory myocardial infarction: defining a new patient population, pages 1698–1706, copyright 2005, with permission from Elsevier)

Table 6.2 Post SVR improvements

- Reduced ventricular size
- Improved ventricular function
  - EF% by echo , MRI, and ventriculography
  - Direct LV measurement
- Neurohormone normalization
- Reduced mechanical dyssynchrony
- Improved ventricular efficiency and energetics
- Improved NYHA functional class
- Improved heart failure scores
  - Functional and psychological

functional capacity (New York Heart Association [NYHA] class) and an excellent 5-year survival in very sick patients [24–33].

Summary

SVR is a procedure that has evolved from the treatment of ventricular aneurysms and has developed into a surgical treatment of CHF in selected patients with ischemic cardiomyopathy. It is not one procedure but several with common surgical goals all of which can successfully help to reverse postinfarction ventricular remodeling and improve ventricular function. It is an excellent treatment option in appropriately selected patients with ischemic cardiomyopathy.

References

1. Gaudron P, Eilles C, Kugler I, Ertl G. Progressive left ventricular dysfunction and remodeling after myocardial infarction: potential mechanisms and early predictors. Circulation. 1993;87:755–63.
2. DiDonato M, Sabatier M, Toso A, et al. Regional myocardial performance of non-ischemic zones remote from anterior wall left ventricular aneurysm. Eur Heart J. 1995;16:1285–92.
3. Fauchier L, Marie O, Cassett D, et al. Intraventriacular and interventricular dyssynchrony in idiopathic dilated cardiomyopathy: a prognostic study with Fournier phase analysis of radionucleotide angioscintigraphy. J Am Coll Cardiol. 2002;40:2022–30.
4. Gheorghiade M, Bonow RO. Chronic heart failure in the United States: a manifestation of coronary artery disease. Circulation. 1998;97:282–9.
5. White HD, Norris RM, Brown PW, et al. Left ventricular end systolic volume as the major determinant of survival after recovery from myocardial infarction. Circulation. 1987;76:44–51.
6. Levy D, Kenchaiah S, Larson MG, Benjamin EJ, Kupka MJ, Ho KKL, et al. Long-term trends in the incidence of and survival with heart failure. N Engl J Med. 2002;347(18):1397–402.
7. Migrin RQ, Young JB, Ellis SG, et al. End-systolic volume index at 90 to 180 minutes into reperfusion therapy for acute myocardial infarction is a strong predictor of early and late mortality: the Global Utilization of Streptokinase and t-PA for Occluded Coronary Arteries (GUSTO)-I Angiographic Investigators. Circulation. 1997;96:116–21.
8. Allman KC, Shaw LJ, Hachamovitch R, Udelson E. Myocardial viability testing and impact of revascularization on prognosis in patients with coronary artery disease and left ventricular dysfunction: a meta-analysis. J Am Coll Cardiol. 2002;39(7):1151–8.
9. Senior R, Lahiri A, Kaul S. Effect of revascularization on left ventricular remodeling in patients with heart failure from severe chronic ischemic left ventricular dysfunction. Am J Cardiol. 2001;88(6):624–9.
10. Dor V, Kreitmann P, Jourdan J. Interest of "physiological" closure of left ventricle after resection and endocardiectomy for aneurysm or akinetic zone comparison with classical technique about a series of 209 left ventricular resections. (abstract). J Cardiovasc Surg. 1985;26:73.
11. Conte JV. Surgical ventricular restoration: technique and outcomes. Congest Heart Fail. 2004;10: 248–51.
12. Menicanti L, Di Donato M, Frigiola A, RESTORE Group, et al. Ischemic mitral regurgitation: intraventricular papillary muscle imbrication without mitral ring during left ventricular restoration. J Thorac Cardiovasc Surg. 2002;123(6):1041–50.
13. Dor V, Saab M, Coste P, Kornaszewska M, Montiglio F. Left ventricular aneurysm: a new surgical approach. J Thorac Cardiovasc Surg. 1989;37:11–9.
14. Dor V. Left ventricular reconstruction: the aim and the reality after twenty years. J Thorac Cardiovasc Surg. 2004;128(1):17–20.
15. Fontan F. Transplantation of knowledge. J Thorac Cardiovasc Surg. 1990;99:387–95.
16. Mickleborough LL. Tech Card Thorac Surg. 1997;2:118–31.
17. Mickleborough LL, Merchant N, Ivanov J, et al. Left ventricular reconstruction: early and late results. J Thorac Cardiovasc Surg. 2004;128:27–37.
18. Jatene AD. Left ventricular aneurysmectomy: resection or reconstruction? J Thorac Cardiovasc Surg. 1985;89:321–31.
19. Cox JL. Surgical management of left ventricular aneurysms: a clarification of the similarities and differences between the Jatene and Dor techniques. Semin Thorac Cardiovasc Surg. 1997;9(2):131–8.
20. Guillmet D, Popoff C, Duboois C, et al. Nouvelle technique qu chiurgicale pur la cure des aneurysms du ventricle gauche. Archive des maladie du cœur. 1984;77:953–8.

21. Calafiore AM, Gallina S, DiMauro M, et al. Left ventricular aneurysmectomy: endoventricular circular patch plasty or Septoexclusion. J Card Surg. 2003;18:93–100.
22. Caldeira C, McCarthy PM. A simple method of left ventricular reconstruction without patch for ischemic cardiomyopathy. Ann Thorac Surg. 2001;72:2148–9.
23. Patel ND, Williams JA, Bonde P, Bluemke D, Waldron M, Barriero C, et al. Surgical ventricular remodeling for multi-territory myocardial infarction: defining a new patient population. J Thorac Cardiovasc Surg. 2005;130:1698–706.
24. Athanasuleas CL, Buckberg GD, Stanley AWH, RESTORE Group, et al. Surgical ventricular restoration in the treatment of congestive heart failure due to post-infarction ventricular dilation. J Am Coll Cardiol. 2004;44:1439–42.
25. Menicanti L, Castelvecchio S, Ranucci M, et al. Surgical therapy for ischemic heart failure: single center experience with surgical anterior ventricular restoration. J Thorac Cardiovasc Surg. 2007;134: 433–41.
26. Di Donato M, Castelvecchio S, Kukulski T, et al. Surgical ventricular restoration: left ventricular shape influence on cardiac function, clinical status, and survival. Ann Thorac Surg. 2009;87:455–61.
27. Schreuder JJ, Castiglioni A, Maisano F, et al. Acute decrease of left ventricular mechanical dyssynchrony and improvement of contractile state and energy efficiency after left ventricular restoration. J Thorac Cardiovasc Surg. 2005;129(1):138–45.
28. Castelvecchio S, Menicanti L, Ranucci M, Di Donato M. Impact of surgical ventricular restoration on diastolic function: implications of shape and residual ventricular size. Ann Thorac Surg. 2008;86(6):1849–54.
29. DiDonato M, Toso A, Dor V, et al. Surgical ventricular restoration improves mechanical ventricular dyssynchrony in ischemic cardiomyopathy. Circulation. 2004;109:2536–43.
30. Schenk S, McCarthy PM, Starling RC, et al. Neurohormonal response to left ventricular reduction surgery in ischemic cardiomyopathy. J Thorac Cardiovasc Surg. 2003;128:38–43.
31. Tulner SA, Steendijk P, Klautz RJ, et al. Clinical efficacy of surgical heart failure therapy by ventricular restoration and restrictive mitral annuloplasty. J Card Fail. 2007;13(3):178–83.
32. Di Donato M, Sabatier M, Dor V, RESTORE group. Surgical ventricular restoration in patients with post-infarction coronary artery disease: effectiveness on spontaneous and inducible ventricular tachycardia. Semin Thorac Cardiovasc Surg. 2001;13:480–5.
33. Di Donato M, Sabatier M, Dor V, Buckberg G, RESTORE group. Ventricular arrhythmias after LV remodelling: surgical ventricular restoration or ICD? Heart Fail Rev. 2004;9:299–306.

Cardiac Resynchronization in Advanced Heart Failure: Biventricular Pacing

7

William T. Abraham and Paul Chacko

Introduction

Heart failure (HF) is the end stage of a cardiac disease and is most often a consequence of hypertension, coronary artery disease, valve disorders, diabetes, and cardiomyopathy. Given the improvement in life expectancy with advances in health care, the incidence and prevalence of HF has dramatically increased [1]. Based on long-term follow-up data from the Framingham heart study, 80 % of men and 70 % of women less than 65 years of age diagnosed with HF die within 8 years [2]. Since the advent of pharmacological therapy with furosemide in 1964, the management of HF utilizing drugs has focused on reduction of myocardial workload and attenuation of the neurohormonal cascade triggered by a fall in cardiac output. Despite optimization of these medications, there still remains a subset of patients who demonstrate no symptomatic improvement or progressively worsen. Though surgical techniques such as left ventricular (LV) volume reduction, ventricular assist devices are often reserved for severely decompensated patients with heart transplantation as a last resort, yet a significant majority are considered high risk for surgery and hence excluded.

In patients suffering from heart failure, replacement of myocardial filaments with fibrotic tissue leads to alteration in morphology and conduction properties [3]. Electrical disturbances such as prolonged atrioventricular (AV) conduction and delayed ventricular activation are fairly common, which begets mechanical dyssynchrony. This can be generally described as AV dyssynchrony, interventricular dyssynchrony, and intraventricular/LV dyssynchrony. This ventricular dyssynchrony due to conduction delay is often manifested on the surface electrocardiogram (EKG) as widened QRS complex (>120 ms), often in the form of left bundle branch block (LBBB). Observed in about third of those with HF, it is also a predictor of mortality along with other parameters such as clinical severity (noted by New York Heart Association or NYHA class), LV ejection fraction, and HF etiology [4, 5]. As a result, LV performance is compromised throughout cardiac cycle due to paradoxical septal motion resulting in increase in LV end-diastolic diameter and reduction in ejection fraction, cardiac output, mean arterial blood pressure, as well as ratio of change in pressure to change in time (dP/dt) [6, 7]. Understanding this pathophysiology has enabled a novel approach to enhance cardiac performance by counteracting this dyssynchrony with atrial synchronized biventricular pacing, otherwise known as cardiac resynchronization therapy (CRT).

W.T. Abraham, M.D., FACP, FACC, FAHA, FESC (✉)
Division of Cardiovascular Medicine, The Ohio State University, 473 W. 12th Avenue–Room 110 P, Columbus, OH 43210-1252, USA
e-mail: william.abraham@osumc.edu

P. Chacko, MBBS
Division of Cardiology, Department of Internal Medicine, The Ohio State University College of Medicine, 473 W. 12th Avenue–Suite 200, Columbus, OH 43210, USA
e-mail: pchacko@metrohealth.org

J.A. Morgan and Y. Naka (eds.), *Surgical Treatment for Advanced Heart Failure*,
DOI 10.1007/978-1-4614-6919-3_7, © Springer Science+Business Media New York 2013

Over the last decade, the improvement noted in symptoms/functional status, exercise capacity measured by six-min walking time (6 MWT), peak oxygen consumption (pVO_2), and quality of life (QoL) with the aid of CRT has been observed through observational studies [8–10]. These have been corroborated by large-scale randomized trials that demonstrated a reversal of ventricular remodeling as well as reduction in morbidity [11–15]. However more recent trials have demonstrated the added benefit of mortality reduction, though the trials were restricted to patients who experienced moderate to severe heart failure as a result of systolic dysfunction as evident by depressed ejection fraction (EF) [16, 17]. In light of these data, the discussion in this chapter will focus on:

- Pathophysiology of dyssynchrony
- Rationale for CRT
- Evidence from the trials
- Challenges following CRT
- Special scenarios and future implication

Pathophysiology of Dyssynchrony

Heart failure is the fastest growing cardiovascular diagnosis with an estimated 37.2 billion dollars spent in direct and indirect costs [18]. It is mainly a clinical diagnosis often characterized by symptoms of cough, dyspnea, fatigue, edema, and weight gain and most often associated with a decreased ejection fraction. Substitution of myocytes with fibrotic tissue results in loss of mechanical and electrical properties leading to dyssynchronous activation.

Dyssynchronous activation noted in HF patients is atrioventricular, interventricular, and left ventricular in nature. Delay in AV conduction results in AV dyssynchrony, causing a suboptimal ventricular filling due to a compromised passive diastolic filling time [19]. However, the more detrimental one is the loss of coordinated contractility due to LV dyssynchrony [20]. Due to the delayed depolarization of the lateral free wall of LV in LBBB, contraction of that segment occurs when the septum is in its relaxation phase, resulting in a paradoxical movement away from the contracting lateral wall and increasing mitral regurgitation (MR) [7]. This inefficient contraction results in poor forward flow into the aortic outflow tract [21]. The prolongation of systole also affects the isovolumic relaxation phase thereby reducing the duration of diastole leading to impaired ventricular filling and reduction in cardiac output (Fig. 7.1).

Typically a widened QRS on the EKG has been considered a surrogate for LV dyssynchrony. Hawkins and their group noted increasing prevalence of dyssynchrony with prolongation of QRS duration [22]. Data from the Vesnarinone (VEST) study has revealed that QRS duration was directly correlated to mortality as noted in Fig. 7.2. Prolongation of QRS (>120 ms) is widely accepted as occurring in about 30 % of patients with HF [23, 24]. It is a significant predictor of LV systolic dysfunction in HF with an inverse correlation between QRS length and left ventricular ejection fraction (LVEF) [24–26]. Xiao et al. showed that early mortality was observed in those with larger increase in QRS duration and the time to death from QRS reaching 160 ms was significantly shorter in those without an implanted pacemaker in comparison to those who had one [27]. Multiple studies have confirmed the higher incidence of sudden cardiac death in HF patients with prolonged QRS complex. In an effort to determine the optimal QRS duration that stratifies HF patients into higher and low risk for increased mortality or need for transplantation, Kalra and his group determined that patients with a QRS duration ≥120 ms were associated with a threefold risk and a significantly low 5-year survival rate [25]. Most large-scale trials have considered QRS length >120 ms as part of their inclusion criteria, thus offering the benefit of application in clinical scenarios.

Rationale for CRT

Given the mounting evidence of dyssynchrony contributing to LV dysfunction, Cazeau and colleagues used CRT to improve the functional status of a patient who presented with HF with conduction abnormalities [28]. This led to further attempts to reverse dyssynchrony with the aid of

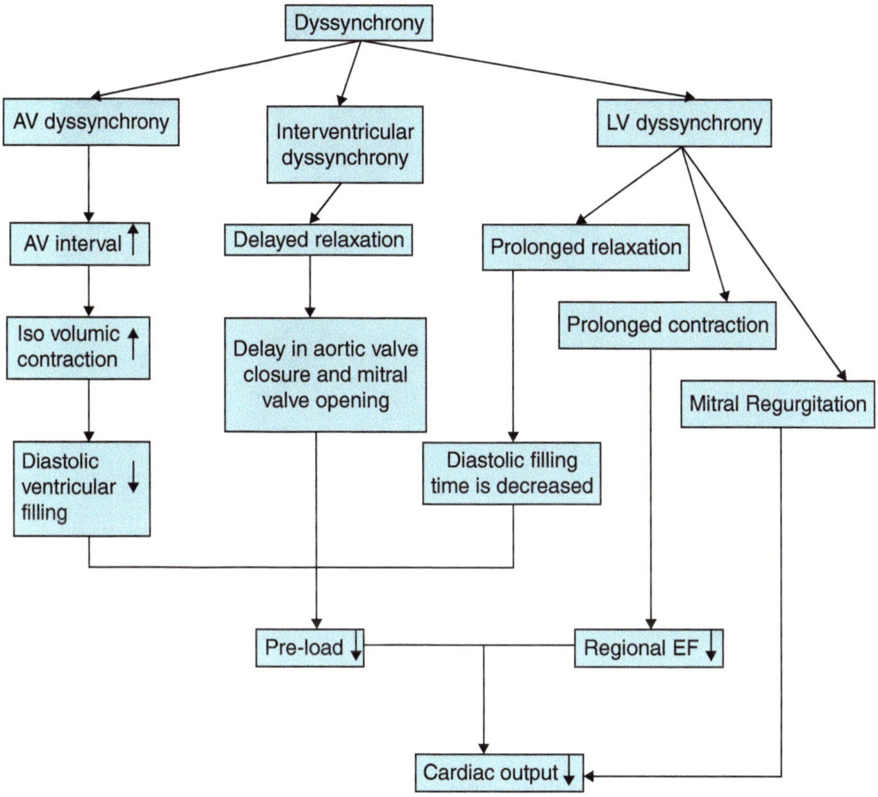

Fig. 7.1 Relation between dyssynchrony and cardiac output

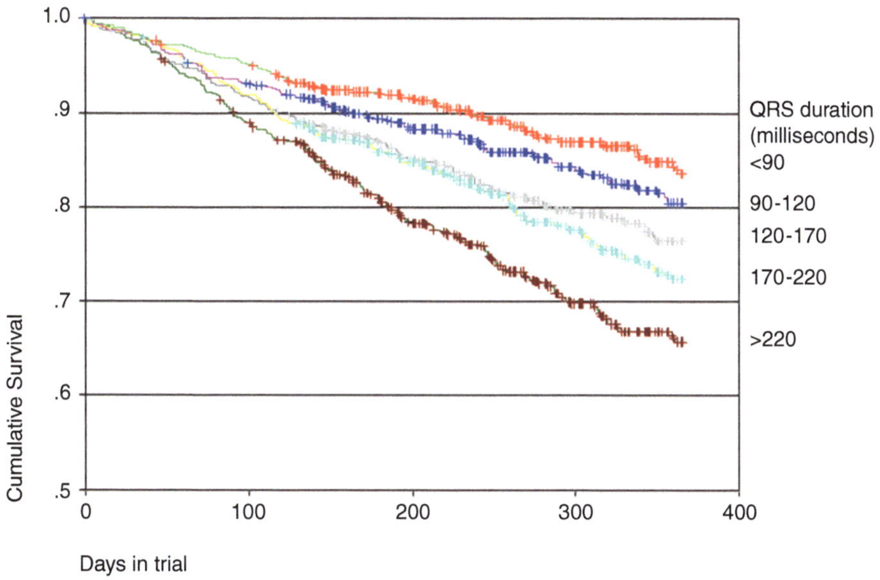

Fig. 7.2 Patient survival stratified by QRS duration (Adapted from Gottipaty V, Krelis S, Lu F, et al. JACC 1999; 33 (2S1):145A)

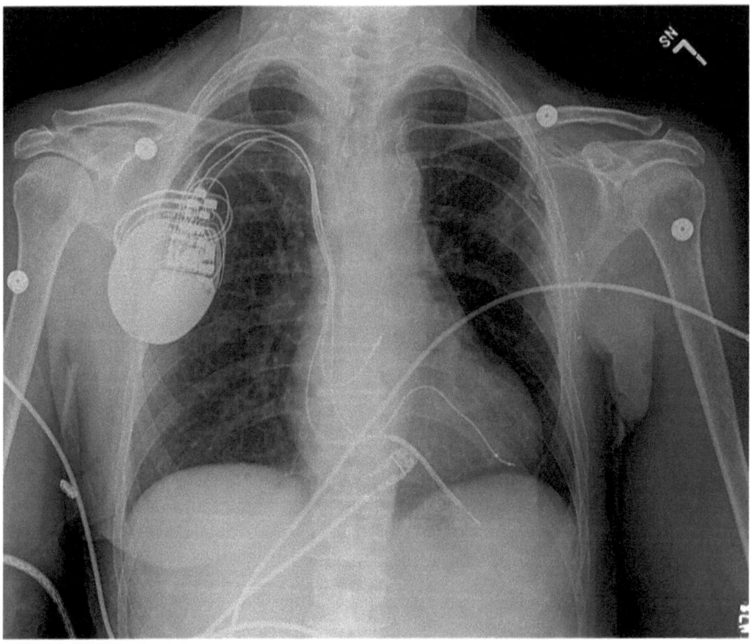

Fig. 7.3 Chest X-ray revealing typical lead placement

pacing leads and spurred a new era of therapeutic application. CRT typically involves placement of pacing leads in the right atrium (RA), right ventricle (RV), and the lateral branch of the coronary sinus (Fig. 7.3). This placement in the branch of the coronary sinus is an attempt to pace the lateral wall of the LV, and hence it is often called the LV lead. With this approach, simultaneous and synchronized pacing of the ventricles can be performed to reduce dyssynchrony so as to simulate a physiological depolarization as seen in a healthy normal myocardium. An alternate approach is to pace the LV lateral wall with appropriate AV delay with the intent to merge with the wave originating through intrinsic activation of the RV, thus resulting in a coordinated contractile movement.

The ability to program the device in a manner such that AV interval can be adjusted so as to pace the ventricles without significant delay has been shown to optimize left ventricular filling (therefore preload) and reduction in presystolic mitral regurgitation [29]. The principle of biventricular pacing is to reverse the intraventricular dyssynchrony by timing the RV and LV pacing so as to encourage simultaneous contractility of the septal and lateral wall segments. The added ability to offset the timing of RV and LV pacing seen in newer devices has been proven to be more beneficial than simultaneous pacing of the ventricular leads [30]. Lateral wall is the site preferred for the LV lead placement since coronary sinus provides easy access to the free wall. Compared to other sites, lateral wall provides best response in terms of percentage change in pulse pressure and LV d*P*/d*t* and the maximal area where this can be effectively achieved [31, 32].

The acute hemodynamic effects are noted shortly after CRT initiation. Improvements in systolic blood pressure, peak d*P*/d*t*, EF, and finally cardiac output with associated decline in pulmonary capillary wedge pressures have been established by invasive hemodynamic monitoring [33]. This is achieved with coordinated contractile function resulting in improvement of ejection fraction as evidenced by improvement in stroke volume and reduction in LV end-systolic volume. The near elimination of functional mitral regurgitation by normalization of mitral valve timing has been known to contribute to reversing the geometrical changes due to disease progression [34, 35].

The clinical effects of these changes were clearly shown in large-scale randomized clinical trials which measured surrogate markers such as NYHA class, QoL, and 6-min walk test [11–13, 16, 35–37].

The long-term benefits of CRT were evident by the progressive reduction in LV cavity volume and LV mass since the initiation of pacing as revealed by the long-term follow-up of several randomized trials (MUSTIC, PATH-CHF, CONTAK-CD, MIRACLE, CARE-HF, REVERSE). The change in hemodynamics with reduction of mitral regurgitation enabled an alteration of LV cavity shape from a globular appearance to more physiological ellipsoid appearance [38]. Importantly, Yu and his group showed the reversal of these changes with discontinuation of CRT thereby highlighting the fact that these changes were independent from that occurs as a result of concomitant use of drugs (β-blockers, angiotensin converting enzyme [ACE] inhibitors, angiotensin receptor blockers [ARB]) [39]. Notably those with depressed EF as a result of nonischemic etiology showed sustained evidence of reversal of ventricular remodeling compared to those with ischemic cardiomyopathy [40]. This is perhaps attributed to the loss of viable myocardium as a result of repeated ischemia. Improvement in these cardiac measures contributed to the reduction in mortality besides the improvement in symptoms that were observed in the COMPANION and CARE-HF trials.

Evidence from the Trials

Since the observation of augmented cardiac performance with CRT, various trials have been undertaken to corroborate those findings. The early observational studies were limited in their sample size where the patient served both as the case as well as the control. The data from the randomized controlled trials have convincingly substantiated the role of CRT in HF management, given that nearly 5,000 patients have been evaluated to date.

A summary of the major trials is noted in Table 7.1, and how they guided standard of care is reviewed below.

Pacing Therapies in Congestive Heart Failure (PATH-CHF) Trial: this European study was the first randomized trial which was single blinded with crossover design where moderate to severe HF patients were allocated to receive RV, LV, or biventricular pacing or no pacing. Acute improvement in hemodynamic parameters was noted in the LV and biventricular categories with reduction in LV end-diastolic volume and LV end-systolic volume observed during chronic pacing in the same group. Besides, PATH-CHF also enabled the identification of mid-lateral epicardial lead as the optimal site for LV lead placement. The study was limited by its small sample size and short follow-up [11].

PATH-CHF II trial evaluated the significance of single-site LV pacing and degree of intraventricular conduction delay to clinical benefits. The patients were divided into two categories based on the QRS duration (short: QRS 120–150 ms, long: QRS > 150 ms). The assumption that CRT response may be linked to degree of QRS duration was driven by the observation that the group with prolonged QRS morphology showed improvement in exercise tolerance and QoL [12].

Multisite Stimulation In Cardiomyopathy In Sinus Rhythm (MUSTIC-SR) trial was similar in design to PATH-CHF II except that biventricular pacing was the intervention planned. There was significant improvement in 6-min walking distance (6 MWD) and pVO_2 which were the primary end points. Significant improvement was seen in QoL measured as secondary end point in the treatment arm. Besides, there was alteration in the structural geometry due to reduction of LV cavity size. The degree of remodeling was more pronounced in HF patients whose etiology was related to nonischemic causes compared to ischemic ones [13].

Multisite Stimulation In Cardiomyopathy In Atrial Fibrillation (MUSTIC-AF) trial was an attempt to extrapolate similar results in patients with atrial fibrillation whose paced QRS > 200 ms. Although the effect was less pronounced than in the sinus rhythm group, it was significant enough to conclude that biventricular pacing was a reasonable option in HF patients with concomitant atrial fibrillation who become pacer dependent due to bradycardia either as a result of ablation or

Table 7.1 Summary of various randomized controlled trials evaluating the efficacy of cardiac resynchronization therapy

		Enrollment criteria					End points		
Trials (year of completion)	Design	zNYHA class	EF	QRS (ms)	Rhythm	ICD	Primary	Secondary	Results (Parameters in bold attained statistical significance)
PATH-CHF (1998)	Crossover	III, IV	<30[a]	≥120	SR	No	6 MWD and pVO_2	NYHA class, QoL	**Improvement in 6 MWD, pVO_2, QoL, and NYHA class**
MUSTIC-SR (1999)	Crossover	III	<35 %	>150	SR	No	6 MWD	QoL, pVO_2, mortality, hospital admissions due to HF	**Improvement in 6 MWD, QoL, pVO_2, and reduction in hospitalization**
MUSTIC-AF (1999)	Crossover	III	<35 %	≥120, Paced QRS≥200	AFib	No	6 MWD	QoL, pVO_2, mortality, hospital admissions due to HF	**Improvement in 6 MWD,** QoL, **pVO_2, and reduction in hospitalization**
MIRACLE (2000)	Parallel	III, IV	≤35 %	≥130	SR	No	6 MWD, QoL, NYHA class	EF, pVO_2, LV volumes, QRS duration, MR severity, and composite clinical response	**Improvement in all end points with statistical significance**
PATH-CHF II (2001)	Crossover	II, III, IV	≤30 %	≥120	SR	No	6 MWD and pVO_2	NYHA class, QoL	**Improvement in QoL, NYHA class, and pVO_2.** Effect more in those with QRS>150 ms
CONTAK-CD (2000)	Parallel[b]	III, IV[c]	≤35 %	≥120	SR	Yes	Progression of HF, 6 MWD, QoL, and pVO_2	Composite response (HF hospitalization, mortality, VT therapy with ICD), 6 MWD, QoL, and pVO_2	**Improvement in QoL, pVO_2** and NYHA class with relative reduction in HF progression
MIRACLE-ICD (2001)	Parallel	III, IV	≤35 %	≥130	SR	Yes	6 MWD, QoL, NYHA class	EF, pVO_2, LV volumes, neurohormones, and clinical composite response	**Improvement in QoL, NYHA class, and pVO_2** and a trend towards better LV volumes and composite score in CRT with no change in 6 MWD

COMPANION (2002)	Parallel	III, IV	≤35 %	≥120	SR	Yes	Time to death from or hospitalization to any cause	Mortality rate	**Improvement in both end points with statistical significance noted in both CRT-P and CRT-D arms**
MIRACLE-ICD II (2002)	Parallel	II	≤35 %	≥130	SR	Yes	pVO_2	NYHA class, EF, 6 MWD, QoL, LV volumes, neurohormones, and clinical composite response	**Improvement of significance noted in LV volumes, EF, NYHA class, and clinical composite response** but no difference in 6 MWD, QoL, and pVO_2
CARE-HF (2003)	Parallel	III, IV	≤35 %	≥120	SR	No	Time to death or hospitalization for cardiovascular events	All cause mortality, composite of mortality and HF hospitalization, NYHA class, QoL, LV volumes, and neurohormones	**Improvement in all end points with improvement of symptoms and mortality benefit**
REVERSE (2007)	Parallel	I, II	≤40 %	≥120	SR	Yes	HF clinical composite response	LV volume end-systolic volume index	**Improvement noted in parameters consistent with reversal of remodeling and time to HF hospitalization in those with NYHA classes I and II**

NYHA New York Heart Association, *EF* ejection fraction, *SR* sinus rhythm, *AFib* atrial fibrillation, *ICD* implantable cardioverter defibrillator, 6*MWD* six-min walking distance, *QoL* quality of life, pVO_2 peak oxygen consumption, *HF* heart failure, *LV* left ventricle, *CRT* cardiac resynchronization therapy

[a]EF data based on baseline data and not an enrollment criteria

[b]Initially a crossover design (phase 1) which was modified to a parallel study design (phase2)

[c]NYHA class II–IV patients enrolled but at randomization included only III and IV

intrinsic conduction disease [14]. The intervention arm in both MUSTIC study groups preferred biventricular pacing and showed reduced hospitalizations in the 12-month follow-up period.

Multicenter InSync Randomized Clinical Evaluation (MIRACLE) trial was the first double-blind randomized control trial to validate the efficacy of CRT. Hence sufficient targets such as 6 MWD, NYHA class, and QoL were included as the primary end points. The patients were divided into two arms and assigned to 6 months of optimal medical therapy with biventricular pacing or medical therapy alone. The CRT group had significant improvement in all primary end points compared to the control. A noteworthy observation was that in those who underwent CRT, 67 % demonstrated improvement in clinical composite end point of NYHA class compared to 39 % in the control [35]. This study paved the way for the US Food and Drug Administration (FDA) to approve the use of InSync® device (Medtronic, Minneapolis, MN) in 2001.

Cardiac Resynchronization Therapy for the Treatment of Heart Failure in Patients With Intraventricular Conduction Delay and Malignant Ventricular Tachyarrhythmias: VENTAK CHF/CONTAK CD Biventricular Pacing Trial: the objective of this study was to assess the safety and effectiveness of CRT in combination with an ICD in patients with HF class II–IV symptoms. The study was unique since HF patients with history of ventricular tachyarrhythmia who were candidates for ICD placement were considered in the inclusion criteria. The primary end point was progression of HF, defined as all cause mortality along with HF hospitalizations and ventricular tachycardia or ventricular fibrillation requiring device intervention. Despite a 15 % reduction in the primary end point, no statistical significance was attained between the two groups. However improvement in secondary end points such as 6 MWT, pVO_2, and EF was noted in NYHA classes III and IV but not so much in class II. Echocardiography demonstration of remodeling effect was evident in the reduction of ventricular dimensions across all NYHA classes studied [41].

MIRACLE-ICD trial was configured to compare the effect of CRT with ICD against ICD alone in terms of QoL and functional capacity. Despite an improvement in NYHA class and QoL, the primary end points and pVO_2, and the secondary end point, no significant difference was noted in terms of 6 MWD. The study established that in those with an indication for ICD, addition of CRT offers symptomatic relief [36].

MIRACLE-ICD II trial was a randomized substudy carried out in HF patients who fit the criteria for MIRACLE-ICD study with the exception of NYHA class being II. Though there was no significant improvement in pVO_2, 6 MWT, and QoL, improvement was noted in LVEF and cardiac dimensions, which are surrogate markers for ventricular remodeling [42].

COMPANION trial is the largest randomized CRT trial to date designed to compare optimal medical therapy against CRT alone and CRT with defibrillator (CRT-D) in advanced heart failure patients who otherwise had no indication for pacemaker or ICD at baseline. The primary end point was all cause mortality or hospitalization, while secondary end points were both all cause mortality and exercise performance. This was the first trial that was powered to evaluate the mortality benefit in a prospective manner. The primary composite end point was reduced by 19 % in the CRT/CRT-D arms with a reduction of total mortality by 15 % and 40 % in the CRT and CRT-D arm, respectively. The benefit offered in terms of reduction in sudden death noted in the CRT-D arm provided compelling evidence for the FDA to approve the CRT-D device for patients who are candidates for CRT implantation [16].

Cardiac Resynchronization in Heart Failure (CARE-HF) trial was a European study designed with the intent to observe morbidity and mortality benefit of CRT in HF patients whose QRS duration was more than 120 ms. The sample was again subdivided based on the QRS width into those with QRS duration more than 150 ms and the other group with QRS duration between 120 and 150 ms. The study was distinctive in its design by requiring to demonstrate the evidence of LV dyssynchrony by echocardiogram (ECHO)

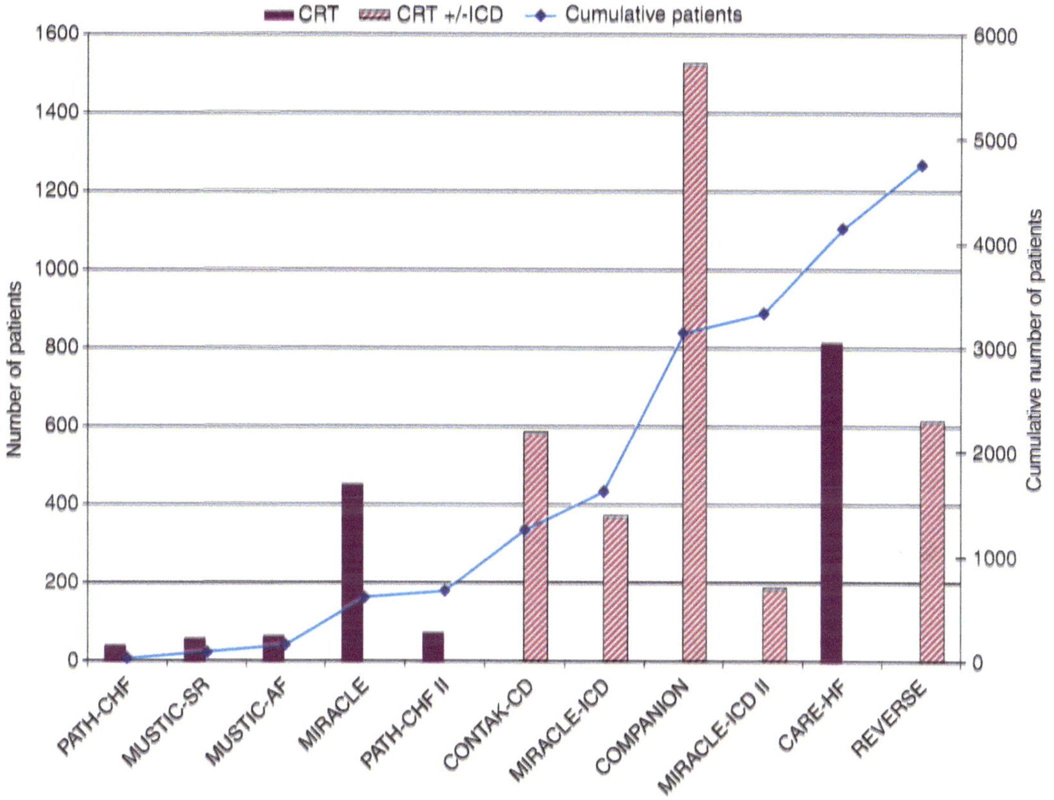

Fig. 7.4 Data spread of various randomized controlled trials on CRT

in the latter group. The primary end point was all cause mortality or any cardiovascular event requiring hospitalization and secondary end point being all cause mortality. CRT was shown to reduce risk of death, intraventricular mechanical delay, mitral regurgitation, and LV end-systolic volume and improve EF, symptoms, and QoL [17]. An extension of the CARE-HF study beyond the initial 29.4 months showed the extension of mortality benefits with long-term follow-up [43].

A recent meta-analysis of pooled data (Fig. 7.5) from 14 randomized controlled trials evaluating the benefit of CRT over 6 months revealed an improvement by at least one NYHA class from baseline in 59 % of patients who underwent CRT implantation in comparison to 37 % among controls with no resynchronization therapy [44]. An augmentation in other parameters such as LVEF, 6 MWD, and QoL was also observed in this study by McAlister and his group. A higher percentage ranging from 63 % to 82 % was noted when 97 observational studies were pooled for analysis by the same group. Only 19 % required hospitalization in the device group compared to 27 % in those without CRT. A notable decrease in all cause mortality was evident in the CRT group (13.2 % in CRT as against 15.5 % with no CRT), and this was expected to increase with duration after CRT. This was in consensus with results of CARE-HF data pertaining to determination of the number needed to prevent one death, which decreased from 13 patients at 2 years to nine patients in 3 years [44]. Figures below demonstrate the response to clinical end points from various randomized controlled trials (Figs. 7.5, 7.6, 7.7, 7.8, 7.9, 7.10 and 7.11).

Given the insurmountable evidence provided by these trials, major cardiology societies (American Heart Association/American College of Cardiology (AHA/ACC), European Society of Cardiology)

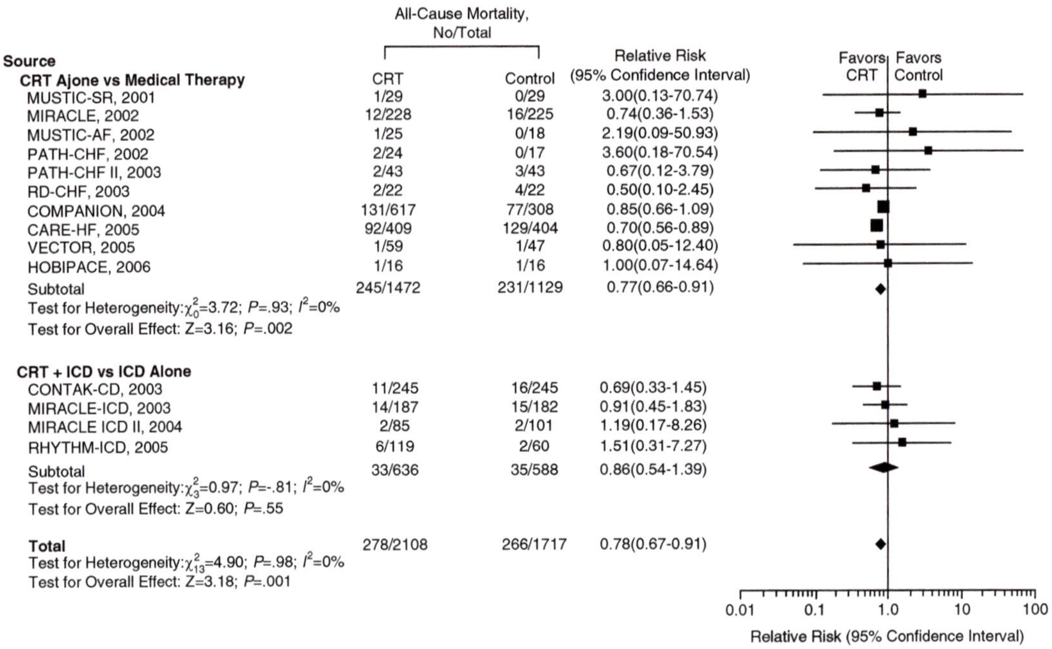

Fig. 7.5 Effect of CRT on all cause mortality (Reprinted with permission from McAlister FA, Ezekowitz J, Hooton N, Vandermeer B, Spooner C, Dryden DM, et al. Cardiac resynchronization therapy for patients with left ventricular systolic dysfunction: a systemic review. JAMA. 2007;297(22):2502–2514). Copyright © (2007) American Medical Association. All rights reserved

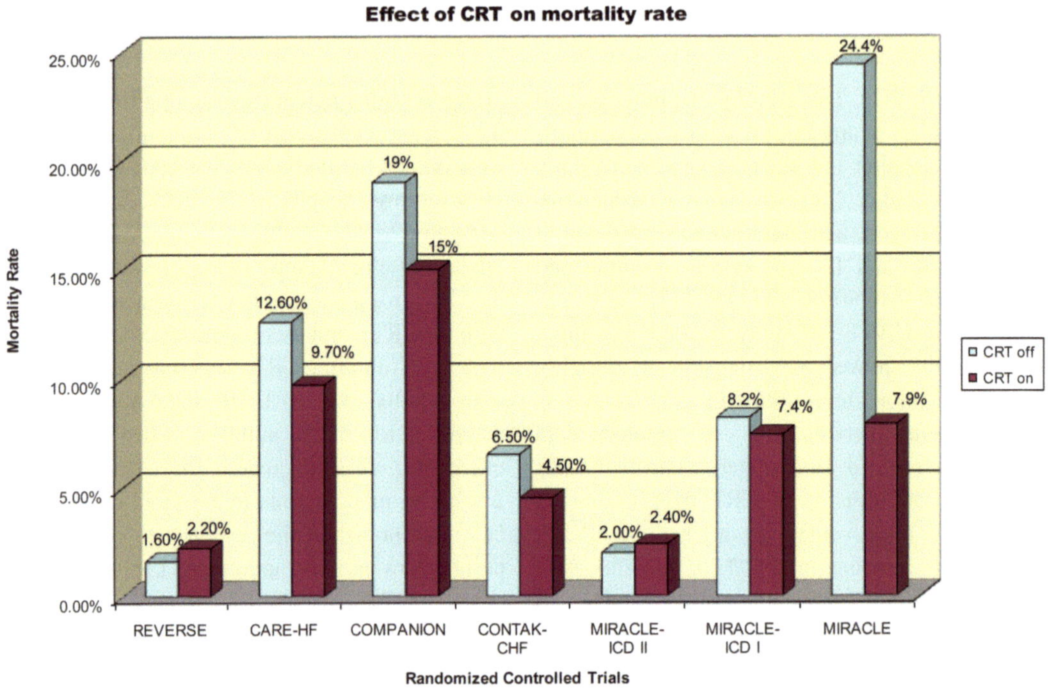

Fig. 7.6 Effect of CRT on mortality rate

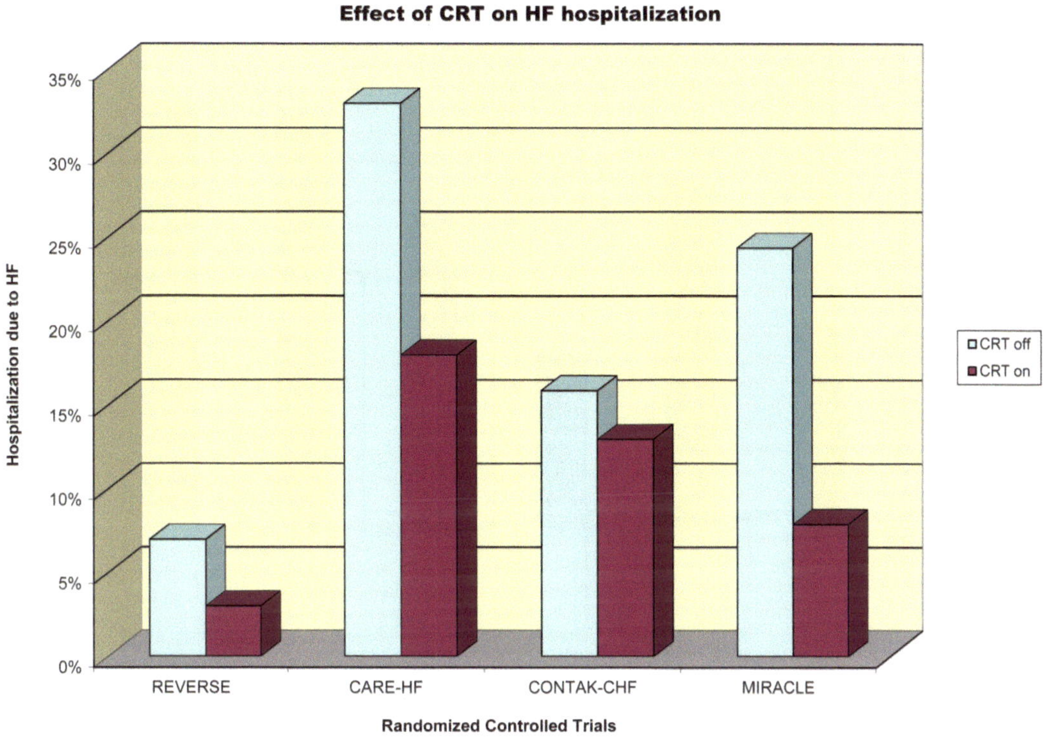

Fig. 7.7 Effect of CRT on HF hospitalization

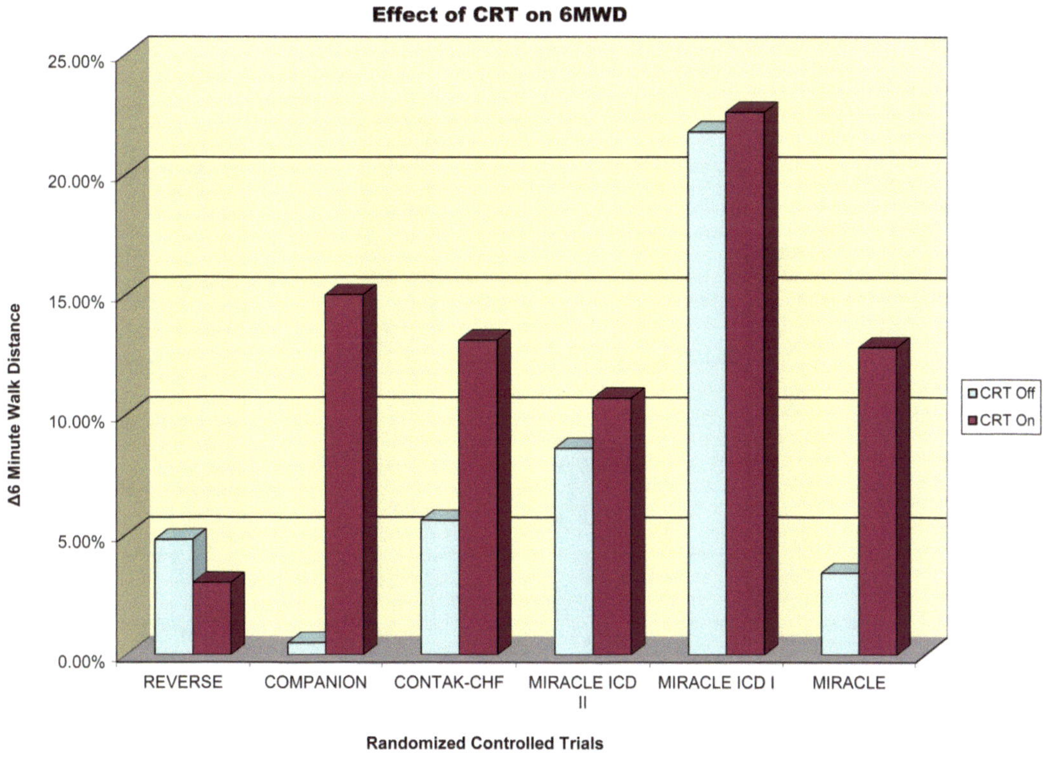

Fig. 7.8 Effect of CRT on 6-min walk distance

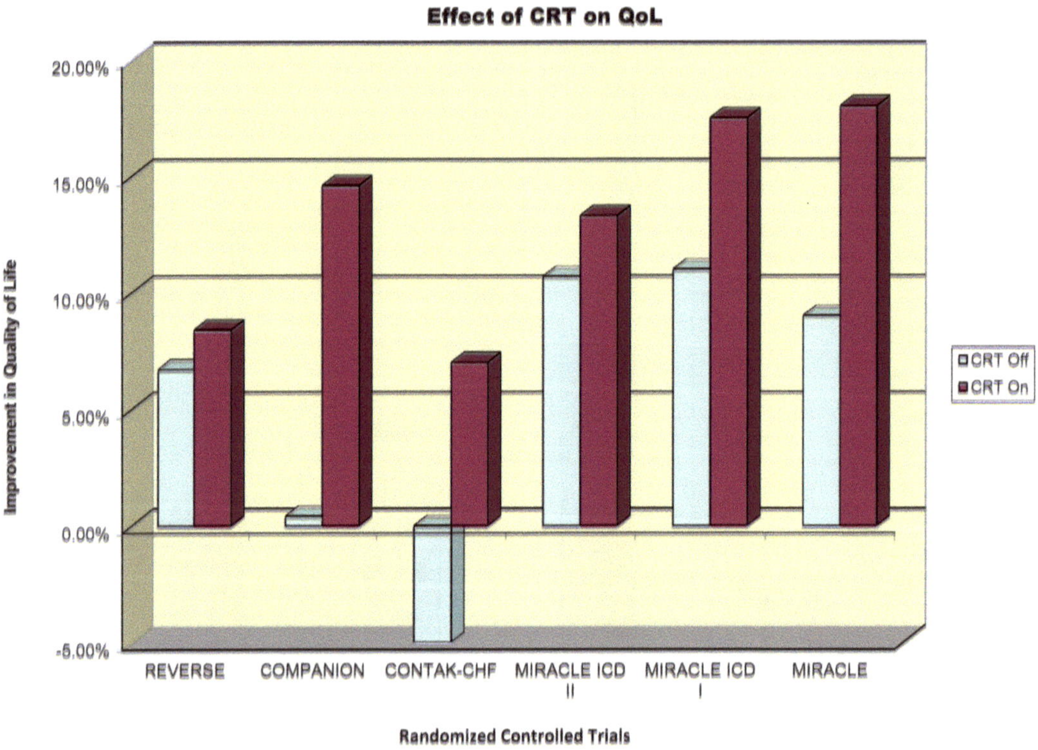

Fig 7.9 Effect of CRT on quality of life

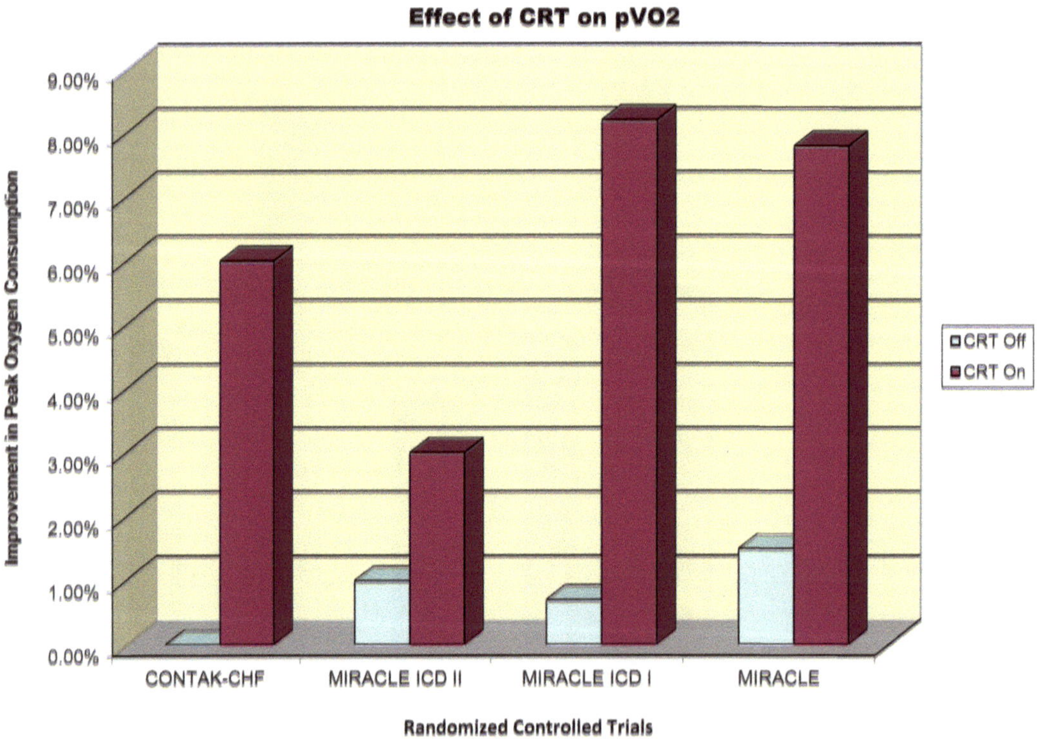

Fig. 7.10 Effect of CRT on pVO_2

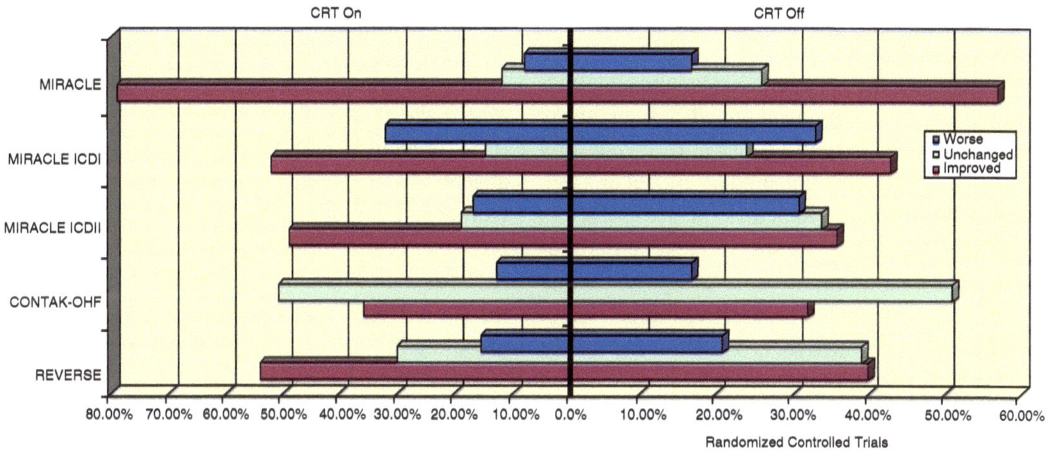

Fig. 7.11 Effect of CRT on HF clinical composite response

have stated CRT as class I indications in heart failure patients who are optimized on medical management and fulfill all of the following:

- A documented EF ≤ 35 %
- In sinus rhythm
- A functional class of NYHA class III or ambulatory NYHA class IV
- Evidence of cardiac dyssynchrony as evidenced by a QRS ≥ 120 ms [45]

Despite these guidelines, a recent study by Hernandez et al. revealed that one in ten patients with CRT implantation has received the devices outside its current recommendations [46]. The researchers hypothesized that a small number of this could be possibly explained by the prophylactic implantation of biventricular pacemaker instead of RV pacing with the intent to prevent systolic dysfunction among those with EF > 35 % as supported by the post AV nodal ablation evaluation (PAVE) trial [47]. Since the update to the AHA/ACC guidelines, results from the "resynchronization reverses remodeling in systolic left ventricular dysfunction" (REVERSE) trial have shed light into the benefit of CRT to patients with HF who are either asymptomatic or have mild symptoms. This randomized control trial evaluated the benefit of CRT (with or without a defibrillator) in patients with systolic HF on optimum drug therapy with an EF ≤ 40 % and QRS duration ≥120 ms who belong to NYHA class I or II. The primary end point in this study was clinical composite response for HF stated as worsened, unchanged, or improved. Due to the inclusion of asymptomatic patients, a proportional analysis was performed as a marker for efficacy. Twenty-one percent in the group with no CRT worsened in comparison to 16 % in the CRT group, but this did not achieve statistical significance. However the time to hospitalization was delayed in the CRT group with added evidence of reversal of LV remodeling noted increasingly in this arm as evidenced by marked improvement in the LV end-systolic volume index [48]. Though this study was not devised to analyze mortality, one can speculate that the evidence of reversal of remodeling may contribute to reduction in mortality. Ongoing trials such as Multicenter Automatic Defibrillator Implantation Trial with CRT (MADIT-CRT) and Resynchronization/Defibrillation for Ambulatory Heart Failure Trial (RAFT) are designed to address mortality benefit in mild HF patients.

Challenges Following CRT Implantation

In spite of the demonstrable effects of CRT, nearly 30 % of those who are suitable for the device do not exhibit clinical improvement and are classically described as "nonresponders." The initial attempt should be to ensure that there is no lead dislodgement and adequate LV lead capture with the help of EKG and chest X-ray.

Interestingly, evidence of LV dyssynchrony was reported in patients with normal QRS duration who were diagnosed with LV systolic dysfunction [23]. Conversely, mechanical dyssynchrony was not associated with electrical dyssynchrony as evident by results published by Bax et al. [49]. Results from the "Predictors of Response to CRT" (PROSPECT) trial showed that no particular echocardiographic measure of dyssynchrony could be recommended to improve patient selection for CRT [50]. Resynchronization therapy in narrow QRS (RethinQ) study was a randomized control trial which failed to show CRT benefit when HF patients with QRS < 130 ms who otherwise met criteria for CRT implantation were selected purely on the basis of mechanical dyssynchrony by ECHO [51]. However there is a rich body of observational trials which shows that echocardiographic criteria for LV dyssynchrony predict CRT response more consistently than QRS duration when applied to responders' and nonresponders' category [52]. Multiple modalities have been attempted to identify mechanical dyssynchrony, the details of which are beyond the scope of this discussion but can be found in reviews elsewhere [52]. In summary, LV dyssynchrony may be measured by applying the following concepts: (1) timing of the valve movement, (2) velocity of aortic-pulmonary flow, and (3) displacement of tissue (wall motion) with respect to reference point or strain of the tissue. Currently trials such as Echocardiography Guided CRT (ECHO-CRT) are underway to determine "responders" to CRT.

In addition, the location of the LV pacing lead and the presence of scar tissue can significantly impede CRT response. Presently the preferred position is the lateral or posterolateral LV region which has yielded the maximum benefit in terms of hemodynamic improvement [53]. Recent work emphasized the need for LV lead placement to be in the area of latest mechanical activation in order to generate the best response in terms of reverse remodeling [54]. In contrast suboptimal lead position was observed to cause deterioration in acute hemodynamic response. In general, accessing the lateral or posterior branches of the coronary sinus via a transvenous approach is successful in approximately 90 % of subjects. Alteration in the cardiac geometry due to underlying cardiac disease progression can occasionally make it a difficult access. Coronary sinus (CS) branches tend to be diminutive or even absent in the areas of previous infarction. Coronary computed tomography (CT) scan with contrast bolus timing and three-dimensional reconstruction imaging can be used to visualize the CS anatomy. Occasionally, fluoroscopic visualization of the venous phase of the coronary angiogram can be used to identify the CS and its tributaries (Fig. 7.12c). Besides use of electrophysiological catheters can aid in identifying the coronary sinus and thus ensure a more successful implant. Alternative approaches are via atrial transseptal route and epicardial placement via sternotomy. The latter has the advantage of avoiding the vascular anatomy and hence minimizes the risk of complications such as perforation or dissection of the coronary sinus. Robotic techniques and minimally invasive access via subxiphoid incision have made epicardial lead implantation safer and appealing than transvenous approach and maybe preferred in the future (Fig. 7.12d).

Presence of viable myocardium is an essential determinant of good CRT response. Bleeker et al. concluded from their study of ischemic cardiomyopathy patients who underwent CRT that presence of scar in the posterolateral segments was a significant factor in being a "nonresponder" [55]. Contrast-enhanced MRI can be a helpful tool to identify and delineate the extent of scar tissue. The extent of myocardial viability identified using myocardial contrast ECHO predicted response to acute and long-term benefit to CRT in comparison to tissue Doppler imaging [56]. Localization of CRT According to Echocardiography (LOCATE) study is a pilot study that is being undertaken so as to evaluate CRT response based on echo-guided lead placement.

Lastly optimization of pacemaker settings in a manner that determines atrioventricular (AV) delay/interventricular (VV) interval so as to generate the best stroke volume can be an approach worth considering in certain subjects. Optimal AV intervals can be chosen with ECHO

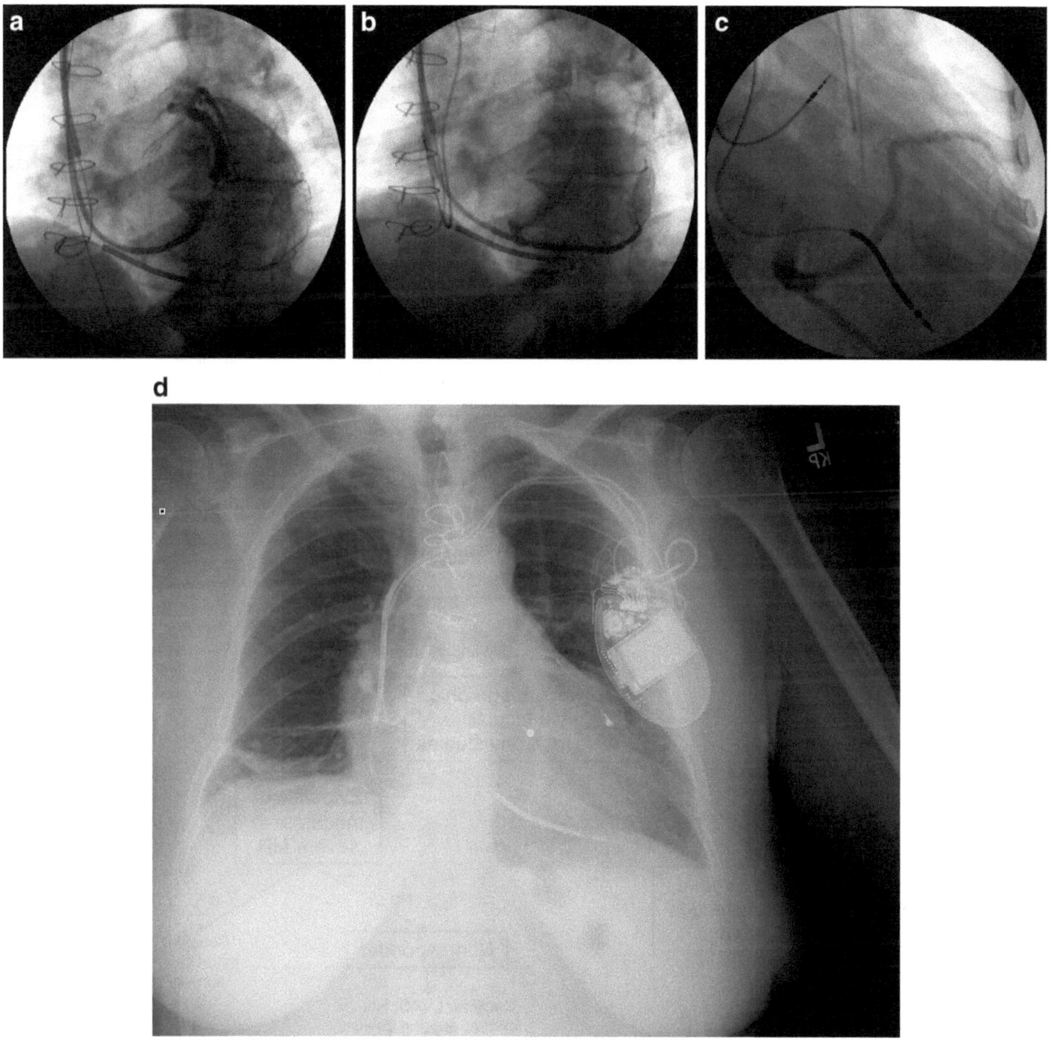

Fig. 7.12 (**a**, **b**) Coronary sinus venogram performed routinely prior to lead placement revealing the various branches. (**c**) Venous phase of coronary angiogram and (**d**) Epicardial lead implantation in a patient who failed transvenous approach

assistance using transmitral flow patterns or surrogate markers for cardiac output (such as aortic outflow velocity) and newer techniques such as tissue tracking. Recent studies have confirmed the initial observations from the PATH-CHF study as to how AV interval determines the degree of dyssynchrony. Data reported from the InSync III Marquis trial showed significant improvement in NYHA class and decrease in LV dyssynchrony in patients who had CRT-D with optimized V-V interval compared to CRT-D alone [57]. Response of CRT Optimization with V-V Timing in Heart Failure Patients (RESPONSE-HF) is an open-label randomized trial underway to evaluate the effect of V-V delay in patients with CRT-D devices. Other ongoing trials such as the Does Echocardiographically Guided Ventriculo-Ventricular Optimization Yield a Sustained Improvement in Echocardiographic Parameters in CRT Patients (DEVISE-CRT) study and The SmartDelay Determined AV Optimization: a Comparison of AV Optimization Methods Used in CRT (SMART-AV) trial are underway to determine

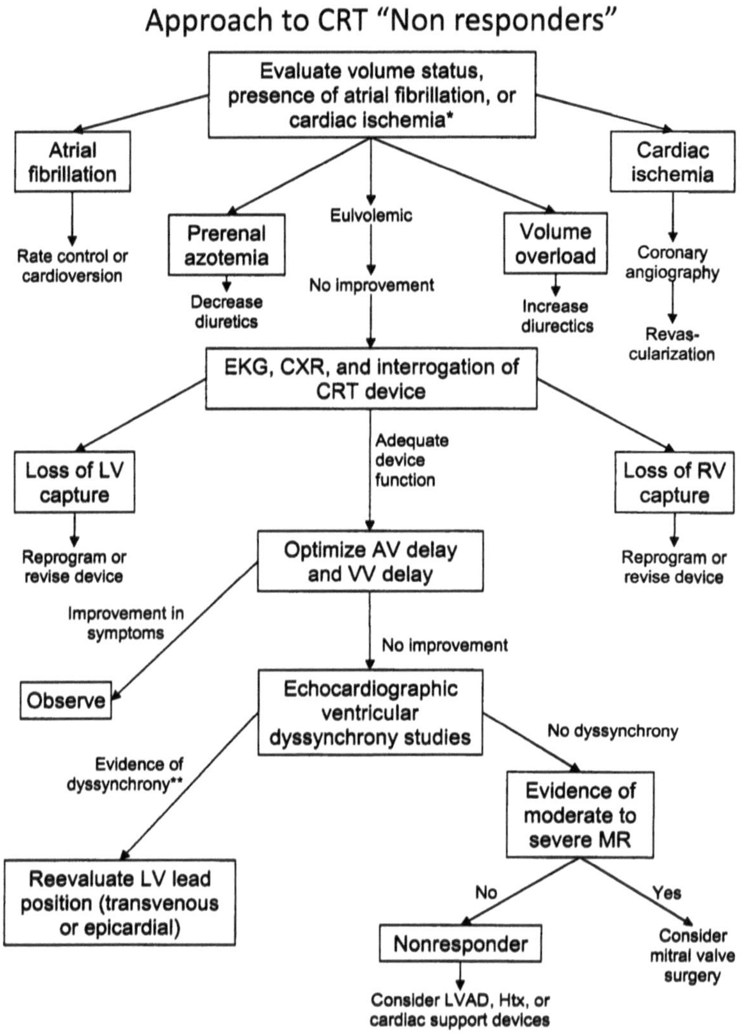

Fig. 7.13 Approach to CRT "nonresponders" (Reprinted from Journal of the American College of Cardiology, Vol. 46, Aranda JM Jr, Woo GW, Schofield RS, Handberg EM, Hill JA, Curtis AB, Sears SF, Goff JS, Pauly DF, Conti JB, Management of heart failure after cardiac resynchronization therapy: integrating advanced heart failure treatment with optimal device function, pages 2193–2198, copyright 2005, with permission from Elsevier)

the ideal modality of pacing to generate the maximum hemodynamic response.

A simplified algorithm has been proposed by Aranda et al. which summarizes the approach to CRT nonresponders [58] (Fig. 7.13).

Of late there has been some concern from reports about CRT rarely potentiating ventricular arrhythmias. Evidence of prolongation of QT interval, R on T phenomenon, and evidence of transmural dispersion of repolarization (TDR) could potentially act as a substrate for Torsade de pointes [59]. In a recent case series report, Shukla et al. demonstrated presence of ventricular tachycardia/ventricular fibrillation (VT/VF) in 5 of 145 consecutive biventricular CRT implants [60]. The resolution of arrhythmia following discontinuation of CRT strengthens the association of these events to CRT. Therefore caution must be exercised when left-sided pacing is considered as an indication for those who require pacemaker, especially in the absence of ICD backup until further studies detailing the underlying mechanism are available.

Special Scenarios and Future Implications

Prevention of HF

With the boundaries of CRT implantation being constantly pushed, clinicians have ventured to determine if CRT could have a role in prevention of HF symptoms. In canine models, biventricular pacing have demonstrated reversal of negative hemodynamic effects and ventricular remodeling attributed to isolated LBBB in the absence of HF. Most randomized trials included patients with NYHA class III/IV, except for MIRACLE-ICD II and CONTAK-CD which incorporated class II patients. Though there was no improvement of significance in clinical parameters (6 MWD, QoL, NYHA class, etc.), ventricular dimensions were superior with an increase in EF in those with mild HF. REVERSE trial was the first prospective randomized trial which evaluated asymptomatic patients who had evidence of low EF and widened QRS complex. A similar observation of no clinical improvement was noted, but considerable evidence of reversal of remodeling was observed in those who received CRT as a prophylaxis. It is debatable if the benefit of delaying the first hospitalization for HF as noted in this study is worthy enough to accept this as standard of care. Furthermore, whether these benefits can be seen long term needs to be adjudicated with larger trials and longer follow-up.

HF with Right Bundle Branch Block (RBBB)

There is scant data regarding the use of CRT in HF patients who show evidence of RBBB. Though there have been case reports which showed benefit, analysis from randomized trials reveal an enrollment of less than 10 %. Conflicting results from MIRACLE and COMPANION trials has not been helpful to allay concerns. Initial data from MIRACLE study revealed that patients with RBBB or IVCD showed benefit from CRT, but COMPANION trial showed a decreased benefit from CRT [61]. A pooled analysis of MIRACLE and CONTAK-CD did not uphold the use of CRT in RBBB [62].

QRS Duration Less Than 120 ms

Widened QRS considered as an evidence of LV dyssynchrony has been inclusive criteria in all major randomized trials. Analysis of data from CARE-HF trial and COMPANION trial revealed the salutary effects of CRT to be strongly correlated with wider QRS complex. Results from the RethinQ study revealed no evidence of improvement with CRT despite echocardiographic evidence of mechanical dyssynchrony in patients who had QRS < 130 ms. The issue to consider is whether all types of contractility problems are related to dyssynchrony or due to dyssynergy. Dyssynergy is mainly an ineffective contraction despite good recruitment which could be due to lack of viable myocardium as a result of underlying ischemic cardiomyopathy or replacement of myofilaments with scar tissue. In this scenario, there is very little CRT can offer given that timing of contraction is not the issue. However in clinical scenario, it is difficult to differentiate between dyssynergy and dyssynchrony, and more imaging modalities need to be evaluated to differentiate these two identities. Given the evidence of remodeling noted in patients with narrow QRS and CRT implant, future research may promise hope to this group of patients who have evidence of HF but do not meet the criteria for CRT implantation as per current guidelines. Results from ECHO-CRT will be helpful in directing treatment guidelines in the future.

Patients with Atrial Fibrillation (AF)

The randomized trials confirming the effect of CRT in HF have mainly included patients with sinus rhythm (SR) except for MUSTIC-AF trial.

The prevalence of AF in HF patients has been observed to be varying from 25 % to 50 %; however only 2 % of patients included in the trials have AF. In general, patients with underlying AF tend to be sicker and older than the subjects included in the trials. Patients with AF pose a challenge since consistent biventricular capture is difficult in the setting of irregularity and intermittent rapid ventricular rate. When rate control was adequately achieved allowing delivery of >85 % biventricular (Bi-V) paced beats, the benefits are comparable to those in sinus rhythm [63]. In those where such a pacing was less successful (<85 % Bi-V pacing), AV junctional ablation is recommended followed by CRT. This was supported by results from the Multicenter Longitudinal Observational Study (MILOS) where similar mortality was noted in both sinus rhythm and AF group but significantly better than those on medical therapy alone [64]. In the absence of long-term follow-up or data from randomized trials, it is a difficult choice to commit a patient to lifetime dependence on pacing, especially given the high proportion of nonresponders to CRT. New treatment options for AF consisting of isolation of pulmonary vein, extensive maze procedure offers alternate options to AV junctional ablation. Hence any randomized trial to evaluate use of CRT in HF patients with AF should be inclusive of all major treatment modalities such as drug therapy, AV junction ablation, and isolation of pulmonary vein. A recent meta-analysis of prospective cohort studies of CRT in AF and SR showed significant improvement in EF but limited change in functional outcomes [65]. PAVE study also noted that in those who undergo AV junctional ablation, biventricular pacing provides significant improvement in function and EF compared to RV pacing. Ablation for Paroxysmal Atrial Fibrillation (APAF) trial is enrolling patients to determine the comparison of echo-guided CRT and right ventricular pacing following AV junction ablation for permanent AF.

Patients with Standard Pacing Indications

RV pacing has been associated with detrimental dyssynchrony as shown in the Dual Chamber and VVI Implantable Defibrillator (DAVID) trial. The Hornburg Biventricular Pacing Evaluation (HOBIPACE) trial was a randomized crossover study that gave evidence to the fact that CRT led to significant improvement in LVEF and LV end-systolic volume as primary end points and reduction in neurohormonal markers for HF and improvement in QoL and EF as secondary gain. However, LV pacing was accepted as a safe and feasible option in comparison to biventricular pacing based on the results from Bi vs Left Ventricular Pacing: an International Pilot Evaluation on Heart Failure Patients with Ventricular Arrhythmias (BELIEVE) trial [66]. Other ongoing trials such as Biventricular Versus Right Ventricular Pacing in Heart Failure Patients with Atrioventricular Block (BLOCK-HF) trial are comparing benefit of CRT versus RV pacing in HF patients who have indications for chronic pacing for bradycardia, while Device Evaluation of CONTAK RENEWAL 2 and EASYTRAK 2: Assessment of Safety and Effectiveness in Heart Failure (DECREASE-HF) study will compare biventricular pacing to permanent left ventricular pacing mode.

Role of Adding ICD to Biventricular Pacemaker

The indication of ICD for primary prevention in advanced HF was based on the reduction of sudden death in chronic HF. COMPANION trial is the only trial that considered drug therapy against ICD (CRT-P) or CRT with a defibrillator (CRT-D). There was survival benefit noted in both arms, but the effect was unchanged beyond the ninth month. MADIT-CRT trial is currently evaluating patients who belong to NYHA classes I and II with a prolonged QRS > 120 ms to assess if there is a mortality benefit with CRT-D.

Advances in pacing technology with possible multiple lead (TRIP-HF trial) placements or multipolar pacing techniques and even consideration of biological pacemaker mediated via transplantation of pacemaker cells are all viable concepts for the future of CRT. While such interests are being pursued, it is important to critically review the strategies already approved to identify areas whereby efficacy can be improved and to identify the ideal subject who can derive maximal benefit.

References

1. Kannel WB, Plehn JF, Cupples LA. Cardiac failure and sudden death in the Framingham Study. Am Heart J. 1988;115:869–75.
2. Lloyd-Jones DM, Larson MG, Leip EP, et al. Lifetime risk for developing congestive heart failure: the Framingham Heart Study. Circulation. 2002;106:3068–72.
3. Weber KT, Brilla CG. Pathological hypertrophy and cardiac interstitium. Fibrosis and renin-angiotensin-aldosterone system. Circulation. 1991;83:1849–65.
4. Farwell D, Patel NR, Hall A, Ralph S, Sulke AN. How many people with heart failure are appropriate for biventricular resynchronization? Eur Heart J. 2000;21:1246–50.
5. Baldasseroni S, Opasich C, Gorini M, et al. Left bundle-branch block is associated with increased 1-year sudden and total mortality rate in 5517 outpatients with congestive heart failure: a report from the Italian network on congestive heart failure. Am Heart J. 2002;143:398–405.
6. Bramlet DA, Morris KG, Coleman RE, Albert D, Cobb FR. Effect of rate-dependent left bundle branch block on global and regional left ventricular function. Circulation. 1983;67:1059–65.
7. Grines CL, Bashore TM, Boudoulas H, Olson S, Shafer P, Wooley CF. Functional abnormalities in isolated left bundle branch block. The effect of interventricular asynchrony. Circulation. 1989;79:845–53.
8. Leclercq C, Cazeau S, Ritter P, et al. A pilot experience with permanent biventricular pacing to treat advanced heart failure. Am Heart J. 2000;140:862–70.
9. Gras D, Leclercq C, Tang AS, Bucknall C, Luttikhuis HO, Kirstein-Pedersen A. Cardiac resynchronization therapy in advanced heart failure the multicenter InSync clinical study. Eur J Heart Fail. 2002;4:311–20.
10. Kuhlkamp V. Initial experience with an implantable cardioverter-defibrillator incorporating cardiac resynchronization therapy. J Am Coll Cardiol. 2002;39:790–7.
11. Auricchio A, Stellbrink C, Sack S, et al. Long-term clinical effect of hemodynamically optimized cardiac resynchronization therapy in patients with heart failure and ventricular conduction delay. J Am Coll Cardiol. 2002;39:2026–33.
12. Auricchio A, Stellbrink C, Butter C, et al. Clinical efficacy of cardiac resynchronization therapy using left ventricular pacing in heart failure patients stratified by severity of ventricular conduction delay. J Am Coll Cardiol. 2003;42:2109–16.
13. Cazeau S, Leclercq C, Lavergne T, et al. Effects of multisite biventricular pacing in patients with heart failure and intraventricular conduction delay. N Engl J Med. 2001;344:873–80.
14. Leclercq C, Walker S, Linde C, et al. Comparative effects of permanent biventricular and right-univentricular pacing in heart failure patients with chronic atrial fibrillation. Eur Heart J. 2002;23:1780–7.
15. Abraham WT. Cardiac resynchronization therapy for the management of chronic heart failure. Am Heart Hosp J. 2003;1:55–61.
16. Bristow MR, Saxon LA, Boehmer J, et al. Cardiac-resynchronization therapy with or without an implantable defibrillator in advanced chronic heart failure. N Engl J Med. 2004;350:2140–50.
17. Cleland JG, Daubert JC, Erdmann E, et al. The effect of cardiac resynchronization on morbidity and mortality in heart failure. N Engl J Med. 2005;352:1539–49.
18. Lloyd-Jones D, Adams R, Carnethon M, et al. Heart disease and stroke statistics—2009 update: a report From the American Heart Association Statistics Committee and Stroke Statistics Subcommittee. Circulation. 2009;119(3):e21–181.
19. Nishimura RA, Hayes DL, Holmes Jr DR, Tajik AJ. Mechanism of hemodynamic improvement by dual-chamber pacing for severe left ventricular dysfunction: an acute Doppler and catheterization hemodynamic study. J Am Coll Cardiol. 1995;25:281–8.
20. Bleeker GB, Schalij MJ, Molhoek SG, et al. Relationship between QRS duration and left ventricular dyssynchrony in patients with end-stage heart failure. J Cardiovasc Electrophysiol. 2004;15:544–9.
21. Kass DA. Ventricular resynchronization: pathophysiology and identification of responders. Rev Cardiovasc Med. 2003;4 Suppl 2Suppl 2:S3–S13.
22. Hawkins NM, Petrie MC, MacDonald MR, Hogg KJ, McMurray JJ. Selecting patients for cardiac resynchronization therapy: electrical or mechanical dyssynchrony? Eur Heart J. 2006;27:1270–81.
23. Bader H, Garrigue S, Lafitte S, et al. Intra-left ventricular electromechanical asynchrony. A new independent predictor of severe cardiac events in heart failure patients. J Am Coll Cardiol. 2004; 43:248–56.
24. Iuliano S, Fisher SG, Karasik PE, Fletcher RD, Singh SN. QRS duration and mortality in patients with congestive heart failure. Am Heart J. 2002;143:1085–91.
25. Kalra PR, Sharma R, Shamim W, et al. Clinical characteristics and survival of patients with chronic heart failure and prolonged QRS duration. Int J Cardiol. 2002;86:225–31.
26. Sandhu R, Bahler RC. Prevalence of QRS prolongation in a community hospital cohort of patients with heart failure and its relation to left ventricular systolic dysfunction. Am J Cardiol. 2004;93:244–6.
27. Xiao HB, Roy C, Fujimoto S, Gibson DG. Natural history of abnormal conduction and its relation to prognosis in patients with dilated cardiomyopathy. Int J Cardiol. 1996;53:163–70.
28. Cazeau S, Ritter P, Bakdach S, et al. Four chamber pacing in dilated cardiomyopathy. Pacing Clin Electrophysiol. 1994;17:1974–9.

29. Auricchio A, Stellbrink C, Block M, et al. Effect of pacing chamber and atrioventricular delay on acute systolic function of paced patients with congestive heart failure. The Pacing Therapies for Congestive Heart Failure Study Group. The Guidant Congestive Heart Failure Research Group. Circulation. 1999;99: 2993–3001.
30. Bordachar P, Lafitte S, Reuter S, et al. Echocardiographic parameters of ventricular dyssynchrony validation in patients with heart failure using sequential biventricular pacing. J Am Coll Cardiol. 2004;44:2157–65.
31. Auricchio A, Klein H, Tockman B, et al. Transvenous biventricular pacing for heart failure: can the obstacles be overcome? Am J Cardiol. 1999;83:136D–42D.
32. Helm RH, Byrne M, Helm PA, et al. Three-dimensional mapping of optimal left ventricular pacing site for cardiac resynchronization. Circulation. 2007;115:953–61.
33. Kass DA, Chen CH, Curry C, et al. Improved left ventricular mechanics from acute VDD pacing in patients with dilated cardiomyopathy and ventricular conduction delay. Circulation. 1999;99:1567–73.
34. Lancellotti P, Melon P, Sakalihasan N, et al. Effect of cardiac resynchronization therapy on functional mitral regurgitation in heart failure. Am J Cardiol. 2004;94:1462–5.
35. Abraham WT, Fisher WG, Smith AL, et al. Cardiac resynchronization in chronic heart failure. N Engl J Med. 2002;346:1845–53.
36. Young JB, Abraham WT, Smith AL, et al. Combined cardiac resynchronization and implantable cardioversion defibrillation in advanced chronic heart failure: the MIRACLE ICD Trial. JAMA. 2003;289:2685–94.
37. Lozano I, Bocchiardo M, Achtelik M, et al. Impact of biventricular pacing on mortality in a randomized crossover study of patients with heart failure and ventricular arrhythmias. Pacing Clin Electrophysiol. 2000;23:1711–2.
38. St John Sutton MG, Plappert T, Abraham WT, et al. Effect of cardiac resynchronization therapy on left ventricular size and function in chronic heart failure. Circulation. 2003;107:1985–90.
39. Yu CM, Chau E, Sanderson JE, et al. Tissue Doppler echocardiographic evidence of reverse remodeling and improved synchronicity by simultaneously delaying regional contraction after biventricular pacing therapy in heart failure. Circulation. 2002;105:438–45.
40. Sutton MG, Plappert T, Hilpisch KE, Abraham WT, Hayes DL, Chinchoy E. Sustained reverse left ventricular structural remodeling with cardiac resynchronization at one year is a function of etiology: quantitative Doppler echocardiographic evidence from the Multicenter InSync Randomized Clinical Evaluation (MIRACLE). Circulation. 2006;113: 266–72.
41. Higgins SL, Hummel JD, Niazi IK, et al. Cardiac resynchronization therapy for the treatment of heart failure in patients with intraventricular conduction delay and malignant ventricular tachyarrhythmias. J Am Coll Cardiol. 2003;42:1454–9.
42. Abraham WT, Young JB, Leon AR, et al. Effects of cardiac resynchronization on disease progression in patients with left ventricular systolic dysfunction, an indication for an implantable cardioverter-defibrillator, and mildly symptomatic chronic heart failure. Circulation. 2004;110:2864–8.
43. Cleland JG, Daubert JC, Erdmann E, et al. Longer-term effects of cardiac resynchronization therapy on mortality in heart failure [the CArdiac REsynchronization-Heart Failure (CARE-HF) trial extension phase]. Eur Heart J. 2006;27:1928–32.
44. McAlister FA, Ezekowitz J, Hooton N, et al. Cardiac resynchronization therapy for patients with left ventricular systolic dysfunction: a systematic review. JAMA. 2007;297:2502–14.
45. Epstein AE, DiMarco JP, Ellenbogen KA, et al. ACC/AHA/HRS 2008 Guidelines for Device-Based Therapy of Cardiac Rhythm Abnormalities: a report of the American College of Cardiology/American Heart Association Task Force on Practice Guidelines (Writing Committee to Revise the ACC/AHA/NASPE 2002 Guideline Update for Implantation of Cardiac Pacemakers and Antiarrhythmia Devices) developed in collaboration with the American Association for Thoracic Surgery and Society of Thoracic Surgeons. J Am Coll Cardiol. 2008;51:e1–62.
46. Piccini JP, Hernandez AF, Dai D, et al. Use of cardiac resynchronization therapy in patients hospitalized with heart failure. Circulation. 2008;118:926–33.
47. Doshi RN, Daoud EG, Fellows C, et al. Left ventricular-based cardiac stimulation post AV nodal ablation evaluation (the PAVE study). J Cardiovasc Electrophysiol. 2005;16:1160–5.
48. Linde C, Abraham WT, Gold MR, St John Sutton M, Ghio S, Daubert C. Randomized trial of cardiac resynchronization in mildly symptomatic heart failure patients and in asymptomatic patients with left ventricular dysfunction and previous heart failure symptoms. J Am Coll Cardiol. 2008;52:1834–43.
49. Bax JJ, Bleeker GB, Marwick TH, et al. Left ventricular dyssynchrony predicts response and prognosis after cardiac resynchronization therapy. J Am Coll Cardiol. 2004;44:1834–40.
50. Chung ES, Leon AR, Tavazzi L, et al. Results of the Predictors of Response to CRT (PROSPECT) trial. Circulation. 2008;117:2608–16.
51. Beshai JF, Grimm RA, Nagueh SF, et al. Cardiac-resynchronization therapy in heart failure with narrow QRS complexes. N Engl J Med. 2007;357:2461–71.
52. Bax JJ, Abraham T, Barold SS, et al. Cardiac resynchronization therapy: part 1–issues before device implantation. J Am Coll Cardiol. 2005;46:2153–67.
53. Rossillo A, Verma A, Saad EB, et al. Impact of coronary sinus lead position on biventricular pacing: mortality and echocardiographic evaluation during long-term follow-up. J Cardiovasc Electrophysiol. 2004;15:1120–5.

54. Murphy RT, Sigurdsson G, Mulamalla S, et al. Tissue synchronization imaging and optimal left ventricular pacing site in cardiac resynchronization therapy. Am J Cardiol. 2006;97:1615–21.
55. Bleeker GB, Kaandorp TA, Lamb HJ, et al. Effect of posterolateral scar tissue on clinical and echocardiographic improvement after cardiac resynchronization therapy. Circulation. 2006;113:969–76.
56. Hummel JP, Lindner JR, Belcik JT, et al. Extent of myocardial viability predicts response to biventricular pacing in ischemic cardiomyopathy. Heart Rhythm. 2005;2:1211–7.
57. William TA, Angel RL, Cole H, William P, Ann F. Results of the InSync III Marquis clinical trial. Heart Rhythm: Official J Heart Rhythm Soc. 2005;2:S65.
58. Aranda Jr JM, Woo GW, Schofield RS, et al. Management of heart failure after cardiac resynchronization therapy: integrating advanced heart failure treatment with optimal device function. J Am Coll Cardiol. 2005;46:2193–8.
59. Medina-Ravell VA, Lankipalli RS, Yan GX, et al. Effect of epicardial or biventricular pacing to prolong QT interval and increase transmural dispersion of repolarization: does resynchronization therapy pose a risk for patients predisposed to long QT or torsade de pointes? Circulation. 2003;107:740–6.
60. Shukla G, Chaudhry GM, Orlov M, Hoffmeister P, Haffajee C. Potential proarrhythmic effect of biventricular pacing: fact or myth? Heart Rhythm. 2005;2:951–6.
61. Aranda Jr JM, Conti JB, Johnson JW, Petersen-Stejskal S, Curtis AB. Cardiac resynchronization therapy in patients with heart failure and conduction abnormalities other than left bundle-branch block: analysis of the Multicenter InSync Randomized Clinical Evaluation (MIRACLE). Clin Cardiol. 2004;27:678–82.
62. Egoavil CA, Ho RT, Greenspon AJ, Pavri BB. Cardiac resynchronization therapy in patients with right bundle branch block: analysis of pooled data from the MIRACLE and Contak CD trials. Heart Rhythm. 2005;2:611–5.
63. Khadjooi K, Foley PW, Chalil S, et al. Long-term effects of cardiac resynchronisation therapy in patients with atrial fibrillation. Heart. 2008;94:879–83.
64. Gasparini M, Auricchio A, Metra M, et al. Long-term survival in patients undergoing cardiac resynchronization therapy: the importance of performing atrio-ventricular junction ablation in patients with permanent atrial fibrillation. Eur Heart J. 2008;29:1644–52.
65. Upadhyay GA, Choudhry NK, Auricchio A, Ruskin J, Singh JP. Cardiac resynchronization in patients with atrial fibrillation: a meta-analysis of prospective cohort studies. J Am Coll Cardiol. 2008;52:1239–46.
66. Gasparini M, Bocchiardo M, Lunati M, et al. Comparison of 1-year effects of left ventricular and biventricular pacing in patients with heart failure who have ventricular arrhythmias and left bundle-branch block: the Bi vs Left Ventricular Pacing: an International Pilot Evaluation on Heart Failure Patients with Ventricular Arrhythmias (BELIEVE) multicenter prospective randomized pilot study. Am Heart J. 2006;152:155. e1-7.

Triage VADs: TandemHeart, Impella, and CentriMag

8

Igor D. Gregoric

Introduction

Considerable progress has been made in recent years for the treatment of acute heart failure syndromes. The management of acute heart failure is challenging due to its diverse etiologies and clinical presentations, which require a multidisciplinary approach to provide appropriate pharmacologic, interventional, and surgical therapy [1]. Many survivors of acute heart failure episodes return to a reasonable state of health, yet a considerable number of patients develop severe cardiogenic shock that is refractory to aggressive therapy. The early mortality in patients with cardiogenic shock ranges from 50 % to 70 %, albeit there is a good long-term prognosis for those who survive the acute phase of the syndrome [2–4]. In the setting of acute profound heart failure with cardiogenic shock while receiving usual medical therapy, rapid stabilization of hemodynamics with mechanical circulatory support (MCS) is necessary to adequately diagnose the underlying cause of heart failure and to formulate the most effective treatment options.

MCS has been used for acute and chronic heart failure with varying success over the past 50 years. Following the introduction of cardiopulmonary bypass during the 1950s, there were a few attempts to support patients with mechanical devices outside of the operating room. Implantable and paracorporeal left ventricular assist devices (LVADs) were first used in the mid-1960s to support patients with postcardiotomy cardiogenic shock [5, 6]. These initial attempts demonstrated that the concept of partial cardiac support for durations of a few days until myocardial function improved was feasible. Total cardiac replacement as a bridge to transplant was also demonstrated clinically in the 1960s; however, at the time, cardiac transplantation did not provide long-term survival due to immune complications [7]. During the 1970s and 1980s, the clinical use of ventricular assist devices (VADs) and total artificial hearts (TAHs) was nominal; however, research and development efforts continued. Today, VAD and TAH systems are used worldwide for bridging to recovery or transplant and for destination therapy.

The immediate goal of therapy upon presentation of cardiogenic shock is to restore circulation to levels that will avoid the development of multiple organ failure due to hypoperfusion. Initial treatment of cardiogenic shock usually consists of inotropes, vasodilators, diuretics, anticoagulants, volume management, and intra-aortic balloon pump (IABP) support. The IABP was the first device developed to provide rapid MCS in the setting of cardiogenic shock [8, 9]. Since its first use in 1969, the IABP has been the most widely

I.D. Gregoric, M.D., FACC (✉)
Center for Advanced Heart Failure,
University of Texas Health Science Center Houston
at Memorial Hermann Hospital, 6410 Fannin St.
UPB Ste. 920, Houston, TX 77030, USA
e-mail: igregoric@hotmail.com;
eva.m.pongratz@uth.tmc.edu

J.A. Morgan and Y. Naka (eds.), *Surgical Treatment for Advanced Heart Failure*,
DOI 10.1007/978-1-4614-6919-3_8, © Springer Science+Business Media New York 2013

used MCS device and continues to be used daily worldwide. However, the amount of circulatory support from an IABP is limited to only 1.5 L/min, which is often less than the amount of cardiac output needed for survival from cardiogenic shock. The Hemopump, another catheter-mounted pump designed for rapid insertion, was developed and tested during the 1980s and was capable of providing up to 3 L/min of cardiac output support [10]. Although this device proved to be useful for the treatment of cardiogenic shock and for support during high-risk interventional procedures, failure to meet regulatory requirements by the manufacturer prevented this device from reaching the market place [11–13]. Consequently, the IABP has remained the mainstay of MCS for cardiogenic shock for almost 50 years.

Other methods of circulatory assist for cardiogenic shock that have been used with varying results include extracorporeal membrane oxygenation (ECMO) and the use of centrifugal pumps without an oxygenator. ECMO has been most effective in treating infants and adults with profound respiratory failure [14, 15], but the complexity of the system has limited its use for extended cardiac support in cardiogenic shock. For patients who failed to wean from cardiopulmonary bypass, extended support beyond the operating room was achieved with the use of centrifugal flow pumps [16, 17]. These techniques of circulatory support offered the advantages of urgent univentricular or biventricular assist in the operating room for postcardiotomy failure; however, the need for high levels of anticoagulation precipitated high rates of bleeding and associated complications [18, 19].

The recent development of MCS devices that are less thrombogenic and more durable, incorporate cannulation techniques for rapid vascular access, and provide higher levels of cardiac output is changing the treatment paradigm for severe cardiogenic shock. A variety of VAD systems have been used for short-term circulatory support and range from complex systems requiring cardiopulmonary bypass for implantation to small catheter-mounted pumps that can be inserted percutaneously in conscious patients. The TandemHeart® system (CardiacAssist, Inc., Pittsburgh, PA) and the Impella® VAD (ABIOMED Inc., Danvers, MA) are two systems that utilize percutaneous techniques for rapid initiation of support and are used for temporary support during high-risk interventions or for support of patients with cardiogenic shock. The CentriMag® system (Levitronix, Waltham, MA) is an extracorporeal VAD that is placed surgically and can provide univentricular or biventricular support. In this chapter, the use of the TandemHeart, Impella, and CentriMag short-term VADs that have been recently introduced into clinical use will be presented. These new VAD systems offer a number of advantages and provide levels of cardiac output support that have the potential to salvage more patients with severe refractory cardiogenic shock.

Short-Term Cardiac Support

The immediate goals of cardiac support for cardiogenic shock are to promptly provide an adequate amount of systemic perfusion to avoid organ damage and to unload the ventricles. The amount of time a patient remains in a severely hypoperfused state plays a major role in outcome. Once patients are stabilized, further diagnostics can take place to accurately determine the best course of therapy, but also time is needed to assess the risks and benefits of further therapy (Fig. 8.1). Usually, several days of support are needed to assess the reversibility of organ dysfunction, determine the likeliness of myocardial recovery, and to consider alternative therapies. Heart transplantation and long-term LVAD support are courses of therapy that are either limited in resources or are very expensive. Patients with neurologic deficit or irreversible end-organ damage may not be suitable candidates for advanced therapy.

The etiology of heart failure plays a major role in determining the ultimate course of therapy for patients with cardiogenic shock. The common etiologies of cardiogenic shock include acute myocardial infarction (AMI), decompensated chronic heart failure, postcardiotomy shock, fulminant myocarditis, peripartum cardiomyopathy, various valve disorders, and congenital defects.

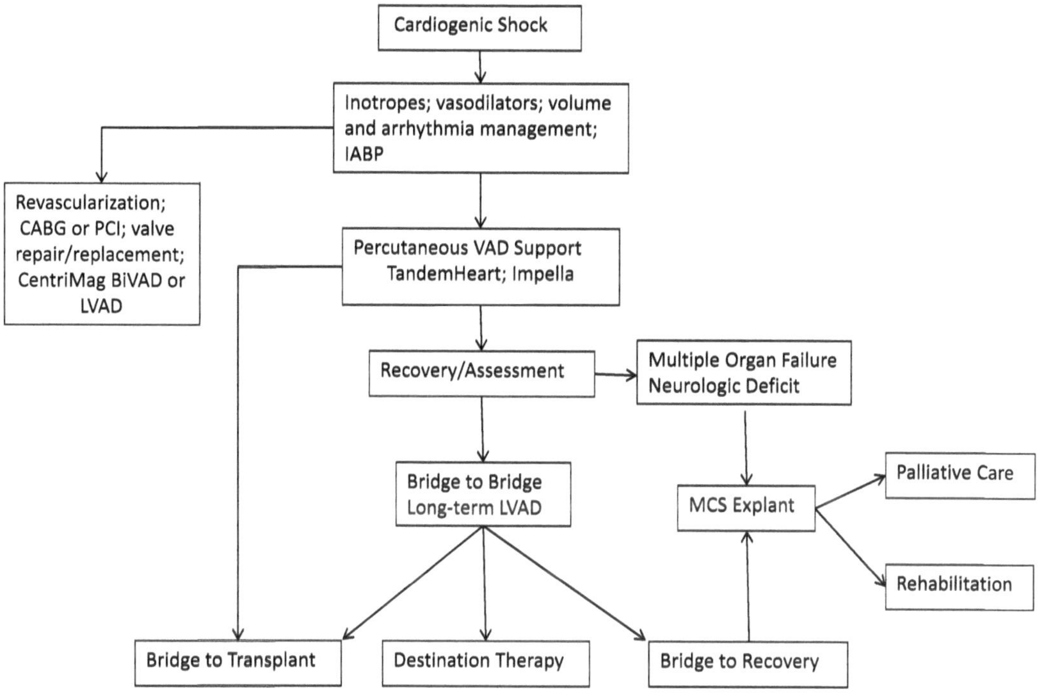

Fig. 8.1 An algorithm depicting the potential courses of care for patients with severe cardiogenic shock

Patients with cardiogenic shock following AMI need to undergo prompt revascularization either by percutaneous coronary intervention (PCI) or coronary artery bypass grafting [20]. For patients with chronic heart failure, temporary VAD support may result in bridging to transplant, recovery of myocardial function, or implantation of a long-term LVAD. The usual goal of temporary postcardiotomy support is to allow time for recovery from the insult of cardiotomy with cardiac arrest. However, the mortality in this group is high, and some will eventually receive a long-term LVAD or heart transplant. Patients with myocarditis or peripartum cardiomyopathy usually require support that ranges in duration from many weeks to a few months until recovery is adequate, which usually requires the use of an intermediate to long-term LVAD or biventricular VAD (BiVAD) [21–24]. Patients presenting with cardiogenic shock secondary to valvular or congenital defects will normally undergo corrective surgery after stabilization.

Once temporary VAD support is initiated and hemodynamics are stabilized, the potential for myocardial recovery is assessed frequently, with the goal of keeping the support duration as minimal as possible. Bleeding, infection, and thromboembolic complications during VAD support contribute considerably to morbidity and mortality. These complications, along with severe ischemia during the acute phase of cardiogenic shock, often lead to multiple organ dysfunction. Aggressive supportive medical therapy and normal hemodynamics may allow for safe weaning and removal of the device. Explant of the VAD is considered when renal, hepatic, pulmonary, and neurologic functions are adequate and the patient can tolerate VAD weaning. Optimally, dialysis, mechanical ventilation, and inotropic medications have been discontinued or are being used minimally at the time of VAD explant.

Availability and Selection of VADS

Several factors influence the choice of which MCS device is most appropriate for individual patients. Age and size of the patient is an important consideration in selection of cannulas or devices. Most contemporary VAD systems are small and can accommodate the majority of patients needing support. However, small children usually require surgical implantation and the use of cannulas suitable for their vessel size. VAD systems that are deployed by percutaneous techniques provide only left ventricular support, and the maximal flow rate ranges from 2.5 to 5.0 L/min. The percutaneous LVADs require expertise for insertion of a transeptal left atrial cannula or for transvalvular left ventricular positioning of a pump and cannula. Severe peripheral vascular disease may preclude the use of both the TandemHeart and Impella VADs because the cannulas or pump are inserted through the femoral vein and artery. Fluoroscopic guidance for proper placement of the cannula is necessary with most implant procedures being performed in the cardiac catheterization laboratory. The percutaneous VADs avoid surgery and associated complications, but support is limited to the left heart only, and the amount of support is limited to 5 L/min at best. A percutaneous VAD may be optimal for patients with severe coagulopathy or other surgical contraindications. These devices are most of the time used for up to 14 days and are usually converted to longer-term devices when continued support is indicated. Because the percutaneous devices are commonly intended for left heart support, surgical placement of a CentriMag VAD may be necessary for patients requiring biventricular support. Early assessment of right heart hemodynamics (central venous pressure, pulmonary artery pressures, and right ventricular stroke work index) or echocardiography may provide sufficient evidence for univentricular versus biventricular support. Patients with prolonged cardiogenic shock with end-organ dysfunction, and those with postcardiotomy shock, are best supported by a surgically placed biventricular support system because of its ability to unload both sides of the heart and to provide a greater flow capacity.

The availability of VAD systems may determine the type of support utilized. Most academic medical centers with a full range of heart failure treatments usually have the ability to fit the proper type of VAD to each patient. These major medical centers also have appropriately trained personnel for the different types of devices. Patients with cardiogenic shock often present at nonacademic community medical centers that do not have multiple VAD systems and trained personnel. Collaborative networks between community and academic hospitals with a hub-and-spoke VAD program offer advanced therapy to those who are not near the full-service heart failure programs [25–27]. Transfer of patients in cardiogenic shock to higher levels of care must be done in a timely fashion before end-organ dysfunction becomes irreversible.

Hub-and-spoke VAD networks between community hospitals and academic medical centers need to have dedicated personnel who are in frequent communication. Specialized transport teams with appropriate personnel and technologies have an important role in the successful transfer of patients with cardiogenic shock [28]. The hub hospital or VAD center must have an available specialist to discuss the care and transport of patients and then, be prepared to provide advance care upon receipt of the patient. The spoke hospital or community center must provide prompt inotropic and IABP support or a higher level of circulatory assist to stabilize hemodynamics for preservation of organ function. Importantly, the spoke hospital must rapidly assess comorbidities, patient viability, and financial issues before transporting the patient to another institution [25]. Multiple transfers of patients with low probability of salvage will become a significant financial burden on the hub facility.

Although there are a number of VAD systems that may be used for short-term circulatory support, three of the most recently developed systems are described in Table 8.1. The TandemHeart and Impella devices are used for support of patients with cardiogenic shock and during risk interventional procedures. The CentriMag is a versatile, surgically placed device that is in use in a variety of clinical scenarios.

Table 8.1 Currently available VAD systems for stabilizing patients with severe cardiogenic shock

VAD system	Type of pump	Cannulation	Amount of support (L/min)	Indications
TandemHeart	Centrifugal flow	Percutaneous (femoral) LA transeptal; femoral artery	Up to 5	Cardiogenic shock, CPR and high-risk PCI
Impella 2.5	Axial flow	Percutaneous femoral insertion; cannula tip in LV, pump in ascending aorta	Up to 2.5	High-risk PCI
Impella 5.0	Axial flow	Surgical femoral insertion; cannula tip in LV, pump in ascending aorta	Up to 5.0	Cardiogenic shock and high-risk PCI
CentriMag	Centrifugal flow	Varies; LA or LV to ascending aorta or femoral artery for LVAD. RA to PA for RVAD	Up to 10	Postcardiotomy

LA left atrium, *PCI* percutaneous coronary intervention, *LV* left ventricle, *PA* pulmonary artery, *RVAD* right ventricular assist device

TandemHeart

The TandemHeart system (CardiacAssist, Inc., Pittsburgh, PA) provides circulatory assist by pumping oxygenated blood continuously from the left atrium to the femoral artery (Fig. 8.2). The goal of support is to reduce cardiac work, oxygen demand, and left ventricular filling pressure. The system consists of a transeptal inflow cannula (Fig. 8.3), a centrifugal flow pump (Fig. 8.4), an outflow cannula (Fig. 8.3), and a bedside control console (Fig. 8.5). The pump can generate up to 5 L/min of blood flow with an impeller speed range of 3,000–7,000 rpm. During support, the pump is positioned near the cannulation sites and usually is secured to the anterior right thigh. Cannulation is usually performed in the cardiac catheterization laboratory with fluoroscopic guidance, or echocardiography may be used in other hospital settings.

With properly trained personnel, support with the TandemHeart system can be initiated in less than 30 minutes of arrival to the catheterization laboratory [29]. The unique feature of the TandemHeart system is the placement of the 21-F polyurethane inflow cannula into the left atrium. From a femoral vein, a septal puncture is performed with a Brockenbrough needle passed through a Mullins sheath into the right atrium. A 0.035-inch pigtail guidewire is introduced into the left atrium, and a two-stage (14-F–21-F) dilator is used to expand the opening in the atrial septum. The tip of the inflow cannula is passed over the wire into the left atrium; this cannula then is attached to the inflow connector of the pump. A 15-F or 17-F cannula is placed in the contralateral femoral artery and connected to the outflow connector of the pump. The pump impeller speed is adjusted with the bedside control console to achieve the desired flow rate. The console monitors pump function and provides audio and visual alerts during abnormal conditions. The console also provides a continuous infusion of heparinized saline to the lower portion of the blood chamber in the pump to prevent clot formation.

The TandemHeart system has been used in a variety of clinical scenarios, but the primary use has been for support of patients with cardiogenic shock [30–34] and during high-risk PCI [35–38]. With modified cannulation techniques, the TandemHeart system has been used as an RVAD and can provide biventricular support in profound cardiogenic shock [39]. When used as a right ventricular assist device (RVAD), cannulation of the right atrium and pulmonary artery is accomplished through the right internal jugular and femoral veins [40]. The TandemHeart system has also been used for support during cardiac surgery and for postcardiotomy failure [41–43]. Direct surgical cannulation may also be employed with the use of shorter cannulas and flow rates up to 8 L/min.

The early randomized clinical trials comparing support between the IABP and TandemHeart system have shown that hemodynamic parameters are consistently better with TandemHeart support; however, 30-day mortality rates were

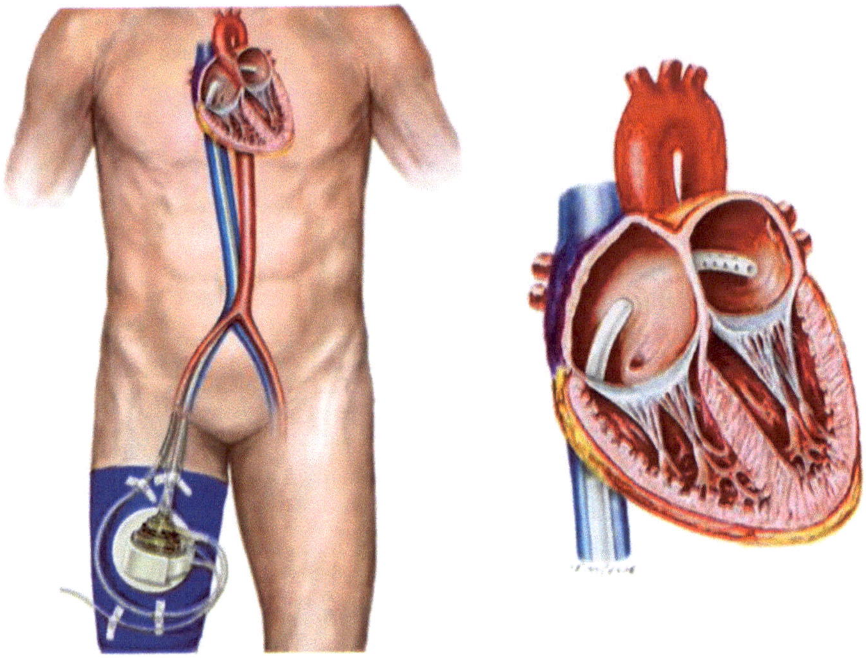

Fig. 8.2 The TandemHeart ventricular assist device (VAD) with view of pump and cannula positioning (*left*) and transeptal inflow cannula tip in the left atrium (*right*)

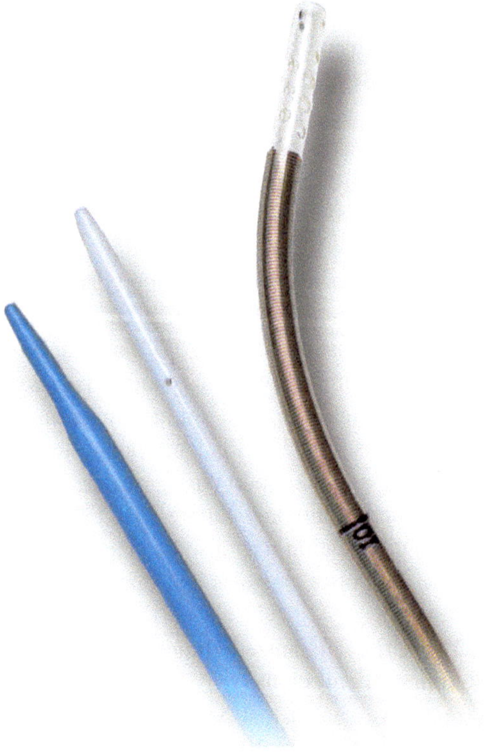

Fig. 8.3 Cannulas for TandemHeart support: transeptal cannula (*right*), femoral outflow cannula (*middle*), and two-stage dilator for dilating the opening in the atrial septum

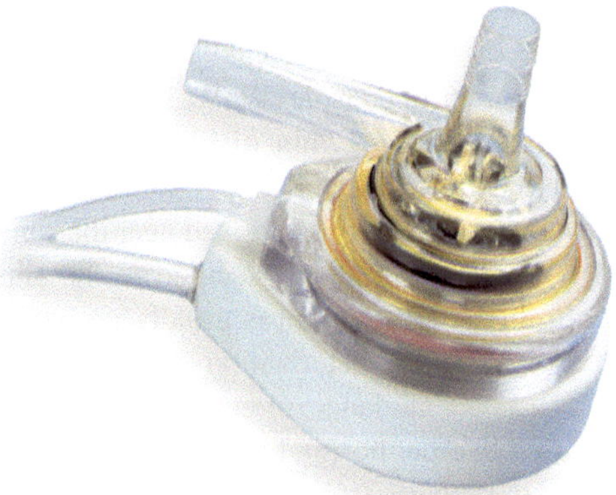

Fig. 8.4 The TandemHeart centrifugal flow blood pump is normally placed on the patient's thigh during support

not different [44, 45]. However, in a recent single-center report of TandemHeart use in 117 patients with severe refractory cardiogenic shock, with nearly 50 % in cardiac arrest and predictive mortality of more than 90 %, improvements in blood pressure, end-organ function, venous oxygen saturation, urine output, and lactic acid levels resulted in a 6-month survival rate of 45 % [46]. In another report involving 22 patients with severe cardiogenic shock supported as a bridge to

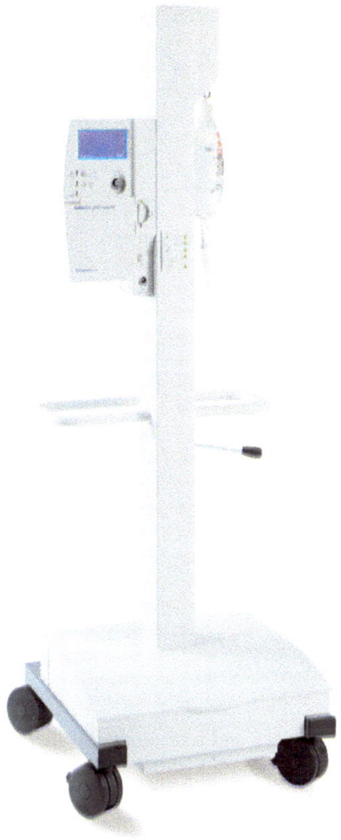

Fig. 8.5 The TandemHeart bedside control console is used to adjust the pump's impeller rotation and to provide a continuous infusion of heparinized glucose solution to the pump

decision, 34 % survived and underwent device explant, transplant, or implantation of a long-term LVAD [47]. The time from the onset of cardiogenic shock to the initiation of support appears to be an important factor in determining outcome. Patients with cardiogenic shock who are successfully stabilized have therapeutic options that may result in long-term survival. Few patients will recover myocardial function without revascularization or corrective surgery. After a period of support and following more definitive therapy, some patients may continue to have good organ function, but poor cardiac function may be suitable for long-term LVAD support [32, 47, 48]. Prolonged TandemHeart support or conversion to an implantable LVAD or BiVAD may be necessary in cases of acute fulminate myocarditis or peripartum cardiomyopathy [49, 50].

Device-related complications, including bleeding from the cannula insertion site, persistent patent foramen ovale, limb ischemia, and thromboembolism, are observed, but these risks do not preclude the use of the TandemHeart system in a population of patients who are facing imminent death [41]. Persistent patent foramen ovale following inflow cannula removal has not been a significant complication [36, 44]. The TandemHeart is the best percutaneous MCS device in cases of ventricular septal defect (VSD) despite the potential for a left to right shunt. Since the inlet cannula is in the left atrium, the blood is aspirated into the cannula prior to reaching the left ventricle and thus avoiding the RV unsaturated blood to be mixed across the VSD. The TandemHeart is contraindicated in patients with severe peripheral vascular disease that prevents cannulation of the femoral vessels [51]. Because the inflow cannula is passed through the inferior vena cava and right atrium, use of this device is contraindicated with the presence of a caval filter. Bleeding from the cannula insertion site results from the requirement to anticoagulate patients during support. Patients are confined to bed and require sedation to prevent dislodgement of the inflow cannula into the right atrium.

Impella

The Impella system (ABIOMED Inc., Danvers, MA) is a catheter-mounted continuous-flow pump and cannula that aspirates blood from the left ventricle into the ascending aorta. A small axial-flow blood pump mounted on the end of a catheter is positioned in the ascending aorta, with its cannula placed across the aortic valve and the tip within the left ventricular cavity. The amount of flow through the pump is determined by the rotor speed, preload (left ventricular pressure), and afterload (aortic pressure). There are two versions of the Impella device; the 2.5 and the 5.0, which are designations indicating the pump's maximum flow rate. The 2.5 version has a 12-F diameter cannula and is inserted percutaneously from the femoral artery (Fig. 8.6). The Impella 5.0 device has a 21-F diameter cannula with versions for femoral insertion (Fig. 8.7) or insertion directly into the ascending aorta through a sternotomy (Fig. 8.8).

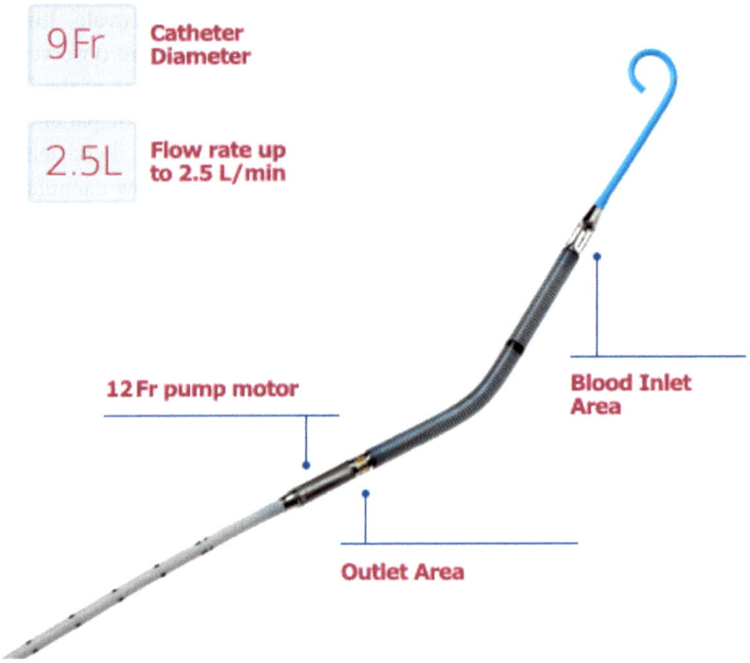

Fig. 8.6 The Impella 2.5 cannula is inserted over a wire via the femoral artery and retrograde through the aorta and across the aortic valve. The blood inlet is within the left ventricle, and the pump outlet is in the ascending aorta

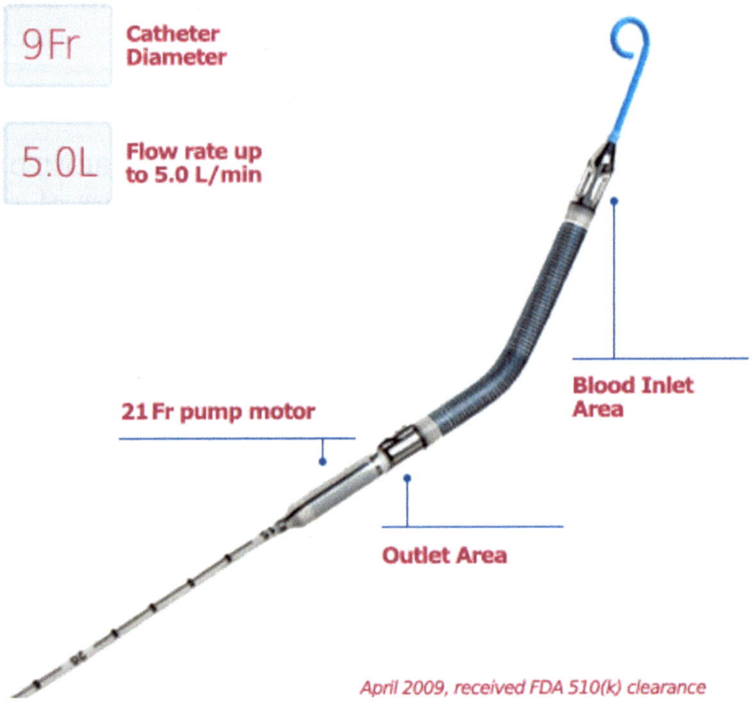

Fig. 8.7 The Impella 5.0 cannula is inserted over a wire via the femoral artery and retrograde through the aorta and across the aortic valve. The blood inlet is within the left ventricle, and the pump outlet is in the ascending aorta

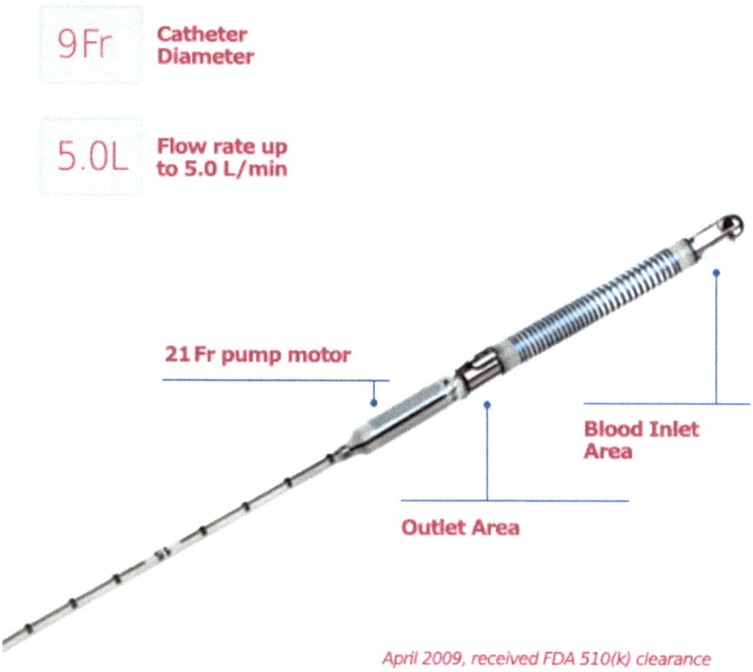

Fig. 8.8 The Impella 5.0 direct (LD) version is inserted through a graft on the ascending aorta with the tip within the left ventricle and the pump in the ascending aorta

Insertion of the Impella 2.5 percutaneous device is normally performed in a cardiac catheterization laboratory with fluoroscopic guidance. This device is used for support of patients with cardiogenic shock or during high-risk PCI. The Impella 2.5 device is inserted percutaneously via the femoral artery through a 13-F sheath. Then a guidewire is passed through the aorta and into the left ventricle, followed by insertion of the pump over the wire until the J-tipped portion enters the left ventricle. Proper placement of the pump is also guided by observation of the pressure waveform, which is detected in the cannula near the pump. The dual-pressure sensor detects the pressure within the cannula and on the outer surface of the cannula. When the cannula crosses the aortic valve, the diastolic pressure within the cannula decreases greatly, indicating entry into the left ventricle, whereas the pressure on the outer portion of the cannula continues to record aortic pressure. Before insertion, the catheter is connected to a bedside console for monitoring and control of the pump speed. A seal within the pump must be continuously purged with a solution of glucose and heparin to prevent clot formation. The bedside console is battery operated for patient transport. Patients must remain supine during support due to the presence of the catheter in the femoral artery.

The Impella 5.0 LD is used intraoperatively to support patients during beating-heart surgery or for postcardiotomy cardiogenic shock. The 21-Fr device is inserted through a graft anastomosed end to side on the ascending aorta. The cannula crosses the aortic valve with the pump just above the valve. If this technique is employed for post-operative support, reoperation is necessary to remove the device and the graft on the aorta.

The Impella 2.5 device has been used for short-term support of patients with cardiogenic shock and during high-risk PCI. Contraindications for the use of this device include the presence of a mechanical aortic valve, severe peripheral vascular disease, and severely calcified aortic valve. Hemodynamic indications for use are a cardiac index <2.0 L/min/m^2, arterial blood pressure <90 mmHg and a pulmonary capillary wedge pressure >18 mmHg, and heart failure that is potentially reversible. There are numerous reports of successful support in patients with postcardiotomy low-cardiac output [52–55], myocardial infarction with cardiogenic shock [33, 56–59], acute myocarditis [60, 61], and severe allograft rejection [62, 63]. The Impella device has been used also to stabilize patients with decompensated chronic heart failure who then undergo heart transplant or implantation of a long-term LVAD [33]. In randomized controlled trials, comparison of the Impella 2.5 and the IABP in patients with cardiogenic shock has shown that the Impella device provides better hemodynamics during support, but there is no difference in 30-day mortality [64]. Support during high-risk PCI is safe and provides adequate hemodynamic support, but superiority over IABP support has not been demonstrated in a randomized trial [65]. Since the Impella 2.5 device provides the maximal flow of 2.5 L/min, it has little benefit for patients in severe refractory cardiogenic shock.

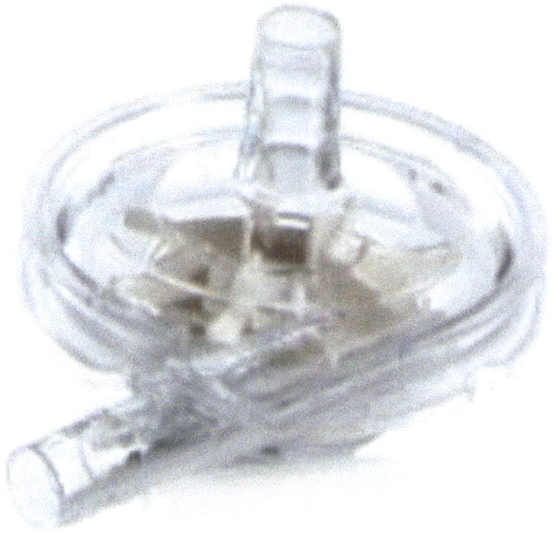

Fig. 8.9 The CentriMag blood pump has a polycarbonate housing with a rotating impeller that is suspended and rotated by magnetic force (Image courtesy of Thoratec Corporation)

CentriMag

The CentriMag Blood Pumping System (Levitronix, Waltham, MA) utilizes a centrifugal flow pump with a magnetically levitated impeller (Fig. 8.9). The impeller is raised away from the pump housing and rotates by magnetic force generated by the motor. This type of impeller rotation improves biocompatibility by eliminating heat from friction, and there is no wear of the moving components. The CentriMag system comprises the pump, an electromagnetic motor, an ultrasonic flow probe, and an external control console. The 3/8-inch diameter inlet and outlet connections accommodate use of standard perfusion tubing. The surgeon determines the cannulas appropriate for the type of support and vessel size. This system is implanted surgically through a sternotomy but also has been adapted for percutaneous use with an oxygenator [66]. Surgical cannulation for univentricular or biventricular support is accomplished with inflow cannulas placed in the left and right atria and with the outflow cannulas placed in the ascending aorta and main pulmonary artery (Fig. 8.10). The maximum flow rate generated by the CentriMag device is 10 L/min at an impeller speed of 5,500 rpm. Blood flow rate is determined using an ultrasonic flow probe attached to the tubing near the pump. The external control console provides a display of impeller speed and pump flow rate and provides audible and visual alerts for abnormal conditions (Fig. 8.11). The control console can be battery operated to provide uninterrupted support during patient transport. Unlike the VAD system with femoral cannula placement, the cannulas used with the CentriMag system may be externalized through the chest or abdominal wall and fixated to allow patient mobility [67, 68].

The CentriMag system is versatile and can be used in numerous clinical scenarios of cardiogenic shock. It can provide univentricular or biventricular support, and it has been used for cardiopulmonary bypass and ECMO [66]. The flow rate range of 0–10 L/min allows its use in children and large adults [69, 70]. The CentriMag system may be used for temporary right ventricular support following LVAD implantation, or in rare cases of isolated right heart failure [71]. An evolving and increasing application of the CentriMag system is used as a bridge to decision for patients whose viability is questionable, and

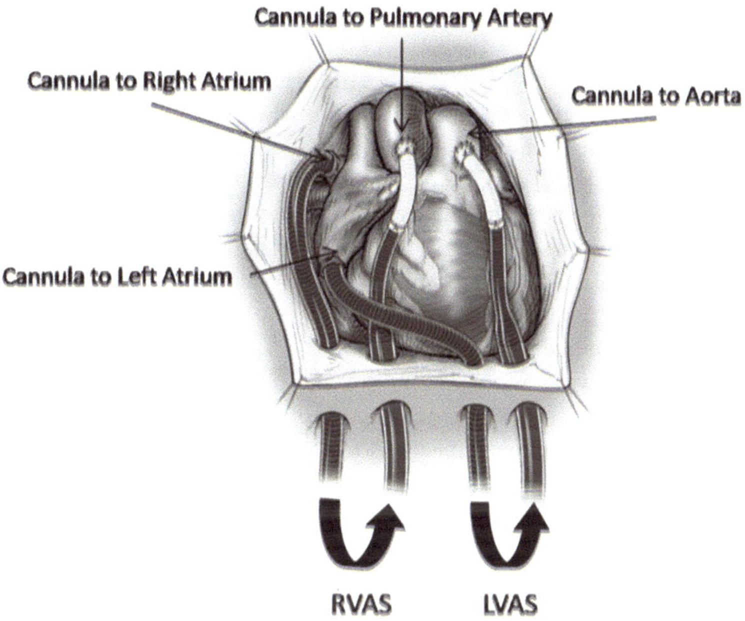

Fig. 8.10 The usual cannulation for biventricular assist with the CentriMag device. For left ventricular assist, the inflow cannula is placed in the left atrium, with the outflow cannula in the ascending aorta. For right ventricular assist, the inflow cannula is placed in the right atrium, and the outflow cannula is in the main pulmonary artery (Image courtesy of Thoratec Corporation)

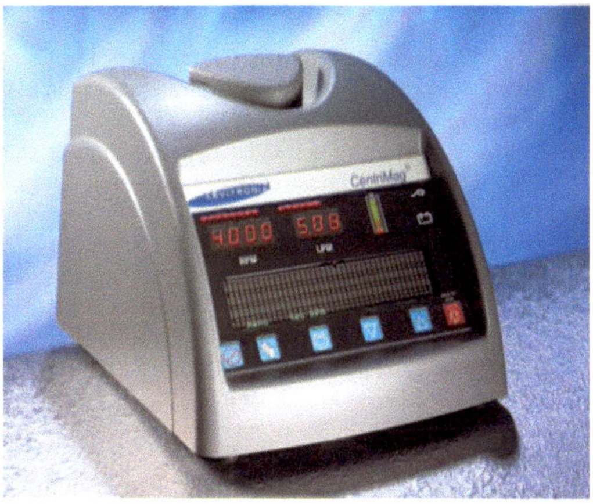

Fig. 8.11 The bedside CentriMag control console displays pump flow and impeller speed and provides audible and visual alerts for abnormal conditions (Image courtesy of Thoratec Corporation)

time is needed to stabilize and assess further treatment options [69, 72–75].

In a multicenter clinical trial evaluating the safety and effectiveness of CentriMag support, 38 patients with cardiogenic shock following myocardial infarction, cardiotomy, and RVAD support following LVAD implant were supported for a mean duration of 13 days (range 1–60 days) with no device failures and a low incidence of device-related complications [76]. In this study, the overall 30-day survival rate was 47 %. When used as a bridge to decision for patients in cardiogenic shock with multiple organ dysfunction and questionable neurologic function following myocardial infarction, most patients are bridged to a long-term implantable LVAD, few tolerate weaning of support, and support is terminated in those with irreversible neurologic function [75]. Extended support (many weeks) may be necessary for patients with cardiogenic shock and organ failure secondary to acutely decompensated chronic heart failure to determine their suitability for heart transplant or long-term LVAD implantation [73]. The most frequent complication during CentriMag support is bleeding, which is secondary to anticoagulation requirements and the need for open chest surgery. Hemolysis has been minimal, and infection occurs in patients with prolonged support.

Comments

Although progress has been made in treatment of acute heart failure and coronary artery disease, outcomes of cardiogenic shock remain poor. Earlier randomized trials of the newer percutaneous cardiac support devices versus the IABP have not shown that higher levels of cardiac output support are having a substantial impact on short-term outcomes. However, the number of patients enrolled in those early trials was low and did not include patients in severe refractory cardiogenic shock, a population where the positive impact of modern percutaneous cardiac support devices has been demonstrated.

The variable of time from the onset of shock to the restoration of adequate systemic perfusion is crucial. The major advantage of the IABP is the ease of insertion and the short time it takes to provide support. The IABP can be inserted in multiple hospital environments, such as the emergency department, intensive care unit, and operating room. The TandemHeart and Impella devices can be inserted rapidly but require fluoroscopic guidance in special facilities as well as specially trained personnel, both of which are not yet widely available in the majority of hospitals where patients with cardiogenic shock present.

The versatility of the CentriMag, Impella, and TandemHeart devices offers the potential to provide prompt and full circulatory support, and it can be applied at the bedside, emergency department, and catheterization laboratory using percutaneous cannulation techniques. Furthermore, these devices are beginning to be used also at community hospitals to rapidly stabilize patients before transport to hospitals with full-service heart failure programs.

The TandemHeart, Impella, and CentriMag short-term VADs are all commercially approved for use for up to 6 h. Because of the diverse clinical presentations of cardiogenic shock and numerous patient variables, these devices have been adapted in different ways in an attempt to meet individual patient needs. The ideal or universal VAD system for treating all forms of heart failure does not exist. MCS technology for acute heart failure has progressed in recent years, but further advances are needed to improve mortality of cardiogenic shock. Blood pumps are capable of providing adequate levels of flow, with limitations mainly in vascular access and highly trained personnel. Continued research and development is needed to improve rapid vascular access along with training on device use and education in patient management.

References

1. Gheorghiade MZF, Sopko G, Klein L, Pina IL, Konstam M, Massie BM, et al. Acute heart failure syndromes: current state and framework for future research. Circulation. 2005;112:3958–68.
2. Reynolds HR, Hochman JS. Cardiogenic shock: current concepts and improving outcomes. Circulation. 2008;117:686–97.
3. Pulido JN, Park SJ, Rihal CS. Percutaneous left ventricular assist devices: clinical uses, future applications, and anesthetic considerations. J Cardiothorac Vasc Anesth. 2010;24:478–86.
4. Babaev A, Frederick PD, Pasta DJ, Every N, Sichrovsky T, Hochman JS. Trends in management and outcomes of patients with acute myocardial infarction complicated by cardiogenic shock. JAMA. 2005;294:448–54.
5. Hall CW, Liotta D, Henly WS, Crawford ES, Debakery ME. Development of artificial intrathoracic circulatory pumps. Am J Surg. 1964;108:685–92.
6. DeBakey ME. Left ventricular bypass pump for cardiac assistance. Clinical experience. Am J Cardiol. 1971;27:3–11.
7. Cooley DA, Liotta D, Hallman GL, Bloodwell RD, Leachman RD, Milam JD. Orthotopic cardiac prosthesis for two-staged cardiac replacement. Am J Cardiol. 1969;24:723–30.
8. Kantrowitz A, Tjonneland S, Freed PS, Phillips SJ, Butner AN, Sherman Jr JL. Initial clinical experience with intra-aortic balloon pumping in cardiogenic shock. JAMA. 1968;203:113–8.
9. Kantrowitz A, Tjonneland S, Krakauer JS, Phillips SJ, Freed PS, Butner AN. Mechanical intra-aortic cardiac assistance in cardiogenic shock. Hemodynamic effects. Arch Surg. 1968;97:1000–4.
10. Butler KC, Moise JC, Wampler RK. The Hemopump–a new cardiac prothesis device. IEEE Trans Biomed Eng. 1990;37:193–6.
11. Wampler RK, Baker BA, Wright WM. Circulatory support of cardiac interventional procedures with the Hemopump cardiac assist system. Cardiology. 1994; 84:194–201.
12. Scholz KH, Figulla HR, Schweda F, Smalling RW, Hellige G, Kreuzer H, et al. Mechanical left ventricular unloading during high risk coronary angioplasty: first

use of a new percutaneous transvalvular left ventricular assist device. Cathet Cardiovasc Diagn. 1994;31: 61–9.
13. Wampler RK, Frazier OH, Lansing AM, Smalling RW, Nicklas JM, Phillips SJ, et al. Treatment of cardiogenic shock with the Hemopump left ventricular assist device. Ann Thorac Surg. 1991;52:506–13.
14. Pennington DG. Artificial heart/circulatory assist gas exchange/ECMO. Trans Am Soc Artif Intern Organs. 1983;29:4–5.
15. Weber TR, Pennington DG, Connors R, Kennan W, Kotagal S, Braun P, et al. Extracorporeal membrane oxygenation for newborn respiratory failure. Ann Thorac Surg. 1986;42:529–35.
16. El-Banayosy A, Posival H, Minami K, Kizner L, Breymann T, Seifert D, et al. Seven years of experience with the centrifugal pump in patients with cardiogenic shock. Thorac Cardiovasc Surg. 1995;43:347–51.
17. Noon GP, Lafuente JA, Irwin S. Acute and temporary ventricular support with Biomedicus centrifugal pump. Ann Thorac Surg. 1999;68:650–4.
18. Willms DC, Atkins PJ, Dembitsky WP, Jaski BE, Gocka I. Analysis of clinical trends in a program of emergent ECLS for cardiovascular collapse. ASAIO J. 1997;43:65–8.
19. Orime Y, Shiono M, Hata H, Yagi S, Tsukamoto S, Okumura H, et al. Clinical experiences of percutaneous cardiopulmonary support: its effectiveness and limit. Artif Organs. 1998;22:498–501.
20. Farkouh ME, Ramanathan K, Aymong ED, Webb JG, Harkness SM, Sleeper LA, et al. An early revascularization strategy is associated with a survival benefit for diabetic patients in cardiogenic shock after acute myocardial infarction. Clin Cardiol. 2006;29:204–10.
21. Gevaert S, Van Belleghem Y, Bouchez S, Herck I, De Somer F, De Block Y, et al. Acute and critically ill peripartum cardiomyopathy and 'bridge to' therapeutic options: a single-center experience with intra-aortic balloon pump, extra corporeal membrane oxygenation and continuous-flow left ventricular assist devices. Crit Care. 2011;15:R93.
22. Oosterom L, de Jonge N, Kirkels J, Klopping C, Lahpor J. Left ventricular assist device as a bridge to recovery in a young woman admitted with peripartum cardiomyopathy. Netherlands Heart J. 2008;16: 426–8.
23. Tandler R, Schmid C, Weyand M, Scheld HH. Novacor LVAD bridge to transplantation in peripartum cardiomyopathy. Eur J Cardiothorac Surg. 1997;11:394–6.
24. Farrar DJ, Holman WR, McBride LR, Kormos RL, Icenogle TB, Hendry PJ, et al. Long-term follow-up of Thoratec ventricular assist device bridge-to-recovery patients successfully removed from support after recovery of ventricular function. J Heart Lung Transplant. 2002;21:516–21.
25. Gonzalez-Stawinski GV, Chang AS, Navia JL, Banbury MK, Buda T, Hoercher K, et al. Regional referral system for patients with acute mechanical support: experience at the Cleveland Clinic Foundation. ASAIO J. 2006;52:445–9.
26. Guirgis M, Kumar K, Zieroth S, Philipp R, Menkis AH, Freed DH. Interprovincial spoke-to-hub transport using the Impella Recover LP 5.0 left ventricular assist device as a bridge to long-term circulatory support. Can J Cardiol. 2010;26:320–2.
27. Griffith KE, Jenkins E. A biomed Impella(R) 2.5 patient transport: lessons learned. Perfusion. 2010;25:381–6.
28. Jaroszewski DE, Kleisli T, Staley L, Pierce C, Scott R, Steidley DE, et al. A traveling team concept to expedite the transfer and management of unstable patients in cardiopulmonary shock. J Heart Lung Transplant. 2011;30:618–23.
29. Kar B, Adkins LE, Civitello AB, Loyalka P, Palanichamy N, Gemmato CJ, et al. Clinical experience with the TandemHeart percutaneous ventricular assist device. Tex Heart Inst J. 2006;33:111–5.
30. Gregoric ID, Loyalka P, Radovancevic R, Jovic Z, Frazier OH, Kar B. TandemHeart as a rescue therapy for patients with critical aortic valve stenosis. Ann Thorac Surg. 2009;88:1822–6.
31. Solomon H, Lim DS, Ragosta M. Percutaneous ventricular assist device to rescue a patient with profound shock from a thrombosed prosthetic mitral valve. J Invasive Cardiol. 2008;20:E320–3.
32. Bruckner BA, Jacob LP, Gregoric ID, Loyalka P, Kar B, Cohn WE, et al. Clinical experience with the TandemHeart percutaneous ventricular assist device as a bridge to cardiac transplantation. Tex Heart Inst J. 2008;35:447–50.
33. Windecker S. Percutaneous left ventricular assist devices for treatment of patients with cardiogenic shock. Curr Opin Crit Care. 2007;13:521–7.
34. Burkhoff D, O'Neill W, Brunckhorst C, Letts D, Lasorda D, Cohen HA. Feasibility study of the use of the TandemHeart percutaneous ventricular assist device for treatment of cardiogenic shock. Catheter Cardiovasc Interv. 2006;68:211–7.
35. Aragon J, Lee MS, Kar S, Makkar RR. Percutaneous left ventricular assist device: " TandemHeart" for high-risk coronary intervention. Catheter Cardiovasc Interv. 2005;65:346–52.
36. Kar B, Forrester M, Gemmato C, Civitello A, Loyalka P, Myers T, et al. Use of the TandemHeart percutaneous ventricular assist device to support patients undergoing high-risk percutaneous coronary intervention. J Invasive Cardiol. 2006;18:93–6.
37. Vranckx P, Schultz CJ, Valgimigli M, Eindhoven JA, Kappetein AP, Regar ES, et al. Assisted circulation using the TandemHeart during very high-risk PCI of the unprotected left main coronary artery in patients declined for CABG. Catheter Cardiovasc Interv. 2009;74:302–10.
38. Vranckx P, Foley DP, de Feijter PJ, Vos J, Smits P, Serruys PW. Clinical introduction of the TandemHeart, a percutaneous left ventricular assist device, for circulatory support during high-risk percutaneous coronary intervention. Int J Cardiovasc Interv. 2003;5:35–9.
39. Kiernan MS, Krishnamurthy B, Kapur NK. Percutaneous right ventricular assist via the internal jugular vein in cardiogenic shock complicating an

acute inferior myocardial infarction. J Invasive Cardiol. 2010;22:E23–6.
40. Goldstein D, Neragi-Miandoab S. Mechanical bridge to decision: what are the options for the management of acute refractory cardiogenic shock? Curr Heart Fail Rep. 2011;8:51–8.
41. Gregoric ID, Bruckner BA, Jacob L, Loyalka P, Kar B, La Francesca S, et al. Techniques and complications of TandemHeart ventricular assist device insertion during cardiac procedures. ASAIO J. 2009;55:251–4.
42. Pitsis AA, Visouli AN, Burkhoff D, Dardas P, Mezilis N, Bougioukas G, et al. Feasibility study of a temporary percutaneous left ventricular assist device in cardiac surgery. Ann Thorac Surg. 2007;84:1993–9.
43. Cohn WE, Morris CD, Reverdin S, Frazier OH, Gregoric ID. Intraoperative TandemHeart implantation as an adjunct to high-risk valve surgery. Tex Heart Inst J. 2007;34:457–8.
44. Thiele H, Sick P, Boudriot E, Diederich KW, Hambrecht R, Niebauer J, et al. Randomized comparison of intra-aortic balloon support with a percutaneous left ventricular assist device in patients with revascularized acute myocardial infarction complicated by cardiogenic shock. Eur Heart J. 2005;26: 1276–83.
45. Burkhoff D, Cohen H, Brunckhorst C, O'Neill WW, TandemHeart Investigators G. A randomized multicenter clinical study to evaluate the safety and efficacy of the TandemHeart percutaneous ventricular assist device versus conventional therapy with intra-aortic balloon pumping for treatment of cardiogenic shock. Am Heart J. 2006;152:E461–8.
46. Kar B, Gregoric ID, Basra SS, Idelchik GM, Loyalka P. The percutaneous ventricular assist device in severe refractory cardiogenic shock. J Am Coll Cardiol. 2011;57:688–96.
47. Brinkman WT, Rosenthal JE, Eichhorn E, Dewey TM, Magee MJ, Savor DS, et al. Role of a percutaneous ventricular assist device in decision making for a cardiac transplant program. Ann Thorac Surg. 2009;88:1462–6.
48. Reverdin S, Gregoric ID, Kar B, Loyalka P, Bieniarz MC, LeMaire SA, et al. Bridge to transplantation with the TandemHeart: bending the indications in a chronic aortic dissection patient with postcardiotomy shock. Tex Heart Inst J. 2008;35:340–1.
49. Khalife WI, Kar B. The TandemHeart pVAD in the treatment of acute fulminant myocarditis. Tex Heart Inst J. 2007;34:209–13.
50. Chandra D, Kar B, Idelchik G, Simpson L, Loyalka P, Gregoric ID, et al. Usefulness of percutaneous left ventricular assist device as a bridge to recovery from myocarditis. Am J Cardiol. 2007;99:1755–6.
51. Lee MS, Makkar RR. Percutaneous left ventricular support devices. Cardiol Clin. 2006;24:265–75.
52. Granfeldt H, Hellgren L, Dellgren G, Myrdal G, Wassberg E, Kjellman U, et al. Experience with the Impella recovery axial-flow system for acute heart failure at three cardiothoracic centers in Sweden. Scand Cardiovasc J. 2009;43:233–9.
53. Lauten A, Franke U, Strauch JT, Kaluza M, Wahlers T. Postocardiotomy failure after ross operation: implantation of intravascular flow pump through pulmonary autograft. Thorac Cardiovasc Surg. 2007;55: 399–400.
54. Siegenthaler MP, Brehm K, Strecker T, Hanke T, Notzold A, Olschewski M, et al. The Impella Recover microaxial left ventricular assist device reduces mortality for postcardiotomy failure: a three-center experience. J Thorac Cardiovasc Surg. 2004;127:812–22.
55. Jurmann MJ, Siniawski H, Erb M, Drews T, Hetzer R. Initial experience with miniature axial flow ventricular assist devices for postcardiotomy heart failure. Ann Thorac Surg. 2004;77:1642–7.
56. Patane F, Centofanti P, Zingarelli E, Sansone F, La Torre M. Potential role of the Impella Recover left ventricular assist device in the management of postinfarct ventricular septal defect. J Thorac Cardiovasc Surg. 2009;137:1288–9.
57. Gupta A, Allaqaband S, Bajwa T. Combined use of Impella device and intra-aortic balloon pump to improve survival in a patient in profound cardiogenic shock post cardiac arrest. Catheter Cardiovasc Interv. 2009;74:975–6.
58. Cheng JM, den Uil CA, Hoeks SE, van der Ent M, Jewbali LS, van Domburg RT, et al. Percutaneous left ventricular assist devices vs. intra-aortic balloon pump counterpulsation for treatment of cardiogenic shock: a meta-analysis of controlled trials. Eur Heart J. 2009;30:2102–8.
59. Meyns B, Stolinski J, Leunens V, Verbeken E, Flameng W. Left ventricular support by catheter-mounted axial flow pump reduces infarct size. J Am Coll Cardiol. 2003;41:1087–95.
60. Garatti A, Colombo T, Russo C, Lanfranconi M, Milazzo F, Catena E, et al. Different applications for left ventricular mechanical support with the Impella Recover 100 microaxial blood pump. J Heart Lung Transplant. 2005;24:481–5.
61. Colombo T, Garatti A, Bruschi G, Lanfranconi M, Russo C, Milazzo F, et al. First successful bridge to recovery with the Impella Recover 100 left ventricular assist device for fulminant acute myocarditis. Ital Heart J. 2003;4:642–5.
62. Rajagopal V, Steahr G, Wilmer CI, Raval NY. A novel percutaneous mechanical biventricular bridge to recovery in severe cardiac allograft rejection. J Heart Lung Transplant. 2010;29:93–5.
63. Beyer AT, Hui PY, Hauesslein E. The Impella 2.5 L for percutaneous mechanical circulatory support in severe humoral allograft rejection. J Invasive Cardiol. 2010;22:E37–9.
64. Seyfarth M, Sibbing D, Bauer I, Frohlich G, Bott-Flugel L, Byrne R, et al. A randomized clinical trial to evaluate the safety and efficacy of a percutaneous left ventricular assist device versus intra-aortic balloon pumping for treatment of cardiogenic shock caused by myocardial infarction. J Am Coll Cardiol. 2008;52:1584–8.
65. Dixon SR, Henriques JP, Mauri L, Sjauw K, Civitello A, Kar B. A prospective feasibility trial investigating

the use of the Impella 2.5 system in patients undergoing high-risk percutaneous coronary intervention (The PROTECT I Trial): initial U.S. experience. JACC Cardiovasc Interv. 2009;2:91–6.
66. Aziz TA, Singh G, Popjes E, Stephenson E, Mulvey S, Pae W, et al. Initial experience with CentriMag extracorporal membrane oxygenation for support of critically ill patients with refractory cardiogenic shock. J Heart Lung Transplant. 2010;29:66–71.
67. Takayama H, Chen JM, Jorde UP, Naka Y. Implantation technique of the CentriMag biventricular assist device allowing ambulatory rehabilitation. Interact Cardiovasc Thorac Surg. 2011;12:110–1.
68. Gregoric ID, Cohn WE, Akay MH, La Francesca S, Myers T, Frazier OH. CentriMag left ventricular assist system: cannulation through a right minithoracotomy. Tex Heart Inst J. 2008;35:184–5.
69. Kouretas PC, Kaza AK, Burch PT, Witte MK, Clayson SE, Everitt MD, et al. Experience with the Levitronix CentriMag in the pediatric population as a bridge to decision and recovery. Artif Organs. 2009;33:1002–4.
70. Hirata Y, Charette K, Mosca RS, Quaegebeur JM, Chen JM. Pediatric application of the Thoratec CentriMag BiVAD as a bridge to heart transplantation. J Thorac Cardiovasc Surg. 2008;136:1386–7.
71. Loforte A, Montalto A, Lilla Della Monica P, Musumeci F. Simultaneous temporary CentriMag right ventricular assist device placement in HeartMate II left ventricular assist system recipients at high risk of right ventricular failure. Interact Cardiovasc Thorac Surg. 2010;10:847–50.
72. Ziemba EA, John R. Mechanical circulatory support for bridge to decision: which device and when to decide. J Card Surg. 2010;25:425–33.
73. Haj-Yahia S, Birks EJ, Amrani M, Petrou M, Bahrami T, Dreyfus G, et al. Bridging patients after salvage from bridge to decision directly to transplant by means of prolonged support with the CentriMag short-term centrifugal pump. J Thorac Cardiovasc Surg. 2009;138:227–30.
74. De Robertis F, Rogers P, Amrani M, Petrou M, Pepper JR, Bahrami T, et al. Bridge to decision using the Levitronix CentriMag short-term ventricular assist device. J Heart Lung Transplant. 2008;27:474–8.
75. John R, Liao K, Lietz K, Kamdar F, Colvin-Adams M, Boyle A, et al. Experience with the Levitronix CentriMag circulatory support system as a bridge to decision in patients with refractory acute cardiogenic shock and multisystem organ failure. J Thorac Cardiovasc Surg. 2007;134:351–8.
76. John R, Long JW, Massey HT, Griffith BP, Sun BC, Tector AJ, et al. Outcomes of a multicenter trial of the Levitronix CentriMag ventricular assist system for short-term circulatory support. J Thorac Cardiovasc Surg. 2010;141:932–9.

Cardiac Transplantation

9

Lucian Lozonschi, Carter T. Smith, and Niloo M. Edwards

Introduction

Heart transplantation has progressed significantly in the 50 years since Lower and Shumway described the technical aspects of the procedure [1]. The progress was though mostly in the perioperative management of donors and recipients and long-term management of the heart transplant patients. Improvements in immunosuppression and postoperative management have led to increasing survival rates and declining complications [2, 3]. The surgical technique progressed in its complexity from the relatively easier biatrial technique to bicaval and to a total orthotopic technique. The latter technique includes a bicaval technique and separate anastomoses for the right and left pulmonary veins. As of 2007, according to the United Network for Organ Sharing (UNOS) database, the standard, biatrial technique was performed in 34.7 % of transplants in the USA, while 62 % underwent bicaval anastomosis [4]. Compared to biatrial and total orthotopic techniques, the use of bicaval technique continues to be used increasingly with improvements in posttransplant survival, atrial geometry, and hemodynamics, as well as decreased valvular insufficiency, arrhythmias, pacing requirements, vasopressor requirements, and hospital stay [5]. We describe in this chapter the bicaval technique as performed at our institution. An orientation figure is shown in each photograph to illustrate patient orientation.

Donor Management and Cardiectomy

In order to achieve a short ischemic time, the coordination between the recipient and donor teams is vital [6]. The surgeon on the donor team should verify (1) the ABO type of the donor and recipient, (2) consent for donation, and (3) a death note. He should take time to review the angiogram and echo. Donor-transmitted coronary atherosclerosis may decrease the 30-day mortality and may be missed without angiographic evaluation [7]. We routinely obtain coronary angiograms on donors over the age of 35 and in those with multiple risk factors for coronary artery disease.

When cardiac donation is undertaken, there is often simultaneous recovery of other organs including the lungs. This presents an additional challenge to the cardiac recovery team. Care must be taken to preserve adequate left atrial tissue while ensuring adequate lengths of pulmonary veins is supplied to the lung recovery team [8].

A median sternotomy and laparotomy are made to give adequate exposure for all surgical

L. Lozonschi, M.D. (✉) • C.T. Smith, M.D.
N.M. Edwards, M.D.
Department of Cardiothoracic Surgery,
University of Wisconsin School of Medicine Hospitals,
H4/348 CSC, 600 Highland Avenue, Madison,
WI 53792, USA
e-mail: lozonschi@surgery.wisc.edu;
CSmith4@uwhealth.org; edwards@surgery.wisc.edu

J.A. Morgan and Y. Naka (eds.), *Surgical Treatment for Advanced Heart Failure*,
DOI 10.1007/978-1-4614-6919-3_9, © Springer Science+Business Media New York 2013

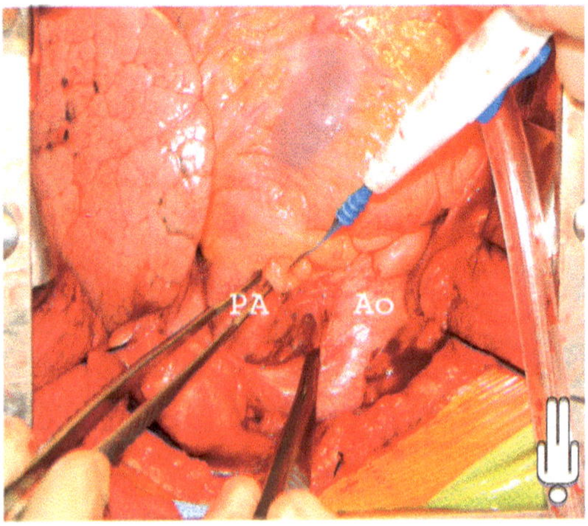

Fig. 9.1 After opening of the pericardium, the aorta and pulmonary artery are isolated and dissected in preparation for division

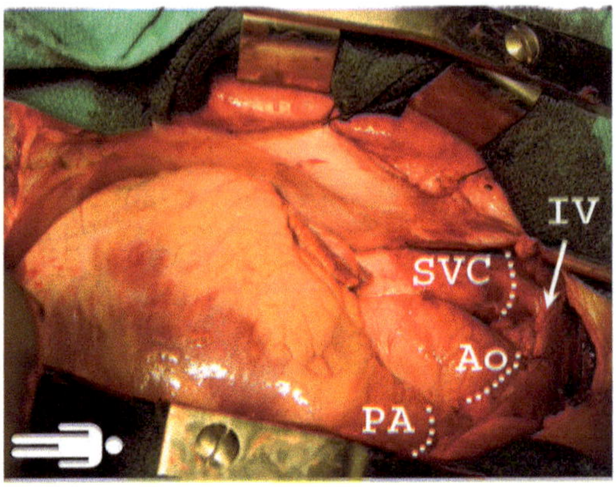

Fig. 9.2 The superior vena cava, pulmonary artery, and aorta shown after their dissection is complete

teams. Examination of the heart prior to cardiectomy should include the coronary arteries by inspection and palpation for evidence of plaques. Care should also be taken to examine the aorta, pulmonary artery (PA), and left atrium (LA) for palpable thrills as well as inspection of the entire heart for contusions [9].

Electrocautery and blunt dissection is used to isolate the aorta and the PA to the level of the arch and bifurcation as seen in Fig. 9.1. Dissection of the superior vena cava (SVC) is carried to the level of or even above the innominate vein. This will assure adequate length of SVC for the redo-sternotomy recipients. Special attention should be paid to the azygous vein ligation to ensure the tie remains with the donor heart. The SVC is dissected free from the right pulmonary artery. Prepare to tie or occlude the SVC with a straight Debakey clamp at the origin of innominate vein. We do not find the need to dissect the pericardial reflection of the inferior vena cava (IVC) at all since this allows an overly eager abdominal surgeon to pull excessively from the intra-abdominal part of IVC. This is prevented by leaving the pericardial reflection on the IVC intact. The cardioplegia needle and its tourniquet are placed in the standard fashion, and we ensure that this will be kept for de-airing during the implantation procedure in the recipient.

Figure 9.2 shows the lines of transaction for the SVC, PA, and aorta. Heparin is administered at 300–400 IU/Kg following the dissection of the abdominal organs [9]. It is important to perform a short briefing session with the recovery teams present in order to avoid any misunderstanding before the initiation of the terminal recovery event and organs perfusion. If the lungs are also being procured, prostaglandin E1 is delivered at this time in the mid-pulmonary artery to reduce vasoconstriction caused by high-potassium concentration, although the efficacy of this remains controversial [10]. As hypotension ensues following the administration of prostaglandin, the inflow is eliminated by clamping the SVC and incising the anterior wall of IVC to allow free flow of the cardioplegia solution. If lungs are recovered, we place a clamp across the LA appendage and amputate it prior to application of cross-clamp. It is essential to make sure to make a large enough egress to allow free flow of the pulmoplegia and prevent LV distention. If the lungs are not recovered, transaction of either the right or left superior pulmonary vein (PV) can allow decompression of the left heart. The LA clamp is opened and the aorta is cross-clamped. Cardioplegia is initiated at 150 mmHg using pressure bags [9]. We use cold storage solution, as developed by F.O. Belzer and James Southard for cardioplegia and storage. This is available as Static Preservation Solution (SPS-1™, Organ Recovery Systems, Chicago, IL). This is cooled between 2 °C and 4 °C. Two liters are hung in pressure bags prior to cross-clamp. Topical cooling

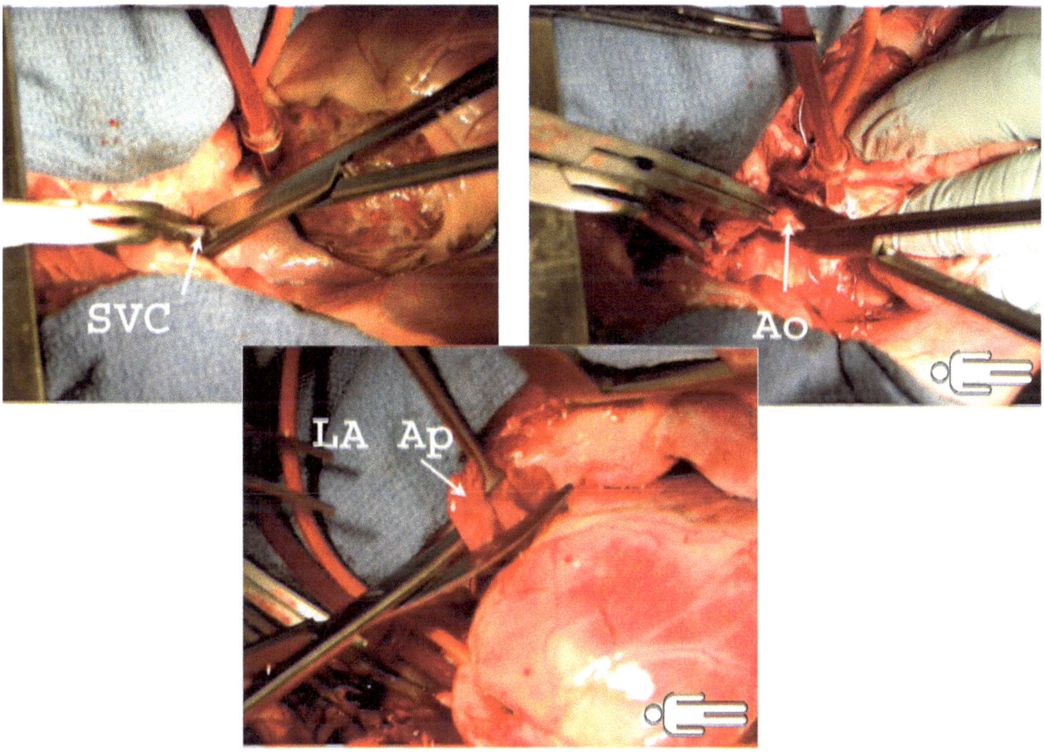

Fig. 9.3 The *upper images* demonstrate division of the superior vena cava and aorta. The *lower images* show amputation of the left atrial appendage. This is followed by division of the left atrium and pulmonary veins

is accomplished with iced saline slush at 4°. It is important to avoid application of large ice blocks on the right ventricle (RV) since this may cause freezing injury to the RV. Once the infusion of preservation solution is complete, the SVC, aorta, and PA are transected along with the SVC.

Figure 9.3 shows transaction of the SVC, aorta, and amputation of the LA appendage.

We routinely leave the aortic vent and cardioplegia needle in for use in the recipient as an aortic de-airing needle. Lastly, the LA or PVs are divided. If lungs are not recovered, then division of right and pulmonary veins is expeditiously achieved. Judicious, left atrial division has to occur when lungs are also recovered. Firstly the Sondergaard's groove has to be developed for at least ½ inch between the right atrium and left atrium in front of the right pulmonary veins. We do prefer to open the left atrium at this level leaving at least 1.5 cm of atrial cuff for the right pulmonary veins to be taken with the right lung.

On the back table in the donor OR room, a sterile bag is placed inside a rigid container and filled with SPS using a bag decanter. The donor heart is inspected for the presence of patent foramen ovale (PFO) and other possible injuries (shown in Fig. 9.4). The container is then placed inside two more sterile bags. The outside bag is labeled with a tag describing its contents and then immersed on ice in a transport cooler [9]. The label includes the organ-specific internal color-coded label provided by UNOS completed with the Organ Procurement and Transplantation Network (OPTN) donor I.D. number, donor ABO type, and description of the specific contents (i.e., heart).

Back Table Preparation of the Donor Heart

Back table preparation is typically undertaken at the removal of the transplant heart from the cooler upon arrival in the recipient operating room.

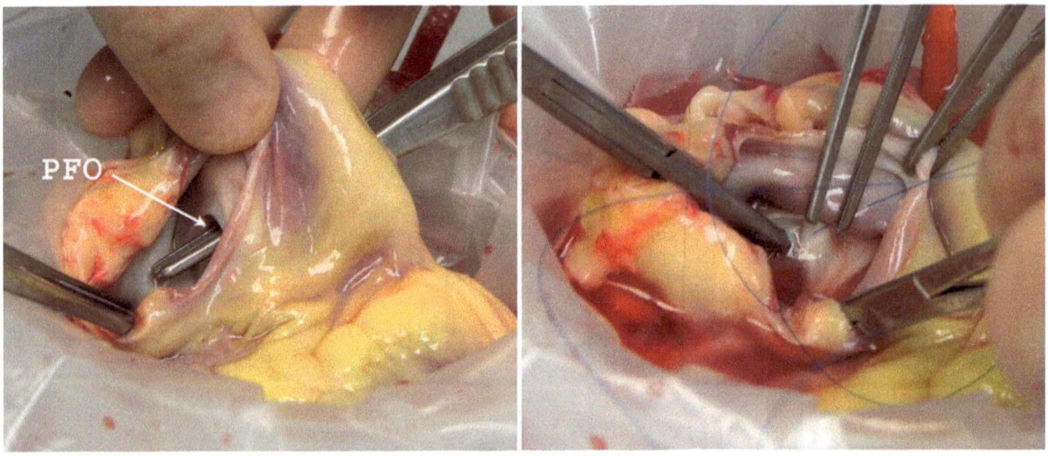

Fig. 9.4 If a patent foramen ovale is found, this is closed on the back table during preparation of the donor heart

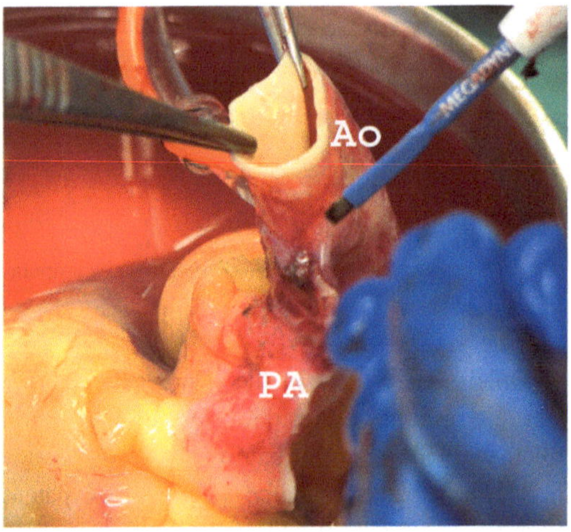

Fig. 9.5 The pulmonary artery and aorta are separated along their length on the back table

When lung recovery did not occur, the LA is left intact, the PVs are opened from between the lower and upper veins on each side and then across [9, 11]. The excess tissue is trimmed in order to provide an atrial cuff to match that of the recipient LA. The atrial wall is inspected for a PFO, and if present this is oversewn [9], usually from the right atrium as depicted in Fig. 9.4.

Electrocautery is used to separate the PA and aorta along its length (Fig. 9.5). The valves are quickly visualized to ensure they were not damaged during the recovery process.

Figure 9.6 illustrates the potential injury to the back wall of the aorta with the cardioplegia needle.

If the venting of the heart was performed through the LA appendage, during heart procurement it should be closed with 4-0 single filament polypropylene running suture. This is illustrated in Fig. 9.7.

Recipient Cardiectomy

Standard preoperative antibiotics are administered. Adequate intravenous access and invasive systemic and pulmonary arterial monitoring are established. The recipient operation is approached most of the time through a median sternotomy, including in re-operative procedures. Occasionally, axillary or femoral cannulation is performed. Sternal adhesions may significantly increase the risk of complications on re-operation [12]. To ensure an easier access for the future redo sternotomy, we routinely reconstruct the pericardium with 2-mm-thick Gore-Tex patch (Gore, Flagstaff, Arizona) at our institution, after left ventricular assist device (LVAD) implantation as bridge to transplantation (Fig. 9.8). We found that this significantly increases the ease of the subsequent sternotomy.

Low-flow carbon dioxide is insufflated into the operative field to reduce the risk of air embolism [13, 14]. The aorta is cannulated as distally as possible in the ascending aorta. The SVC and IVC are

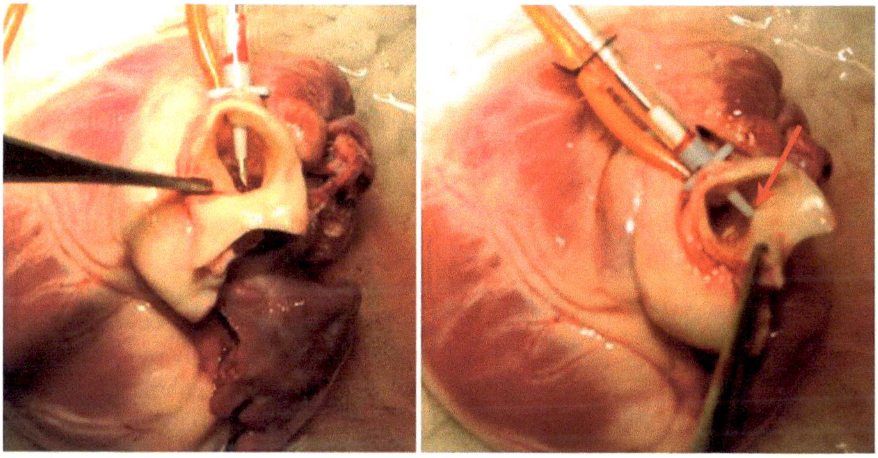

Fig. 9.6 Care must be taken to prevent and look for back wall injury to the aorta from the cardioplegia needle

Fig. 9.7 The site of the left atrial appendage is closed on the back table using 4-0 monofilament suture

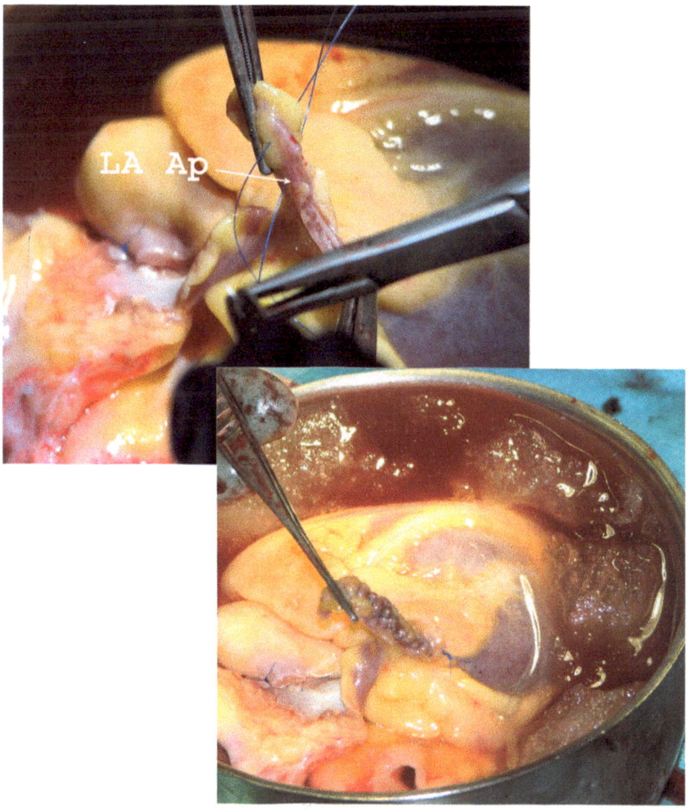

cannulated with right-angle 24–28 F and 28 F cannulas, respectively. Cardiopulmonary bypass is initiated and moderate hypothermia is employed.

Snares are placed around both SVC and IVC cannulae. The aorta is mobilized off of the PA to allow enough room for and safe placement of the aortic cross-clamp. This is particularly important in re-operative surgery when dense scarring may be present between the aorta and pulmonary artery. We initiate the terminal cardiectomy when we

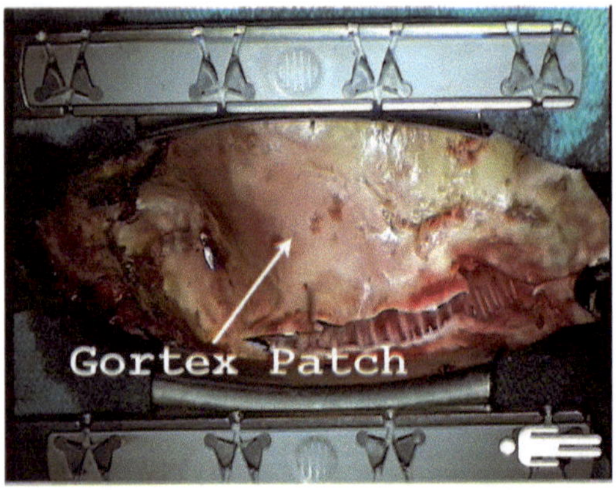

Fig. 9.8 A 2-mm-thick Gore-Tex patch used to reconstruct the pericardium at the time of left ventricular assist device implantation is of great help during the subsequent sternotomy at the time of transplant

ensure that the donor team has safely landed. This allows us approximately 20 min for the recipient cardiectomy. This is initiated by tightening the snares around each vena cava followed by application of cross-clamp after temporarily lowering the flow on cardiopulmonary bypass. We divide the upper and lower parts of the right atrium contiguous with the SVC and IVC leaving a cuff of right atrium of at least 2–3 cm on each vena cava. Care is taken during this procedure to avoid injury of the left atrium especially with re-operative surgery. Preexisting pacing/defibrillator wires are pulled intrapericardially and cut flush with the SVC snare with a wire cutter. Swan–Ganz catheter is removed from the recipient heart at this point and retracted out of the mediastinum and secured to the drapes.

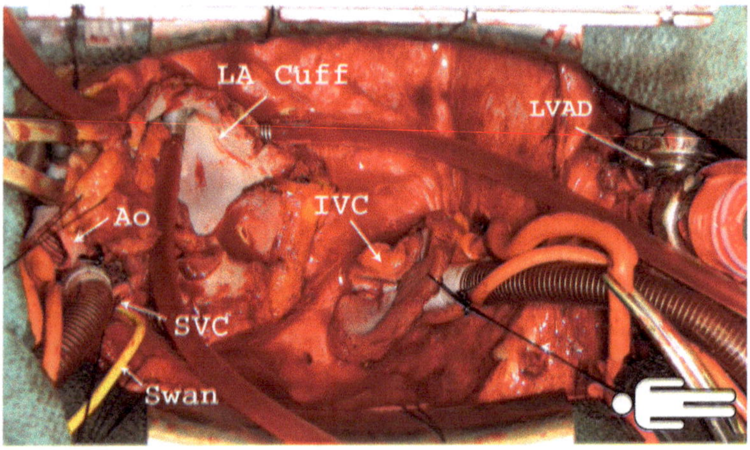

Fig. 9.9 Recipient cardiectomy is completed and shown are the snared stumps of the superior and inferior vena cava and left atrial cuff with the pulmonary veins

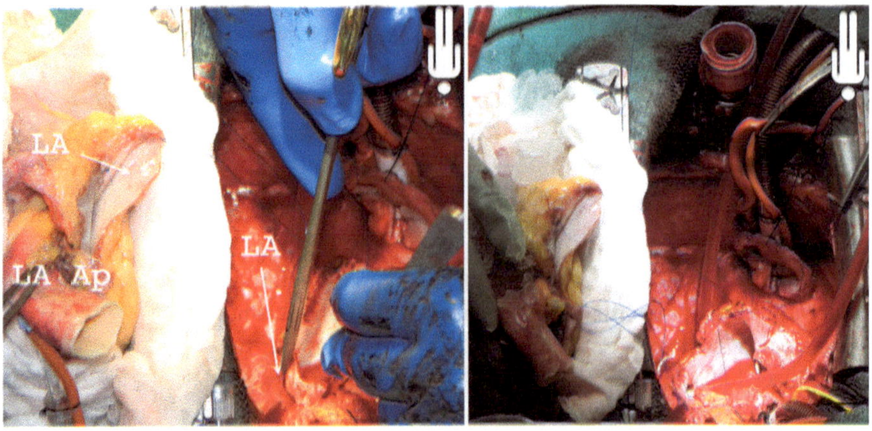

Fig. 9.10 The donor heart is brought into the field, and the back wall of the left atrial anastomosis is begun using a long 3-0 Prolene suture on an M-H needle in a running fashion

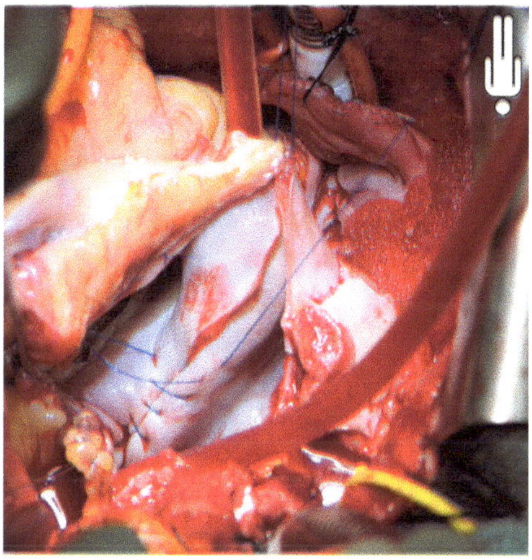

Fig. 9.11 The left atria of the donor and recipient are aligned, and the posterior atrial walls are sutured using everting, full-thickness bites

Aorta and the PA are both divided at the level of the valve commissures. Lastly, the LA is divided along the atrioventricular groove. If an LVAD is present, the left ventricle can be amputated close to the apex and LVAD cannula oriented outside of the pericardial cavity and removed after completion of all anastomoses.

Figure 9.9 shows the empty pericardium after the recipient cardiectomy, showing a large cuff of atrium with the SVC and IVC. Note the pulmonary artery catheter exiting the SVC, the LVAD outflow graft left on the recipient aorta, and the LVAD (HeartMate II, Thoratec Corporation, Pleasanton, CA) in the preperitoneal space.

Allograft Implantation

Left Atrial Anastomosis

The donor cardiac allograft is brought in to the operative field and placed on an ice slush sponge on the left side of the sternotomy retractor. Correct orientation of the donor heart and best matching of the donor and recipient atria is essential at this point to enable optimal positioning of the subsequent anastomosis. The donor left atrium is oriented so the atrial appendage and the medial aspect of the IVC stump will match those of the recipient. Two 54-inch, 3-0, single-stranded, double-armed, polypropylene sutures are used as stay sutures to mark the landmarks mentioned above [11]. This is illustrated in Figs. 9.10 and 9.11.

The cranial suture, placed near the left atrial appendage, is run along the posterior atrial walls. Care is taken to run this posterior atrial wall using everting, full-thickness bites through the endocardium. This everting stitch with apposition of the intimal layers may reduce the risk of clot formation and possible embolization during the early postoperative period [11]. After all the length of the suture is used, the heart is "parachuted" from the left hemi-sternum in the pericardial cavity. Ice slush is added as needed to provide continued cooling to the graft once it is lowered into the pericardium. The posterior wall is run until the inferior stay suture is encountered, and the other end of the cranial suture is then run anteriorly using a simple over–over suture technique. We frequently do not use the inferior stay suture for this anastomosis. We tie this suture without employing special maneuvers to de-air the left atrium.

IVC Anastomosis

The IVC anastomosis is completed next using 4-0 single-stranded polypropylene suture [9]. To aid in visualization of the field, a floppy pump sucker can be threaded through the SVC into the IVC in front of the coronary sinus while the posterior wall of the IVC anastomosis is completed. One can leave the anterior wall of the IVC anastomosis to be completed after the removal of the cross-clamp, and the aortic anastomosis can be completed at this point. However, if IVC is completed at this time, care is taken to match the almost universal size discrepancy between the small donor and large recipient IVC stumps as depicted in Fig. 9.12. The recipient RA is usually incised anteriorly for 1–2 cm as to match the larger recipient IVC. Attention to this fact is essential in preventing strictures or torsion [11]. Additionally the excess IVC tissue can be plicated and oversewn anteriorly when the anastomosis is nearly complete.

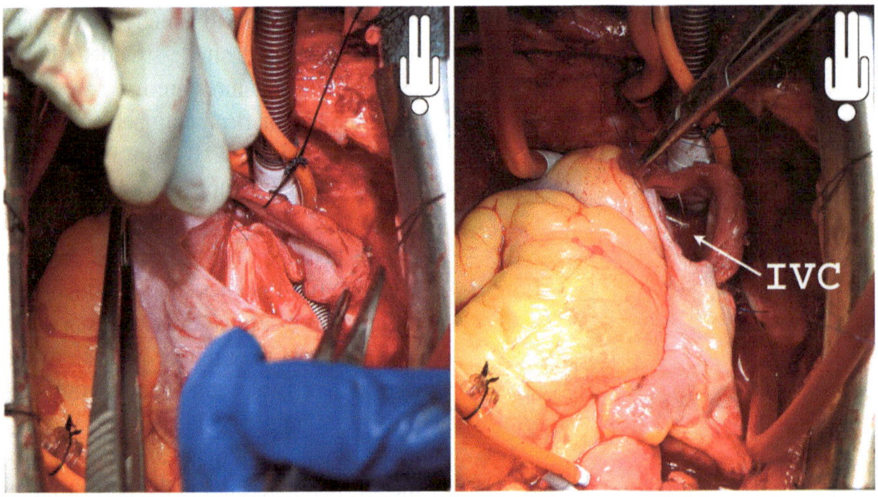

Fig. 9.12 The donor right atrium is commonly incised anteriorly for 1–2 cm to account for the common size discrepancy between the small inferior vena cava in the donor and the large one in the recipient

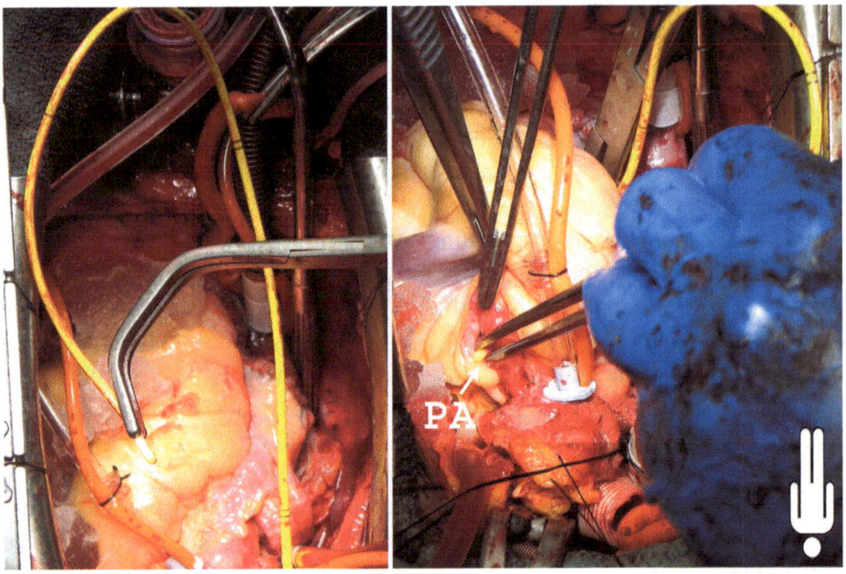

Fig. 9.13 A Satinsky clamp may aid in passage of the pulmonary artery catheter from the recipient vena cava through the donor right atrium and ventricle towards the pulmonary artery

SVC Anastomosis

The pulmonary artery catheter should be threaded from the recipient SVC through the donor SVC, RA, and RV towards the PA prior to completing the anastomosis as illustrated in Fig. 9.13. We routinely use a Satinsky clamp to enable passage of the pulmonary catheter antegrade through the right heart. Afterwards, the SVC anastomosis is completed using 4-0 single-stranded polypropylene suture.

Special care must be taken not to narrow ("purse-string") the SVC, and it is recommended to tie the suture very loosely at the end. A technique where open forceps are used to prevent overtightening the SVC anastomosis is shown in Fig. 9.14 (insert).

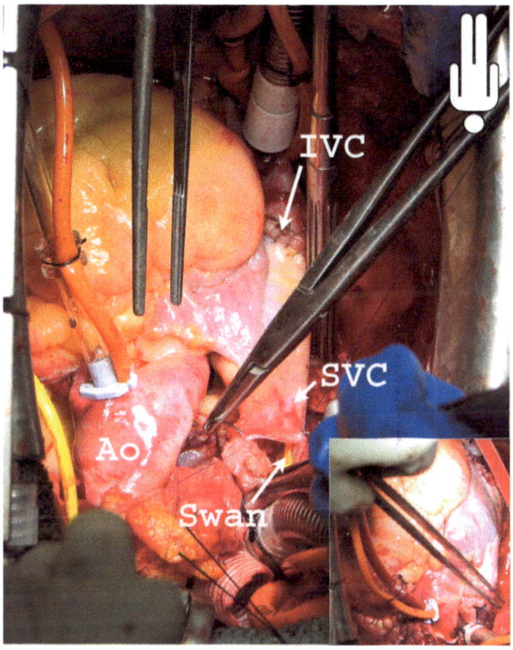

Fig. 9.14 Care must be taken to avoid purse-stringing the superior vena cava anastomosis; tying over and instrument such as forceps can prevent overtightening the anastomosis

Aortic Anastomosis

Aortic anastomosis can be completed right after LA anastomosis when an earlier release of cross-clamp is anticipated or in the order preferred. An end-to-end anastomosis is completed with 3-0 or 4-0 single-stranded polypropylene suture according to individual preference. It's our choice to use 4-0 single-stranded polypropylene suture and a strip of bovine pericardium during the completion of both the aortic and PA anastomosis. Larger size discrepancy between the larger recipient and smaller donor aortic ends is dealt by either more pronounced beveling of the donor (usually) longer aorta or by reducing the size of the recipient aorta by excising a 1–2 cm triangular piece from its anterior aspect and closing the defect transversely. If an LVAD stump graft is present, as seen in Fig. 9.15, it is preferable to remove it, but occasionally it can be stapled off depending on length of aorta needed for anastomosis.

Finally, an interposition graft can be used between the two aortic ends when additional length is needed. Once the aortic anastomosis is completed, the aortic cross-clamp can be removed and rewarming started. We usually keep and use the same aortic de-airing needle, along with its tourniquet, that was placed at the time of recovery for delivery of preservation solution.

PA Anastomosis

The pulmonary anastomosis is completed lastly before or after removal of the cross-clamp. Adequate matching of optimal length as well as approximation of the best orientation of the two pulmonary artery ends is again essential to prevent kinking of this anastomosis [9, 11]. The adventitial fat from donor and recipient is matched to avoid twisting. Both ends are also trimmed to avoid any possible redundancy. The pulmonary artery catheter is passed into the recipient PA at this point, as seen in Fig. 9.16. We use 4-0 single-stranded polypropylene suture and a 1-cm wide strip of bovine pericardium to complete this anastomosis.

Reperfusion

Once the atrial and aortic anastomoses are complete, the standard de-airing maneuvers are accomplished [15], the immunosuppressive steroid dose is given along with the antiarrhythmic agents, and cross-clamp is removed. We do not administer any cardioplegia to the donor heart during implantation. Instead we do perform frequent applications of ice slush and attempt to minimize the implantation time by removing the cross-clamp after the completion of only LA and aortic anastomoses if needed. Rewarming is continued until bypass is discontinued. The disconnected LVAD device, if not removed earlier, (Fig. 9.9) is removed at this point by dissecting it out of its pocket and cutting off its driveline as distal as possible. It is our routine to place a Betadine impregnated lap in the LVAD pocket. Atrial and ventricular pacing wires are placed and passed through the skin below the

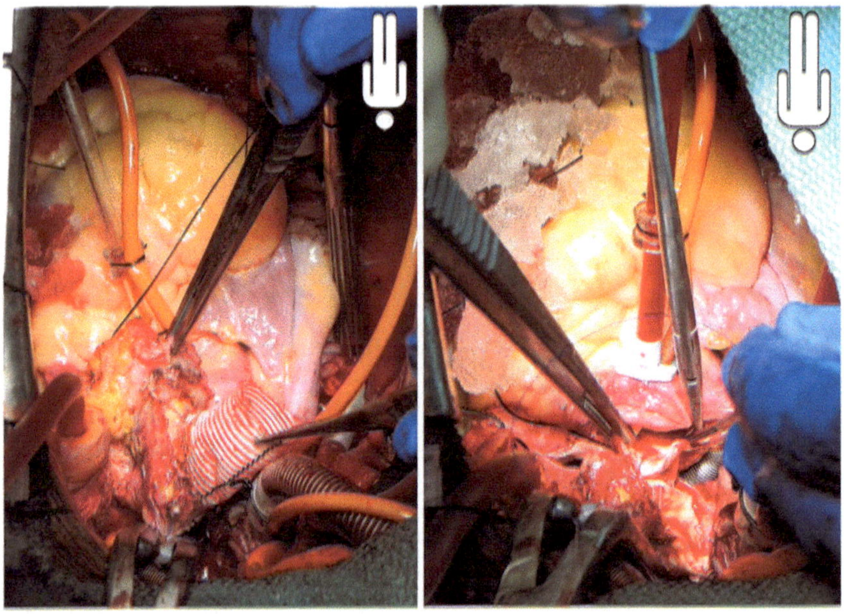

Fig. 9.15 If present, an LVAD stump graft is removed prior to completion of the end-to-end aortic anastomosis. In rare cases it may be stapled off and left in place if removing it will result in insufficient length of the aorta

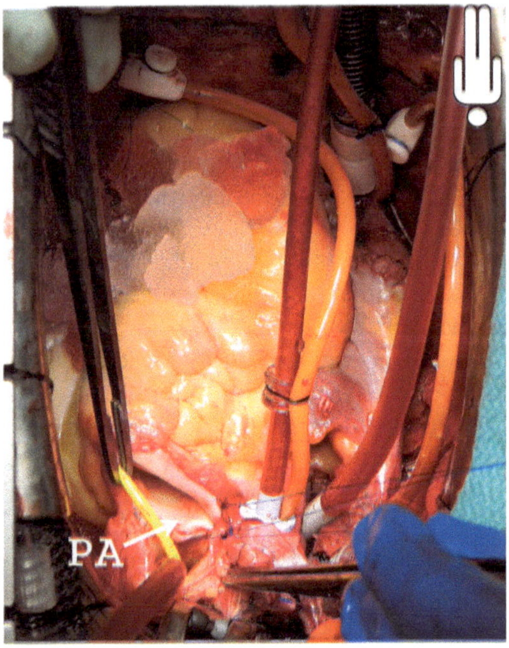

Fig. 9.16 The pulmonary arterial anastomosis is completed using single-stranded polypropylene suture after the pulmonary artery catheter is passed into the recipient pulmonary artery

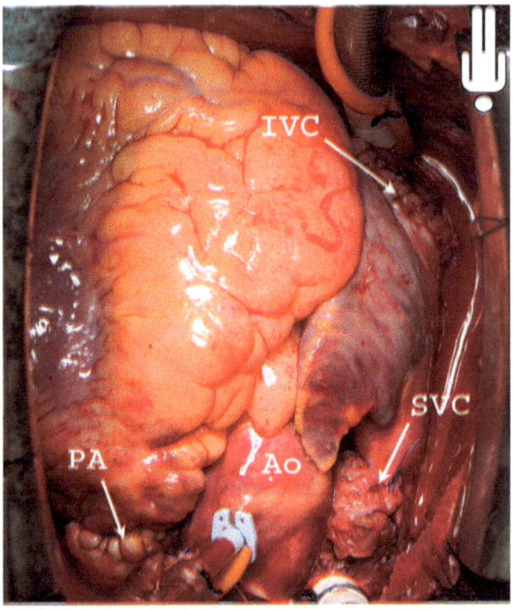

Fig. 9.17 The completed heart transplantation procedure showing inferior and superior vena caval anastomoses, the aorta with cardioplegia needle still in place and used for de-airing and pulmonary artery anastomosis

costal margin. Figure 9.17 shows the completed anastomoses. After skin closure the ICD/pacer generator if present is removed along with the remaining pacemaker wires. If these have been in place for an extended period of time or several attempts to remove them are unsuccessful, they may be left in situ. The external part of LVAD driveline is also removed once the sternotomy incision is closed.

References

1. Lower RR, Shumway NE. Studies on orthotopic homotransplantation of the canine heart. Surg Forum. 1960;11:18–9.
2. Kirklin JK, Pambukian SV, McGiffin DC, Benza RL. Current outcomes following heart transplantation. Semin Thorac Cardiovasc Surg. 2004;16(4):395–403.
3. Johnson MR, Meyer KH, Haft J, Kinder D, Webber SA, Dyke DB. Heart transplantation in the United States, 1999–2008. Am J Transplant. 2010;10(4 Pt 2): 1035–46.
4. Davies RR, Russo MJ, Morgan JA, Sorabella RA, Naka Y, Chen JM. Standard versus bicaval techniques for orthotopic heart transplantation: an analysis of the United Network for Organ Sharing database. J Thorac Cardiovasc Surg. 2010;140(3):700–8, 708.e1-2.
5. Morgan JA, Edwards NM. Orthotopic cardiac transplantation: comparison of outcome using biatrial, bicaval, and total techniques. J Card Surg. 2005; 20(1):102–6.
6. Hakim MG, Gill SS. Heart transplantation: operative techniques and postoperative management. J La State Med Soc. 1993;145(5):233–40.
7. Grauhan O, Siniawski H, Dandel M, et al. Coronary atherosclerosis of the donor heart–impact on early graft failure. Eur J Cardiothorac Surg. 2007;32(4): 634–8.
8. Bolman 3rd RM. Heart transplantation technique. Oper Tech Thorac Cardiovasc Surg. 1999;4(2):98–113.
9. Baumgartner WA. Atlas of cardiac surgery. Philadelphia: Hanley and Belfus; 2000.
10. Novick RJ, Menkis AH, McKenzie FN. New trends in lung preservation: a collective review. J Heart Lung Transplant. 1992;11(2 Pt 1):377–92.
11. Fleischer KJ, Baumgartner WA. Modified cardiac transplantation. Oper Tech Thorac Cardiovasc Surg. 1999;4(2):114–23.
12. Yamauchi T, Miyamoto Y, Ichikawa H, Takano H, Sawa Y. Large vessel—sternum adhesion after cardiac surgery; a risk-factor analysis. Surg Today. 2006; 36(7):596–601.
13. Martens S, Neumann K, Sodemann C, Deschka H, Wimmer-Greinecker G, Moritz A. Carbon dioxide field flooding reduces neurologic impairment after open heart surgery. Ann Thorac Surg. 2008;85(2):543–7.
14. Selman MW, McAlpine WA, Albregt H, Tatan R. An effective method of replacing air in the chest with CO_2 during open-heart surgery. J Thorac Cardiovasc Surg. 1967;53(5):618–22.
15. Sadowsky HS. Cardiac transplantation: a review. Phys Ther. 1996;76(5):498–515.

Mechanical Circulatory Support as a Bridge to Transplantation

10

Jeffrey A. Morgan and Yoshifumi Naka

Introduction

Left ventricular assist devices (LVADs) have become the standard of care for patients with refractory, end-stage heart failure [1, 2]. Several studies have demonstrated the superiority of mechanical support over optimal medical therapy with respect to improving survival as well as quality of life in this subgroup of patients [3–5]. Over the last decade, there has been a significant evolution in VAD-related technologies. Devices have undergone substantial modifications in an effort to improve survival while on support, increase durability, and limit device-related infections, device thrombosis, device malfunction, and perioperative bleeding [6, 7]. Improvements in device design have also yielded devices that can be implanted as destination therapy.

There are currently several broad differentiating features of devices which can be used to separate devices into various subcategories, including short-term vs. long-term devices, paracorporeal vs. intracorporeal devices, pulsatile vs. continuous flow devices, full vs. partial support devices, and assist device vs. complete heart replacement (i.e., total artificial heart). The indications for implantation of a mechanical device have expanded over time and include acute cardiogenic shock, bridge to transplant (BTT), bridge to decision, and destination therapy (DT) [8–15]. This chapter will focus on VADs for long-term support as a BTT, including important factors relating to patient selection, types of devices, results using mechanical support, surgical technique, postoperative management, and complications.

Chronic Heart Failure as a Bridge to Transplant

Progression of chronic heart failure encompasses the largest subgroup of patients who receive LVADs [16, 17]. These patients are typically well known to the heart failure group and are already listed and waiting for a heart transplant. While most of these patients chronically deteriorate to the point that they require mechanical support, a subset of these patients will have an acute exacerbation of chronic heart failure due to the presence of a new, acute infection, arrhythmia, or new area of myocardial ischemia. These patients typically do well after placement of a long-term VAD, such as the HeartMate II (Thoratec Corp., Pleasanton, CA) [1, 2, 18–20]. They are often discharged from the hospital after their VAD and return at a later date for their transplant [4, 5].

J.A. Morgan, M.D. (✉)
Division of Cardiothoracic Surgery,
Henry Ford Hospital, 2799 W. Grand Blvd.,
K-14, Rm. 1439, Detroit, MI 48202, USA
e-mail: jmorgan2@hfhs.org

Y. Naka, M.D., Ph.D.
Department of Cardiothoracic Surgery,
New York Presbyterian Hospital,
177 Fort Washington Ave., Milstein 7GN-435,
New York, NY 10032, USA
e-mail: yn33@columbia.edu

J.A. Morgan and Y. Naka (eds.), *Surgical Treatment for Advanced Heart Failure*,
DOI 10.1007/978-1-4614-6919-3_10, © Springer Science+Business Media New York 2013

Patient Selection

Cardiac Factors

Prudent patient selection is a critical element in achieving good clinical results with LVADs. Numerous studies have identified independent predictors of adverse outcome after LVAD implantation [21–23]. The common denominator among these independent predictors of mortality is end-organ failure, such as respiratory failure requiring mechanical ventilation, renal failure requiring dialysis, shock liver with markedly elevated transaminases, and diffuse coagulopathy due to malfunctioning clotting mechanisms. It is important to implant mechanical support in patients prior to development of end-organ failure. This applies to patients with chronic heart failure with an acute decompensation who are receiving long-term VADs [22, 23].

It is important to identify those patients with significant right ventricular (RV) dysfunction prior to LVAD implantation, as RV failure post-LVAD implantation could be a fatal complication [24, 25]. Preoperative predictive factors for RV failure after LVAD implantation include low preoperative mean pulmonary artery pressure and low right ventricular stroke work index (RVSWI). RVSWI = CI/HR × 1,000 × [(MPAP − RAP) ×0.0136][25]. Normal RVSWI is 8–10. A lower RVSWI implies increased chance for RV failure post-LVAD implantation [25]. These patients should be considered for biventricular assist device (BIVAD) implantation instead of an isolated LVAD.

Noncardiac Factors

Contraindications for device implantation include irreversible end-organ failure, particularly renal, hepatic, and respiratory, which are uniformally independent predictors of poor outcome [21–23, 26, 27]. Severe, unrecoverable neurologic injury is also a contraindication for device implantation. Systemic sepsis poses a significant risk to patients undergoing LVAD implantation for its ability to cause a profound, refractory vasodilatory state as well as the increased incidence of device-related infections, such as device endocarditis [28, 29].

A patient's neurologic status should be evaluated thoroughly before implantation of a mechanical device. This is sometimes not practical or possible in certain situations, such as an unstable patient transferred from an outside institution. However, in relatively stable patients, it is prudent to rule out an irreversible head injury or a large stroke prior to VAD implantation.

Preoperative renal failure is a significant independent predictor of mortality after VAD implantation [22, 23, 26]. It is for this reason that we attempt to avoid placing VADs in patients with renal failure requiring dialysis. This is particularly true for patients in the category of acute exacerbation of chronic heart failure. Renal failure constitutes less of a contraindication for a patient presenting with acute cardiogenic shock without a history of heart failure, such as post-acute myocardial infarction (AMI) or from acute myocarditis. Several indicators of poor renal function that have been identified as predictors of outcome include urine output less than 0.5 cm^3/kg/h despite diuretics and creatinine >5 mg/dL.

Active infection represents a relative contraindication for LVAD implantation [28, 29]. Ideally, patients should have two negative blood cultures over a 1-week period prior to LVAD implantation, which demonstrates that they cleared their bloodstream of the infection.

Poor preoperative hepatic function has also been demonstrated to be an independent predictor of mortality after LVAD implantation [21–23]. Prothrombin time of greater than 16 s is indicative of significantly decreased hepatic synthetic function and increases the chances for developing a diffuse coagulopathy intraoperatively and postoperatively. Diffuse coagulopathy can cause right heart failure (RHF) secondary to increased transfusion requirements of blood and blood products, such as platelets, FFP, cryoprecipitate, as well as factor VII, that may need to be administered to the patient [24, 25]. Development of RHF post-LVAD implantation increases mortality [30]. Other markers of hepatic function that have been correlated with survival after LVAD implantation include preoperative bilirubin [21–23].

Other relative contraindications to LVAD implantation include the presence of a malignancy with a life expectancy of ≤2 years. Each of these cases requires individual attention and evaluation for appropriate decision-making. A patient with human immunodeficiency virus (HIV) who is compliant with medical therapy, has a normal CD4 count, and has undetectable viral load should be considered for an LVAD [21–23].

Although it is important not to delay VAD implantation to the point when there is significant end-organ dysfunction, in a relatively stable patient, it is beneficial to optimize the patient preoperatively. This may include optimizing the patient's hemodynamics with inotropes, pressors, and an IABP; correcting a coagulopathy with vitamin K, platelets, and/or FFP; and diuresing the patient as tolerated. With appropriate patient selection and timing of LVAD implantation, it is possible to achieve excellent results with relatively low associated morbidity and mortality.

Types of Devices

Devices for Long-Term Mechanical Support

Pulsatile Devices for Long-Term Mechanical Support

Thoratec HeartMate XVE

The HeartMate (HM) XVE LVAD (Thoratec Corp., Pleasanton, CA) is Food and Drug Administration (FDA) approved both for BTT and for DT (Fig. 10.1). The device is electrically vented and contains a portable console and batteries, affording patients the opportunity to ambulate easily, as well as the ability to be discharged from the hospital with their device [1, 2, 4].

The device employs pusher plate technology to produce pulsatile flow with a stroke volume of 83 cm^3 and a maximal flow of 10 L/min. The device can be inserted intra-abdominally or extraperitoneally in the preperitoneal space of the left upper quadrant. The inflow cannula is placed in the LV apex and the outflow graft is anastomosed to the ascending aorta. The driveline for the

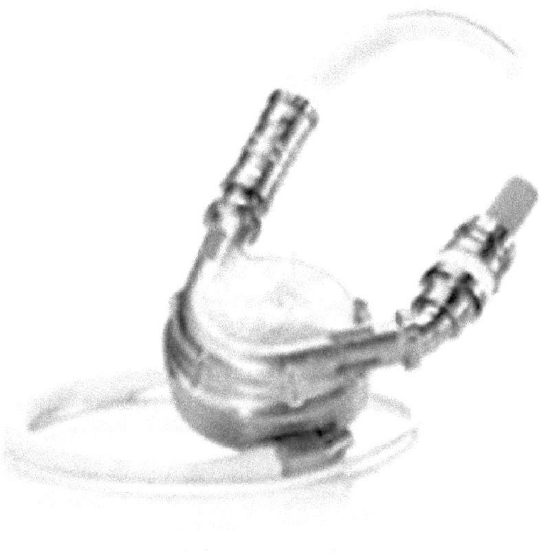

Fig. 10.1 HeartMate I XVE (courtesy of Thoratec Corp., used with permission)

device is tunneled subcutaneously and exits via the right upper quadrant. Due to the relatively large size of the device, the minimum body surface area (BSA) of the patient being implanted with the HM XVE must be 1.5 m^2 [1, 2, 4, 5, 8].

The blood-contacting portion of the device incorporates titanium microspheres, and the flexible diaphragm is covered with textured polyurethane. This promotes formation of a pseudointimal layer; decreases the risk of thromboembolic events, such as strokes; and obviates the need for systemic anticoagulation. Patients are maintained only on aspirin therapy [1, 2, 4].

In 2004, we published our 12-year experience with 236 patients who underwent implantation of a Thoratec HeartMate device as a bridge to transplantation [1]. This included 52 (22.0 %) pneumatic (PNEUM), 17 (7.2 %) dual-lead vented electric (DLVE), and 167 (70.8 %) single-lead vented electric (SLVE) devices. SLVE patients were analyzed pre and post February 1999, when United Network for Organ Sharing (UNOS) changed its regulations and designated SLVE 1 and SLVE 2. Overall transplantation rate increased from 63.5 % ($n=33$) for PNEUM, to 64.7 % ($n=11$) for DLVE, to 70.3 % ($n=52$) for SLVE 1, to 77.4 % ($n=72$) for SLVE 2. Post-transplant 1-year survival increased from 87.5 %

in pneumatics to 92.5 % in SLVE 2, while 3-year survival increased from 78.1 % to 87.6 %, respectively. Device infection and regurgitation occurred in 16.5 % ($n=39$) and 2.1 % ($n=5$), respectively [1].

Thoratec PVAD

The Thoratec paracorporeal VAD (PVAD; Thoratec Corp., Pleasanton, CA) is a versatile device that has been used extensively for uni-ventricular and/or biventricular support (Fig. 10.2) [1]. Its paracorporeal placement of the pumping chamber allows the device to be implanted in patients with BSAs of less than 1.5 m^2. It consists of a polyurethane blood sac contained within a polycarbonate housing. It is associated with a large pneumatic console, which is used to generate pulsatile flow with a maximum stroke volume of 65 cm^3. The device is capable of flowing up to 7.2 L/min. Tilting disc mechanical valves maintain unidirectional flow. Because the device is placed paracorporeally, less dissection is required. Inflow for the LVAD is from the left atrium (LA) or LV apex with outflow to the ascending aorta. Inflow for the RVAD is from the right atrium (RA) or right ventricle (RV) with outflow to the pulmonary artery. The device requires systemic anticoagulation with either heparin or warfarin. With the introduction of the TLC-II portable driver, the system has become less cumbersome to patients and caretakers and has improved patient's mobility and ability to participate in rehabilitation programs [31, 32].

Thoratec IVAD

The Thoratec intracorporeal VAD (IVAD; Thoratec Corp., Pleasanton, CA), like the PVAD, is a versatile device that can provide isolated left, right, or biventricular support (Fig. 10.3) [33]. It is the first FDA-approved implantable VAD with biventricular capability for BTT and for postcardiotomy shock.

Slaughter and colleagues recently reported the results of the multicenter IVAD trial. 24 patients received an LVAD and 15 patients received a BIVAD IVAD as a BTT or for postcardiotomy shock [34]. Mean duration of support was 101 days. Support was successful outcomes occurred in 70 % of BTT patients and 67 % for postcardiotomy patients as compared to 69 %

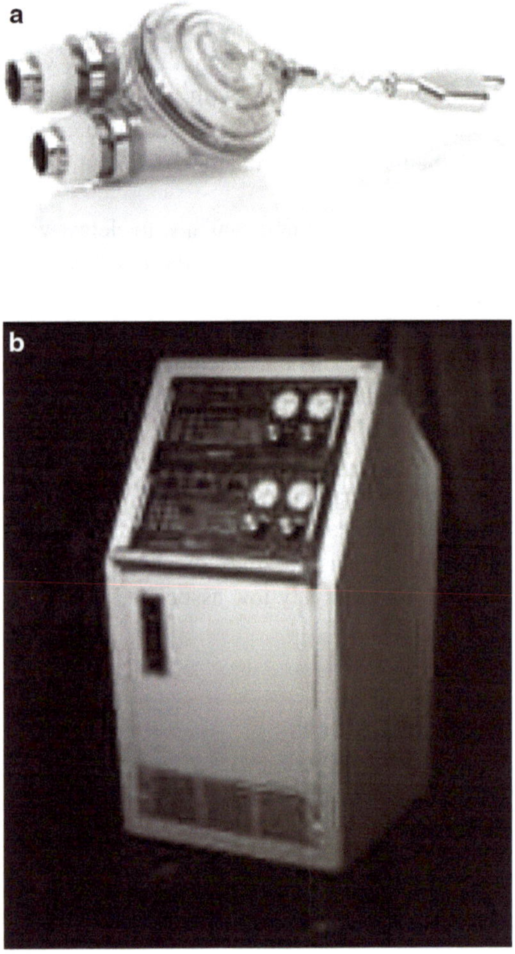

Fig. 10.2 Thoratec PVAD (courtesy of Thoratec Corp., used with permission)

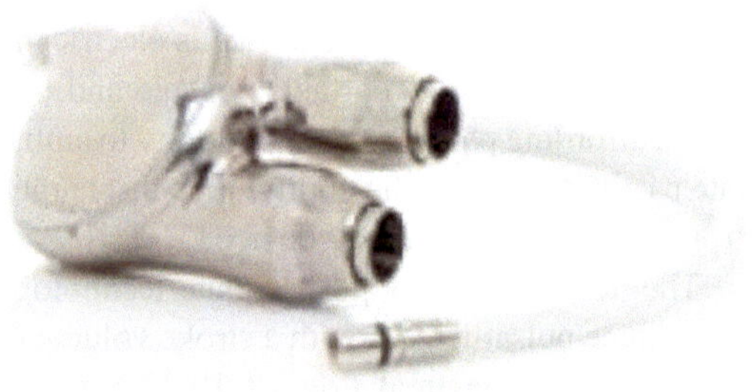

Fig. 10.3 Thoratec IVAD (courtesy of Thoratec Corp., used with permission)

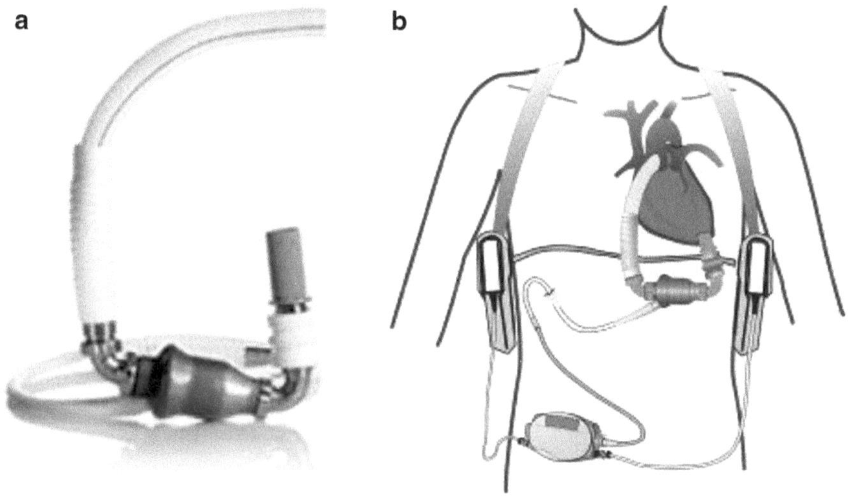

Fig. 10.4 Thoratec HeartMate II (courtesy of Thoratec Corp., used with permission)

and 48 %, respectively, for historical controls using the PVAD. Eighteen of the IVAD patients were discharged home on IVAD support. There were no device failures [34].

Axial Flow Pumps for Long-Term Mechanical Support: Second-Generation Devices

Axial flow pumps are continuous flow pumps that operate with a propeller rotating to a set number of revelations per minute (RPM). Advantages over pulsatile pumps include that they operate more quietly and have enhanced durability, the latter being due to having a decreased number of moving parts and contact bearings. The smaller size of these pumps also allows the device to be inserted with less dissection since the size of the pocket is minimized and sometimes eliminated completely [35]. Disadvantages of an axial flow pump include the lack of a mechanical backup mechanism if there is a major device malfunction, hemolysis as a result of shear forces, and the potential for creating negative intraventricular pressure, with resulting device thrombosis, air embolism, and/or arrhythmias. Optimizing preload and perfect LV apical inflow cannula placement are key factors in avoiding creating negative intraventricular pressure [35].

Several papers have evaluated the potential adverse effects of low-pulsatile continuous flow pumps on end-organ perfusion and function. Based on the current body of data, it seems that adequate end-organ perfusion and function can be maintained with low-pulsatile continuous blood flow [35, 36].

Thoratec HeartMate II

The Thoratec HeartMate II ventricular assist device (Thoratec Corp., Pleasanton, CA) is an axial flow rotary pump constructed of titanium (Fig. 10.4) and is the pump used most commonly at our institution. It is substantially smaller than the HeartMate XVE and requires a less invasive operative approach. It can generate flows up to 10 L/min operating at pump speeds of 6,000–15,000 RPM. Inflow is via the LV apex and outflow is via the ascending aorta. The pump housing is implanted in the preperitoneal space, and given its small size, only a small pocket is necessary. A small percutaneous driveline exits the skin in the right upper abdomen. Systemic anticoagulation is necessary. The HM II is approved by the FDA for BTT and DT [37].

Dr. Miller and colleagues recently reported the results of the prospective, multicenter HeartMate II trial [38]. Of the 133 patients with end-stage heart failure who underwent implantation of a HM II, the primary endpoint, which was defined as the proportion of patients, who, at 180 days, had undergone transplantation, had undergone cardiac

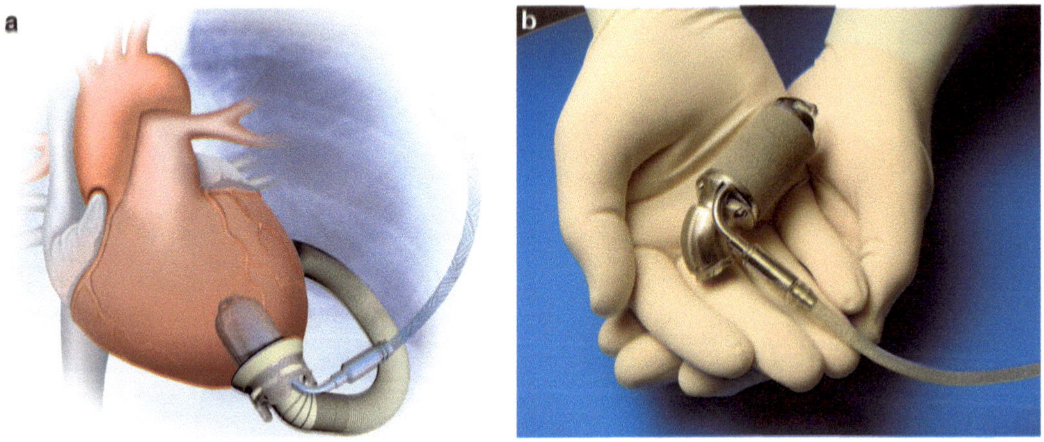

Fig. 10.5 Jarvik 2000 (courtesy of Texas Heart Institute, used with permission)

recovery, or had ongoing mechanical support while remaining eligible for transplant, was reached in 100 patients (75 %). The median duration of support was 126 days. The survival rate during support was 75 % at 6 months and 68 % at 12 months. There was also significant improvement in functional status as well as quality of life. Adverse events included postoperative bleeding, stroke, RHF, and percutaneous lead infection. Pump thrombosis occurred in two patients [38].

Dr. Pagani and colleagues reported in 2009 18-month follow-up on 281 patients who underwent a HM II implantation as a BTT. Of the 281 patients, 222 (79 %) underwent transplantation, underwent LVAD removal for cardiac recovery, or had ongoing LVAD support [39]. Actuarial survival on support was 72 % at 18 months. At 6 months, there were significant improvements in functional status and 6-min walk test and in quality of life.

Jarvik 2000

The Jarvik 2000 (Jarvik Heart Inc., New York, NY) is an electromagnetically actuated pump, which is constructed of titanium, measures 2.5 cm in diameter, and weighs 90 g (Fig. 10.5). It has a displacement of approximately 25 cm^3. Titanium impeller blades are held in place by ceramic bearings. The impeller rotates at speeds of between 8,000 and 12,000 RPM and can generate flow of up to 7 L/min. A unique feature of this device is that the actual pumping chamber is implanted within the left ventricle. The outflow graft is anastomosed to the descending thoracic aorta. Surgical implantation of the device is typically accomplished through a left thoracotomy [40]. The pump can be operated via a fixed-rate analogue system or a variable-speed microprocessor-controlled system.

There are several versions of the Jarvik 2000 device, which are differentiated by their energy source. There is a percutaneous model that has a single driveline that exits through the patient's anterior abdominal wall. There is a version that contains skull-mounted pedestals used with cochlear implants, where a titanium pedestal is screwed into the skull with a transcutaneous connector that attaches to the power cord. There is also a completely implantable version that utilizes a transcutaneous energy transfer system for recharging of the battery [40, 41].

Dr. Siegenthaler and colleagues reported on 102 patients implanted with the Jarvik 2000 Heart between 2000 and 2004. Mean support time for BTT patients was 159 days. No implantable component failures occurred [42].

Newer (Third)-Generation Pumps and Future Devices

Newer-generation devices, so-called third-generation devices, have been designed to address several shortcomings of second-generation axial flow pumps, such as thromboembolic complications and limited device durability. Many of these devices operate based on magnetic levitation technology, in which the rotating propeller is magnetically suspended within a column of blood, obviating the need for contact-bearing moving parts, and providing the theoretical benefit of enhanced durability. Continuous flow pumps are generally smaller, can be inserted with only a small-sized device pocket or no pocket at all, are less traumatic, and may have a decreased associated risk of infection. Some have been designed to be completely implantable with a transcutaneous energy transfer system. Along with smaller control consoles, these devices allow patients to be readily discharged from the hospital, increase a patient's ability to ambulate, and will likely be associated with a significant improvement in quality of life for patients.

Thoratec HeartMate III

The Thoratec HeartMate III (Thoratec Corp., Pleasanton, CA) device is also a magnetically suspended centrifugal pump, which is powered by a magnetically levitated centrifugal impeller. It uses a transcutaneous energy transfer system for battery charging and is totally implantable [43–45]. This device has not begun clinical testing to date.

HeartWare

The HeartWare HVAD (HeartWare, Inc., Sydney, Australia) is a centrifugal pump with no mechanical bearings that weighs 145 g, has a displaced stroke volume of 45 cm^3, and can flow up to 10 L/min at 2,000–3,000 RPM (Fig. 10.6). The inflow cannula is integrated into the left ventricle. The device is implanted in the pericardial space without the need for an abdominal incision. A single, flexible driveline that is 4.2 mm in diameter exits the anterior abdomen. The device has been tested in several centers throughout Europe with good preliminary results [45, 46]. The HVAD was recently approved for BTT in the Unites States and there is currently a DT trial underway.

CircuLite Synergy

CircuLite (CircuLite, Inc., Hackensack, NJ) Synergy is a partial support LVAD that can be placed intravascularly (Fig. 10.7). An inflow cannula is placed through the subclavian vein, into the right atrium, and across the interatrial septum into the left atrium. Outflow is to the subclavian artery. Computer simulation models have demonstrated that partial support devices can increase cardiac output (native heart cardiac output + LVAD) and decrease left ventricular end diastolic pressure (LVEDP) in moderate to severe heart failure [47]. Clinical trials are currently ongoing to evaluate the safety and efficacy of this device.

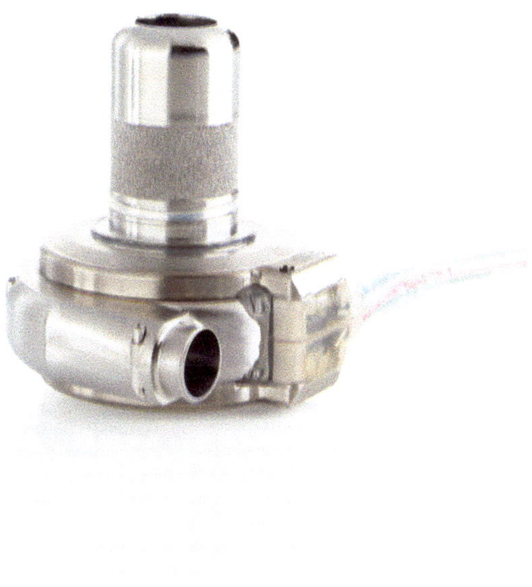

Fig. 10.6 HeartWare (courtesy of HeartWare, Inc., used with permission)

Surgical Technique of LVAD Implantation

Although technique for LVAD implantation varies depending on the institution and individual surgeon, there are certain common steps in the operation that can be summarized as follows:

1. Skin incision
2. Creation of a preperitoneal pocket
3. Tunneling of the device
4. Mediastinal exposure
5. Cannulation of the aorta and venous system
6. Outflow graft anastomosis to ascending aorta

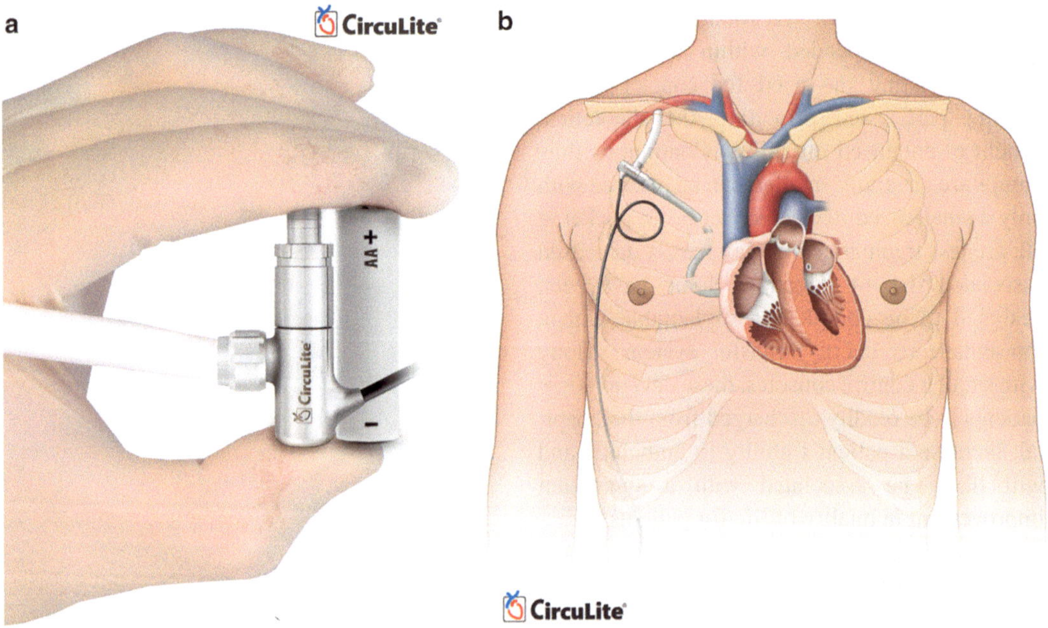

Fig. 10.7 CircuLite synergy (courtesy of CircuLite, Inc., used with permission)

7. Going on cardiopulmonary bypass (CPB)
8. Coring left ventricle (LV), placing core sutures on LV, and inserting inflow core into LV apex
9. Deairing the device
10. Weaning off CPB and actuating LVAD
11. Establishing hemostasis
12. Closing sternotomy and preperitoneal pocket

Incision

A vertical midline incision is made beginning just below the sternal notch with variable extension below the xiphoid depending on the type of device being implanted and the corresponding required pocket size. The Bovie electrocautery is used for hemostasis. A sternotomy is made. Care is taken to avoid getting into the pleural spaces unless there are pleural effusions that need to be drained. Likewise, the peritoneal cavity is not entered.

Development of LVAD Pocket

The LVAD pocket is developed posterior to the posterior rectus sheath in the preperitoneal space. Alternatively, the LVAD pocket can be developed between the posterior rectus sheath and the muscle. A portion of the left hemidiaphragm is taken down to accommodate for the LVAD. Careful attention is given to hemostasis. The device is then placed in the preperitoneal pocket (Fig. 10.8).

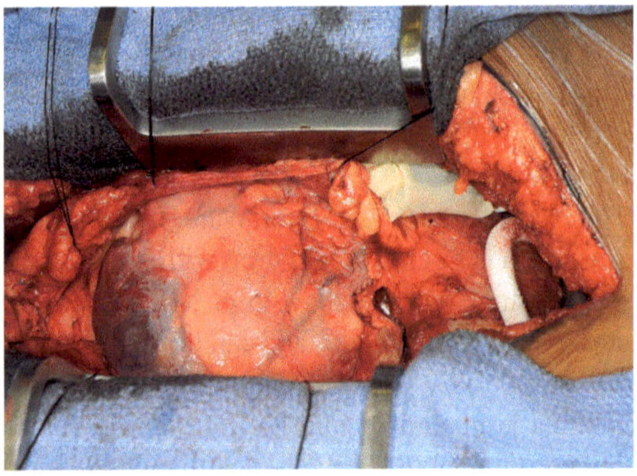

Fig. 10.8 Placement of HM II LVAD into pocket

Tunneling of the Device

The device is screwed onto the tunneler. The spear end of the tunneler is then brought into the incision, pierces through the fascia just to the left of the midline in the pocket, and is tunneled to exit the skin through a previously placed circular incision in the right upper quadrant (Fig. 10.9). The exit point is generally halfway between the umbilicus and anterior superior iliac spine. The driveline is pulled though the exit site. All felt is kept on the inside. The LVAD is then positioned in the pocket.

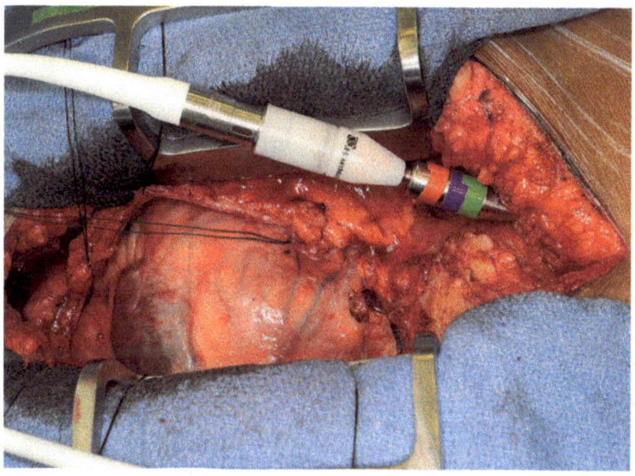

Fig. 10.9 Tunneling of HM II driveline

Mediastinal Exposure

The retrosternal fat and perithymic tissue are divided in a hemostatic fashion using the Bovie and clips. The pericardium is opened along the right side of the heart, down to the diaphragm, and then over to the left by the apex of the heart. Superiorly, the pericardium is opened up just above the aorta until the pericardial reflection. Retraction sutures are placed, creating a pericardial well for exposure of the heart.

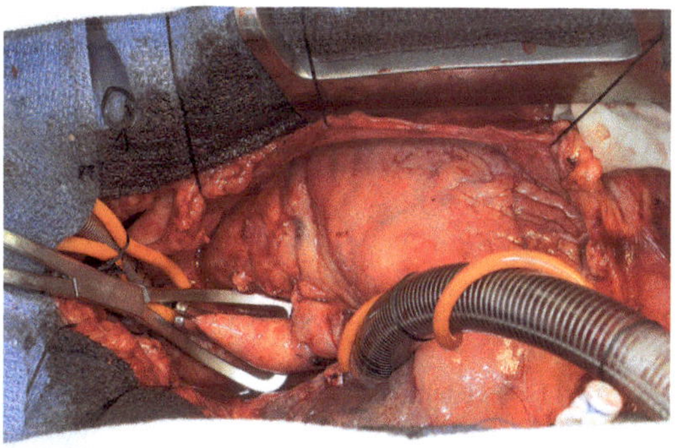

Fig. 10.10 Partial occlusion clamp on proximal ascending aorta

Cannulation

The patient is fully heparinized. Two purse strings are placed on the distal ascending aorta using 3-0 Prolene suture. A purse-string suture is then placed on the anterior portion of the right atrial appendage. When the ACT is 400 s or higher, the ascending aorta is cannulated at the level of the pericardial reflection. The cannula is deaired and secured, and the line is tested. The RA is then cannulated and connected to the bypass circuit. If a tricuspid valve repair or closure of an ASD is planned, the patient is bicavally cannulated with vessel loops and snares placed around the SVC and IVC cannulas. CO_2 is also brought onto the field.

Outflow Graft Anastomosis

The outflow graft is measured and cut appropriately to be anastomosed to the proximal ascending aorta. It is cut with a slight bevel. A partial occlusion side-biting clamp is then applied to the proximal ascending aorta and secured to the drape (Fig. 10.10). An aortotomy is made with a 15 blade and the aortotomy is then extended with a Potts or Iris scissors. The graft is then anastomosed to the proximal ascending aorta using two 4-0 Prolene sutures. Mattress sutures are placed at the heel and toe of the graft and corresponding aorta. The graft is parachuted down (Fig. 10.11). The sutures are tied. A single-layer running anastomosis is then performed followed by application of BioGlue (CryoLife Inc., Kennesaw, GA) (Fig. 10.12). The graft is then deaired and clamped, and the anastomosis is inspected for bleeding.

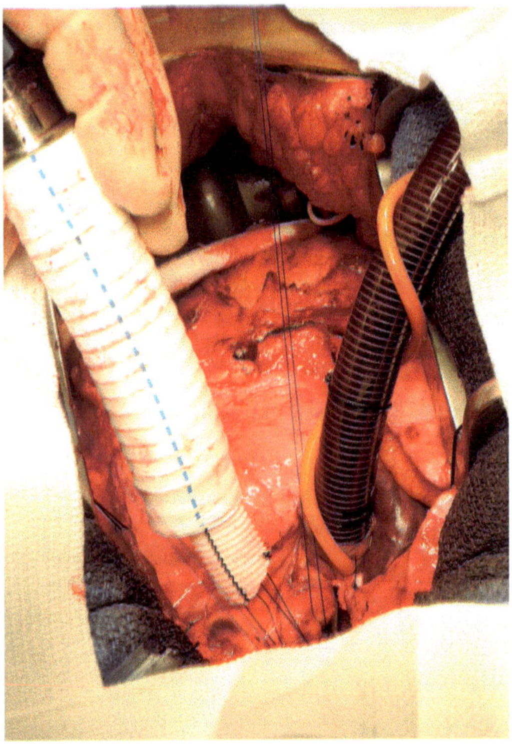

Fig. 10.11 Parachuting outflow graft down onto ascending aorta

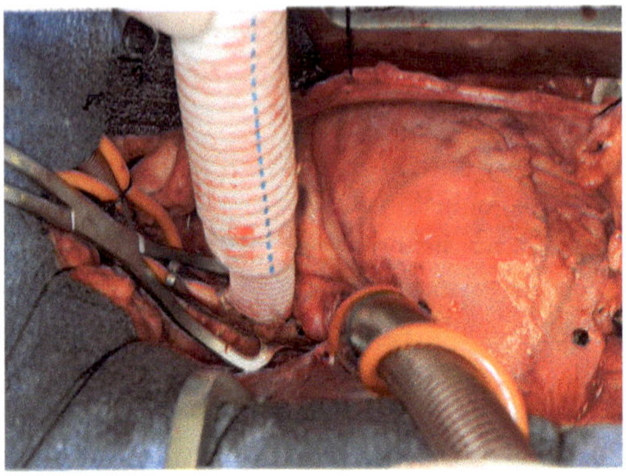

Fig. 10.12 Outflow graft anastomosis to ascending aorta after application of partial aortic clamp

Initiating Cardiopulmonary Bypass

The patient is then placed on CPB and kept warm. Volume is taken out of the heart. The carbon dioxide is turned on so that the field is flooded with CO_2.

Coring LV, Placing Core Sutures on LV, and Inserting Inflow Core into LV Apex

After CPB is commenced, the LV apex is exposed by placing several lap pads in the posterior pericardial space, elevating the heart and bringing the apex to the middle of the field. The LV is then incised at the apex, precisely where the dimpling of the heart occurs. This is generally 2 cm to the left of the left anterior descending artery. A Foley catheter is inserted into the LV, the balloon is inflated, and the Foley is lifted up, abutting the balloon against the coring site. Coring is performed using a 14 Fr coring knife, directing the knife to the LV cavity and not the septum (Fig. 10.13). The LV is then inspected for trabeculations. Prominent trabeculations are excised and any thrombus is removed. Full thickness 2-0 Tevdek pledget sutures are placed in a horizontal mattress fashion around the circumference of the ventriculotomy (Fig. 10.14). The sutures are placed through the sewing ring of the inflow cuff, the sewing ring is seated, and the sutures are tied and cut. BioGlue (CryoLife Inc., Kennesaw, GA) is then applied onto the pledgets of the sutures and around the inflow cuff. The cannula is then inserted into the inflow housing and secured with a tie and 2–3 umbilical tapes (Fig. 10.15). The lap pads are removed, the heart is placed back in its normal position, and the LVAD is placed back in the pocket.

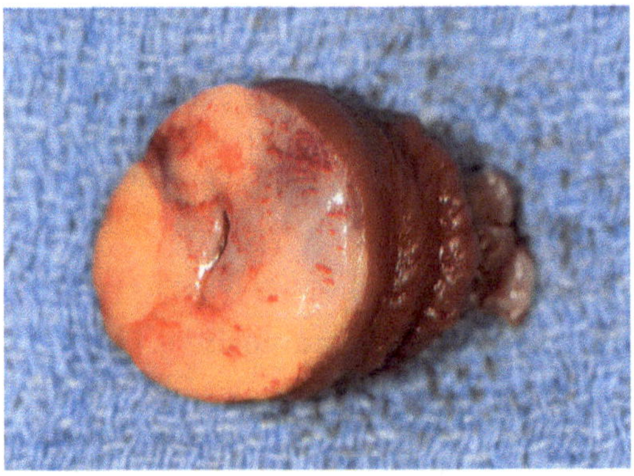

Fig. 10.13 Apical core from LV

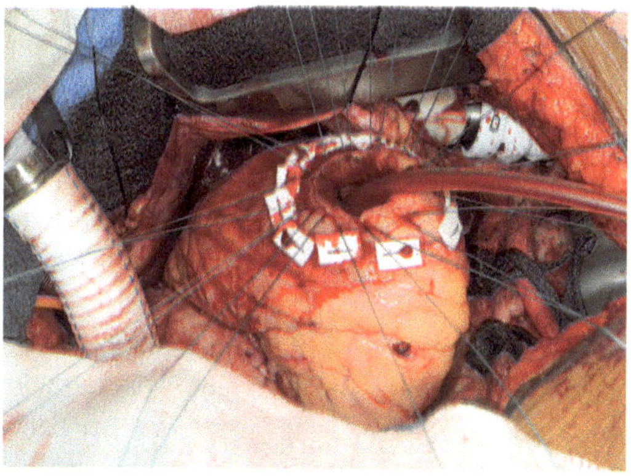

Fig. 10.14 Mattress sutures placed around cored LV apex

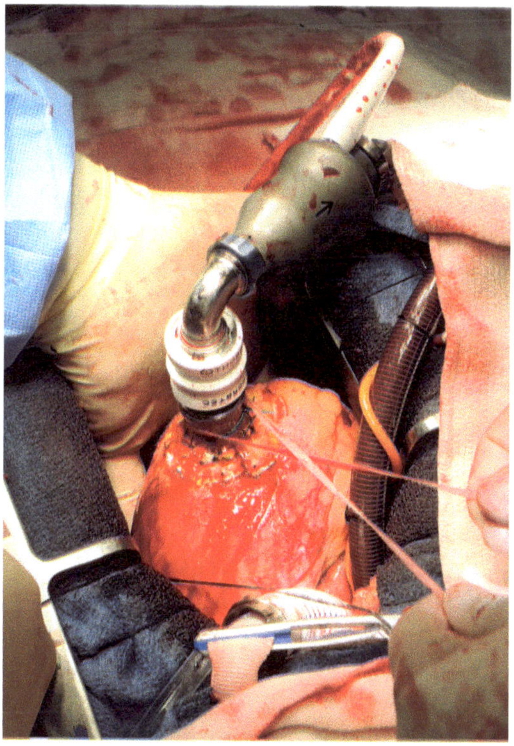

Fig. 10.15 Inflow cannula attached to inflow housing and secured in place

Dearing

The dearing process is then begun by opening the outflow housing (Fig. 10.16). The heart is allowed to fill by having perfusion put volume in. The patient is ventilated. The position of the operating table is also altered by putting the head up and the left side of the table down. Eventually, the outflow graft is connected to the outflow

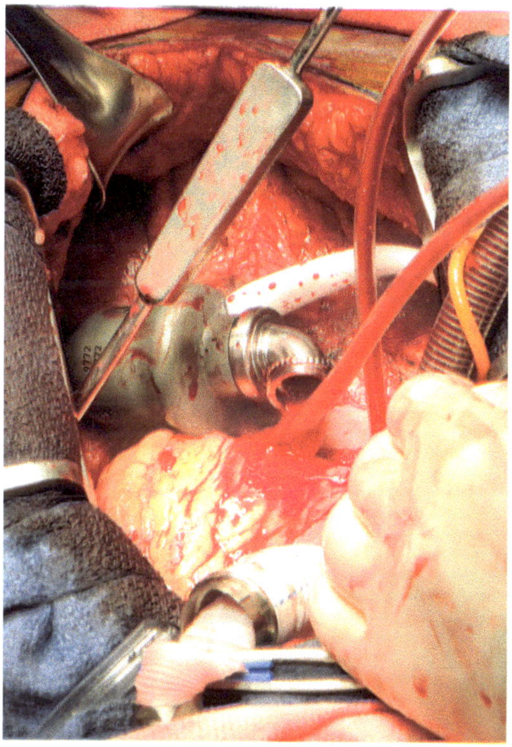

Fig. 10.16 Deairing of device through outflow housing

housing, and a deairing hole is made in the outflow graft. The cross clamp is kept on the outflow graft distal to the deairing hole (Fig. 10.17). Adequacy of deairing is assessed by transesophageal echocardiography.

Dobutamine and milrinone are started at this point to optimize right heart function. Additionally, pressors (Levophed and vasopressin) are started to maintain a MAP of 60–80 mmHg.

Weaning Off CPB and Actuating LVAD

CPB is weaned. With the HeartMate II, the device is begun at 6,000 RPM when the CPB flow is down to 2 L. The cross clamp on the outflow graft is released to allow for forward flow (Fig. 10.18). The device RPM is increased as CPB is weaned. The RPM is generally increased to between 8,800 and 9,600 RPM. The deairing hole in the outflow graft is kept open to allow for additional deairing.

The transesophageal echocardiogram is viewed to assess the degree of decompression of

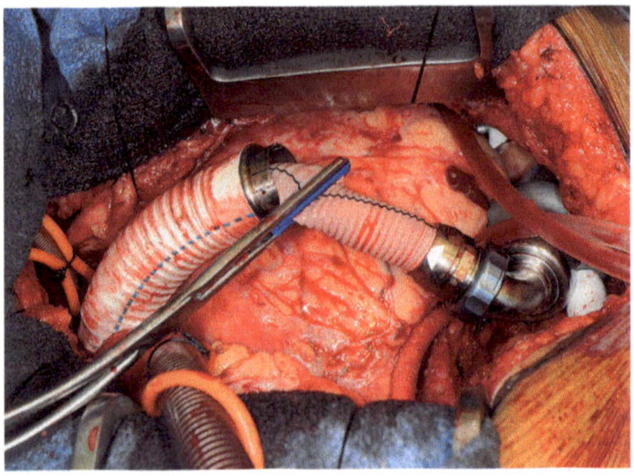

Fig. 10.17 Device connected to outflow housing and deaired through hole in outflow graft

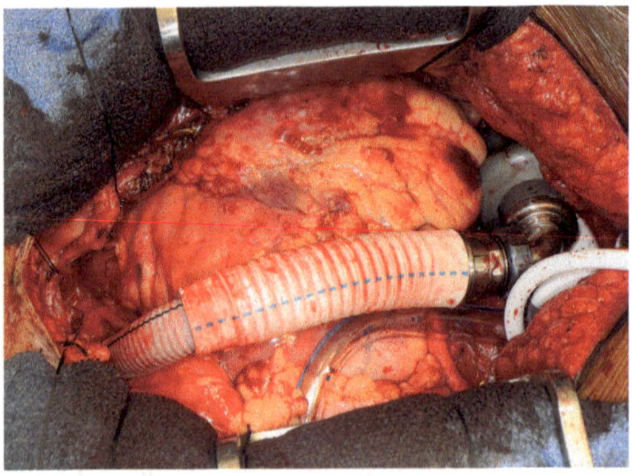

Fig. 10.18 Clamp removed from outflow housing with device in final position

the LV and degree of mitral regurgitation, evaluate the flow across the inflow and outflow cannulae, rule out aortic insufficiency, assess right ventricular function, and evaluate the interventricular septum to make sure it is not bowing. The echocardiographic findings guide the RPM setting of the LVAD, whether to take more volume and/or increase inotropes.

Establishing Hemostasis

It is crucial to establish meticulous hemostasis. All surgical sites including the inflow and outflow graft anatomoses as well as cannulation sites are examined for bleeding. Surgical bleeding is addressed with sutures, usually pledgeded. Nonsurgical bleeding is reevaluated after protamine is fully reversed and the ACT has returned to baseline. These sites will generally respond favorably to repetitive, light packing with gauze and/or usage of topical hemostatic agents, such as Surgicel or thrombin gel foam. The electrocautery is used for the soft tissue, LVAD pocket, and sternum. The LVAD pocket should be examined thoroughly and bleeding controlled.

In the event of a diffuse coagulopathy with excess bleeding, the mediastinum is packed with gauze along with suturing of a Gore-Tex patch onto the skin. The patient is then brought back to the operating room after adequate resuscitation and when the coagulopathy has resolved, which generally occurs 24 h after the initial surgery.

Closing Sternotomy and Preperitoneal Pocket

A Gore-Tex pericardial membrane (Gore Medical Products, Flagstaff, AZ) is sutured to the pericardial edges to minimize reentry injury on the reoperation. Mediastinal and pleural tubes are placed. The sternum is closed in the standard fashion. The abdominal portion of the incision is closed with interrupted figure of eight #1 Prolene sutures. The superficial soft tissue and skin are closed in the standard fashion.

Concomitant Procedures Along with Implantation of LVAD

If the patient has a PFO, it must be closed at the time of LVAD implantation. This requires bicaval cannulation, cross clamping of the aorta, cardioplegic arrest, and primary suture closure of the PFO. This is generally performed after the aortic anastomosis but before the LV inflow anastomosis. In this case, the aorta can be unclamped after the PFO is closed, and the LV inflow anastomosis can be performed with the heart beating. Likewise, aortic valve insufficiency that is moderate or greater should also be addressed with an aortic valve replacement using a bioprosthetic or with central closure of the valve. Finally, severe tricuspid valve regurgitation should be repaired, generally with a tricuspid valve ring annuloplasty at the time of LVAD implant.

Postoperative Management

Early Postoperative Management

RHF is treated with milrinone, dobutamine, and nitric oxide [48, 49]. Vasodilatory hypotension is treated with norepinephrine and arginine vasopressin [50]. Ventricular and atrial arrhythmias are managed with the standard antiarrhythmic agents, such as amiodarone and lidocaine.

Late Postoperative Management

Late postoperative management focuses on encouraging ambulation and rehabilitation, as well as monitoring patients for signs of infection. Median length of hospital stay is 14 days [4, 5]. Patients are then followed at the outpatient LVAD clinic weekly for the first month after discharge from the hospital and then less frequently thereafter.

Anticoagulation

HeartMate II, Thoratec IVAD, and Thoratec PVAD all require anticoagulation with Coumadin, as well as antiplatelet therapy with aspirin in order to prevent thromboembolic complications. Anticoagulation and antiplatelet therapies, however, are generally not administered in the first 2 days postoperatively. The decision as to when to start anticoagulation is individualized for each patient based on device type, risk of thromboembolism, chest tube output, coagulation profile, and treatment plan for the patient.

Complications

Bleeding

Bleeding post-VAD insertion can be excessive and may be due to surgical causes or a diffuse coagulopathy. Coagulopathy can result from alterations in the hemostatic system, including dilutional thrombocytopenia and exposure to long-acting antiplatelet or antithrombotic agents. For bleeding due to a diffuse coagulopathy, platelets, FFP, and/or cryoprecipitate may be administered. The decision as to whether to administer these products is made based on the PT/PTT/INR/fibrinogen profile. For bleeding due to a coagulopathy that is unresponsive to products, concentrated factor VII (Novo 7) should be considered. However, one must be very judicious with its usage given its ability to induce RHF as well as to create a prothrombotic state. Coagulopathic patients are often hypothermic and should be warmed up with heating blankets.

Patients whose chest tubes cumulatively have outputs >200 cm^3/h should be evaluated for re-exploration. Our policy is to re-explore patients earlier rather than later to avoid excessive administration of blood and blood products, which can induce RHF. Additionally, patients with excessive bleeding benefit from being "washed out" to prevent accumulation of blood/fluid and subsequent infection.

A bleeding patient with a rising CVP, downward trending VAD flows, increasing pressor requirements, and decreasing urine output should be presumed to be tamponading and should be taken to the OR immediately for re-exploration.

Infection

Infection, one of the most common complications in LVAD patients, can manifest as driveline, pocket, blood, or device endocarditis [51, 52]. Sepsis occurs in 11–26 % of LVAD patients, accounts for 21–25 % of LVAD deaths, and represents a major driver of overall cost [53, 54]. It is important to prophylactically begin antibiotics preoperatively, as previously described, as well as to treat infections aggressively with antibiotics when they do occur. The only way to definitively eradicate device endocarditis is to explant the device. Infection is generally not a contraindication to heart transplantation.

Thromboembolism

Thromboembolic complications are a major concern in LVAD patients because of the blood-device interface. The prevalence varies depending on the device and ranges from 7 % to 47 % [55]. Thromboembolic events with the HM II have been reported to be 8 % [38].

Device Malfunction

The severity of a device malfunction varies from minor to fatal. With improvement in device design and engineering, the overall incidence of serious device malfunctions has decreased significantly over time [37, 38].

Right Heart Failure

The incidence of RHF after LVAD implantation is 20 % [24, 25, 30]. There are different degrees of severity of RV dysfunction and a spectrum of interventions ranging from diuresis, to inotropic support, to implantation of an RVAD. Patients can develop RHF from volume overload with excess volume administered to them in the form of blood, blood products, colloids, and crystalloid. It is for this reason that it is critical to avoid excess volume resuscitation in LVAD recipients.

Early signs of RHF include elevated CVP over 16 mmHg, marginal VAD flows equal or less than a device flow index of 2.2 L/min/m^2, and decreased urine output. Later signs include decreased LVAD flows on high-dose inotropes and pressors, acidosis, and elevated lactate. Treatment of early RHF involves stopping/limiting all infusions, aggressive diuresis with Lasix, and starting or increasing milrinone and/or dobutamine [30]. Nitric oxide at 20 ppM may be added as well [48, 49]. A Lasix drip may follow bolus doses of Lasix as the diuresing process may be more uniform and may avoid hemodynamic lability due to excessive diuresis. Diuril and/or Zaroxolyn may be given in addition to Lasix if Lasix yields an inadequate response.

Signs of an appropriate response to treatment of RHF and improvement in right heart function include a decreasing CVP, improvement in LVAD flows, and normalization of the patient's MVO2. A small percentage of patients will not respond and will require implantation of an RVAD [30].

Multisystem Organ Failure

Despite effective restoration of adequate cardiac output for tissue perfusion, some patients progress to develop multisystem organ failure. This is related to the preoperative severity of organ dysfunction. Multisystem organ failure is often due to a cascade of events, such as bleeding, sepsis, RHF, and other events. It accounts for 11–29 % of VAD deaths [51].

Summary

LVADs represent the standard of care for patients with end-stage heart failure due to a variety of etiologies as a BTT. Significant progress has been made over the last 10 years with respect to evolution of devices, patient selection, surgical techniques, and postoperative management of patients with LVADs. Limitations of current devices have stimulated research and innovation in an attempt to reduce device size, minimize the invasiveness of the surgical approach, increase device durability, decrease infection, reduce associated thromboembolic complications, and enhance quality of life of patients with LVADs. Outcomes will likely continue to improve with additional technological evolution.

References

1. Morgan JA, John R, Rao V, et al. Bridging to transplant with the Heartmate left ventricular assist device: the Columbia Presbyterian twelve-year experience. J Thorac Cardiovasc Surg. 2004;127(5):1309–16.
2. Dang NC, Topkara VK, Kim BT, et al. Clinical outcomes in patients with chronic congestive heart failure who undergo left ventricular assist device implantation. J Thorac Cardiovasc Surg. 2005;130(5):1302–9.
3. Rose EA, Gelijns AC, Moskowitz AJ, Randomized Evaluation of Mechanical Assistance for the Treatment

of Congestive Heart Failure (REMATCH) Study Group, et al. Long-term mechanical left ventricular assistance for end-stage heart failure. N Engl J Med. 2001;345(20):1435–43.
4. DeRose JJ, Umana JP, Argenziano M, et al. Implantable left ventricular assist devices provide an excellent outpatient bridge to transplantation and recovery. J Am Coll Cardiol. 1997;30:1773–7.
5. Morales DL, Catanese KA, Helman DN, et al. Six-year experience of caring for forty four patients with a left ventricular assist device at home: safe, economical, necessary. J Thorac Cardiovasc Surg. 2000;119:251–9.
6. Dowling RD, Park SJ, Pagani FD, et al. Heartmate VE LVAS design enhancements and its impact on device reliability. Eur J Cardiothorac Surg. 2004;25(6): 958–63.
7. Frazier OH. The development of an implantable, portable, electrically powered left ventricular assist device. Semin Thorac Cardiovasc Surg. 1994;6:181–7.
8. Oz MC, Rose EA, Levin HR. Selection criteria for placement of left ventricular assist devices. Am Heart J. 1995;129:173–7.
9. Deng MC, Loebe M, El Banayosy A, et al. Mechanical circulatory support for advanced heart failure: effect of patient selection on outcome. Circulation. 2001;103:231–7.
10. Dang NC, Topkara VK, Leacche M, et al. Left ventricular assist device implantation after acute anterior wall myocardial infarction and cardiogenic shock: a two-center study. J Thorac Cardiovasc Surg. 2005;130(3):693–8.
11. Topkara VK, Dang NC, Barili F, et al. Ventricular assist device use for the treatment of acute viral myocarditis. J Thorac Cardiovasc Surg. 2006;131(5):1190–1.
12. Farrar DJ, Hill JD, Gray LA, et al. Successful biventricular circulatory support as a bridge to cardiac transplantation during prolonged ventricular fibrillation and asystole. Circulation. 1989;80: III147–51.
13. Kherani AR, Cheema FH, Oz MC, et al. Implantation of a left ventricular assist device and the hub-and-spoke system in treating acute cardiogenic shock: who survives? J Thorac Cardiovasc Surg. 2003;126(5):1634–5.
14. Oz MC, Argenziano M, Catanese KA, et al. Bridge experience with long-term implantable left ventricular assist devices. Are they an alternative to transplantation? Circulation. 1997;95:1844–52.
15. Park SJ, Tector A, Piccioni W, et al. Left ventricular assist devices as destination therapy: a new look at survival. J Thorac Cardiovasc Surg. 2005;129(1): 9–17.
16. Kormos RL, Murali S, Dew MA, et al. Chronic mechanical circulatory support: rehabilitation, low morbidity, and superior survival. Ann Thorac Surg. 1994;57:51–7.
17. Sun BC, Catanese KA, Spanier TB, et al. 100 long-term implantable left ventricular assist devices: the Columbia Presbyterian interim experience. Ann Thorac Surg. 1999;68:688–94.
18. Ashton RC, Goldstein DJ, Rose EA, et al. Duration of left ventricular assist device support affects transplant survival. J Heart Lung Transplant. 1996;15:1151–7.
19. Morgan JA, Flannery MF, Kherani AR, et al. Effects of changes in UNOS policy regarding left ventricular assist devices. J Heart Lung Transplant. 2004;23(5): 621–3.
20. Morgan JA, Park Y, Kherani AR, et al. Does bridging to transplant with a left ventricular assist device adversely affect post-transplant survival? A comparative analysis of mechanical versus inotropic support. J Thorac Cardiovasc Surg. 2003;126(4):1188–90.
21. Deng MC, Weyand M, Hammel D, et al. Selection and outcome of ventricular assist device patients: the Muenster experience. J Heart Lung Transplant. 1998; 17:817–25.
22. Oz MC, Goldstein DJ, Pepino P, et al. Screening scale predicts patients successfully receiving long-term implantable left ventricular assist devices. Circulation. 1995;92:II169–73.
23. Rao V, Oz MC, Flannery MA, et al. Revised screening scale to predict survival after insertion of a left ventricular assist device. J Thorac Cardiovasc Surg. 2003;125:855–62.
24. Dang NC, Topkara VK, Mercando M, et al. Right heart failure after left ventricular assist device implantation in patients with chronic congestive heart failure. J Heart Lung Transplant. 2006;25(1):1–6.
25. Fukamachi K, McCarthy PM, Smedira NG, et al. Preoperative risk factors for right ventricular failure after implantable left ventricular assist device insertion. Ann Thorac Surg. 1999;68:2181–4.
26. Topkara VK, Dang NC, Barili F, et al. Predictors and outcomes of continuous veno-venous hemodialysis use after implantation of a left ventricular assist device. J Heart Lung Transplant. 2006;25(4):404–8.
27. Topkara VK, Dang NC, Martens TP, et al. Bridging to transplantation with left ventricular assist devices: outcomes in patients aged 60 years and older. J Thorac Cardiovasc Surg. 2005;130(3):881–2.
28. Schulman AR, Martens TP, Christos PJ, et al. Comparisons of infection complications between continuous flow and pulsatile flow left ventricular assist devices. J Thorac Cardiovasc Surg. 2007;133(3):841–2.
29. Argenziano M, Catanese KA, Moazami N, et al. The influence of infection on survival and successful transplantation in patients with left ventricular assist devices. J Heart Lung Transplant. 1997;16:822–31.
30. Morgan JA, John R, Lee BJ, et al. Is severe right ventricular failure in LVAD recipients a risk factor for unsuccessful bridging to transplant and post-transplant mortality. Ann Thorac Surg. 2004;77(3):859–63.
31. Farrar DJ. The thoratec ventricular assist device: a paracorporeal pump for treating acute and chronic heart failure. Semin Thorac Cardiovasc Surg. 2000; 12:243–50.
32. Farrar DJ, Hill JD, Pennington DG, et al. Preoperative and postoperative comparison of patients with univentricular and biventricular support with the thoratec ventricular assist device as a bridge to cardiac

transplantation. J Thorac Cardiovasc Surg. 1997;113: 202–9.
33. Samuels LE, Holmes EC, Hagan K, et al. The Thoratec Implantable Ventricular Assist Device (IVAD): initial clinical experience. Heart Surg Forum. 2006;9(4): E690–2.
34. Slaughter MS, Tsui SS, El-Banayosy A, et al. Results of a multicenter clinical trial with the Thoratec Implantable Ventricular Assist Device. J Thorac Cardiovasc Surg. 2007;133(6):1573–80.
35. Sezai A, Shiono M, Orime Y, et al. Major organ function under mechanical support: comparative studies of pulsatile and nonpulsatile circulation. Artif Organs. 1999;23:280–5.
36. Feller ED, Sorensen EN, Haddad M, et al. Clinical outcomes are similar in pulsatile and nonpulsatile left ventricular assist device recipients. Ann Thorac Surg. 2007;83(3):1082–8.
37. Frazier OH, Gemmato C, Myers TJ, et al. Initial clinical experience with the HeartMate II axial-flow left ventricular assist device. Tex Heart Inst J. 2007; 34(3):275–81.
38. Miller LW, Pagani FD, Russell SD, et al. HeartMate II clinical investigators. Use of a continuous-flow device in patients awaiting heart transplantation. N Engl J Med. 2007;357(9):885–96.
39. Pagani FD, Miller LW, Russell SD, et al. Extended mechanical circulatory support with a continuous flow rotary left ventricular assist device. J Am Coll Cardiol. 2009;54(9):312–21.
40. Frazier OH, Gregoric ID, Cohn WE. Initial experience with non-thoracic, extraperitoneal, off-pump insertion of the Jarvik 2000 Heart in patients with previous median sternotomy. J Heart Lung Transplant. 2006;25(5):499–503.
41. Frazier OH, Shah NA, Myers TJ, et al. Use of the Flowmaker (Jarvik 2000) left ventricular assist device for destination therapy and bridging to transplantation. Cardiology. 2004;101(1–3):111–6.
42. Siegenthaler MP, Frazier OH, Beyersdorf F, et al. Mechanical reliability of the Jarvik 2000 Heart. Ann Thorac Surg. 2006;81(5):1752–9.
43. Farrar DJ, Bourque K, Dague CP, et al. Design features, developmental status, and experimental results with the Heartmate III centrifugal left ventricular assist system with a magnetically levitated rotor. ASAIO J. 2007;53(3):310–5.
44. Bourque K, Gernes DB, Loree HM, et al. HeartMate III: pump design for a centrifugal LVAD with a magnetically levitated rotor. ASAIO J. 2001;47(4):401–5.
45. Wood C, Maiorana A, Larbalestier R, et al. First successful bridge to myocardial recovery with a HeartWare HVAD. J Heart Lung Transplant. 2008; 27(6):695–7.
46. Tuzun E, Roberts K, Cohn WE, et al. In vivo evaluation of the HeartWare centrifugal ventricular assist device. Tex Heart Inst J. 2007;34(4):406–11.
47. Morley D, Litwak K, Ferber P, et al. Hemodynamic effects of partial ventricular support in chronic heart failure: results of simulation validated with in vivo data. J Thorac Cardiovasc Surg. 2007;133(1):21–8.
48. Chang JC, Sawa Y, Ohtake S, et al. Hemodynamic effect of inhaled nitric oxide in dilated cardiomyopathy patients on LVAD support. ASAIO J. 1997;43:M418–21.
49. Salamonsen RF, Kaye D, Esmore DS. Inhalation of nitric oxide provides selective pulmonary vasodilatation, aiding mechanical cardiac assist with thoratec left ventricular assist device. Anaesth Intensive Care. 1994;22:209–10.
50. Argenziano M, Choudhri AF, Oz MC, et al. A prospective randomized trial of arginine vasopressin in the treatment of vasodilatory shock after left ventricular assist device placement. Circulation. 1997;96:II90.
51. Pennock JL, Pierce WS, Wisman CB, et al. Survival and complications following ventricular assist pumping for cardiogenic shock. Ann Surg. 1983;198:469–78.
52. Morgan JA, Park Y, Oz MC, et al. Device-related infections while on LVAD support do not adversely impact bridging to transplant or post-transplant survival. ASAIO J. 2003;49(6):748–50.
53. Morgan JA, Oz MC. Cost-effectiveness of ventricular assist devices. Expert Rev Pharmacoecon Outcomes Res. 2003;3(4):427–32.
54. DiGiorgi PL, Reel MS, Thornton B, et al. Heart transplant and left ventricular assist device costs. J Heart Lung Transplant. 2005;24(2):200–4.
55. Rose EA, Levin HR, Oz MC, et al. Artificial circulatory support with textured interior surfaces. A counterintuitive approach to minimizing thromboembolism. Circulation. 1994;90:II87–91.

Ventricular Assist Devices for Destination Therapy

11

Sanjeev Aggarwal and Mark S. Slaughter

Introduction

Heart failure continues to be an ever-growing public health concern facing our country today. The continued aging of the population has contributed to the increasing incidence and prevalence of heart failure. Presently, approximately five million people are affected, with over 500,000 new cases diagnosed each year. Economically, this represents over 30 billion dollars in health-care spending annually [1, 2].

Despite advances in the understanding of the neurohormonal changes involved in the progression of heart failure and improvements in medical management, the natural history of the disease dictates a dismal prognosis. In the Framingham Study cohort, overt congestive heart failure led to a median survival of 1.7 years in men and 3.2 years in women, with 5-year survival rates in men and women of 25 % and 38 %, respectively [3]. In patients suffering from American Heart Association (AHA) Stage D heart failure who are inotrope dependent, Hershberger and colleagues reported a median survival of 3.4 months and a 12-month survival of only 6 % [4]. Overall, it is estimated that congestive heart failure is responsible for approximately 250,000 deaths per year [5]. Cardiac transplantation has been regarded as the "gold standard" treatment for end-stage heart failure. However, limitations of donor organs have relegated transplantation as a viable option for only a very small percentage of this growing population. Over the past decade, the number of transplants being performed annually has remained between 3,000 and 4,000 worldwide, with a decreasing trend noted in recent years [6]. In addition, cardiac transplant is typically offered to patients less than 65 years of age. Heart failure is seen in all age groups but is increasingly common with older age having a prevalence of over 10 % in patients greater than 65 years. Demographic studies indicate that the continued aging of the population will lead to a doubling of this sector of the population over the next 20 years. Cardiac transplant is a viable option for only a minority of patients needing cardiac replacement therapy and will likely continue to have a limited impact on the epidemiology of heart failure in the future.

Ventricular assist device (VAD) therapy has emerged as an important modality in the treatment of end-stage heart failure, both as a bridge to transplantation (BTT) and as permanent or "destination" therapy for patients who are not candidates for cardiac transplantation. While there has been widespread use of devices for

S. Aggarwal, M.D.
Department of Cardiothoracic Surgery, Saint Luke's Mid America Heart Institute, 4320 Wornall Road, Suite 50-II, Kansas City, MO 64111, USA
e-mail: saggarwal@mahls.com

M.S. Slaughter, M.D. (✉)
Division Thoracic and Cardiovascular Surgery, University of Louisville, 201 Abraham Flexner Way, Suite 1200, Louisville, KY 40202, USA
e-mail: mscabg@gmail.com

J.A. Morgan and Y. Naka (eds.), *Surgical Treatment for Advanced Heart Failure*, DOI 10.1007/978-1-4614-6919-3_11,

BTT, the experience with destination therapy has been more limited. The feasibility of a mechanical-based approach to the treatment of end-stage heart failure was validated by the REMATCH (Randomized Evaluation of Mechanical Assistance for the Treatment of Congestive Heart Failure) trial in 2001 [7]. This prospective trial randomized 129 patients suffering from New York Heart Association class IV heart failure to receive either optimal medical management or implantation of a first-generation pulsatile left ventricular assist device (LVAD). Patients receiving an LVAD demonstrated a significant survival benefit in patients receiving an LVAD for the treatment of end-stage heart failure when compared to medical management alone. At the same time, the limitations of device technology were highlighted by the incidence of adverse events related to mechanical support, such as infection, device failure, and thromboembolic events.

Other trials comparing LVAD therapy with optimal medical management have shown a similar survival benefit [8, 9]. Since the conclusion of REMATCH trial, improvements in survival have been achieved through improvements in first-generation device design, patient selection, and management [10–13]. A recent report by Long and colleagues describes more contemporary results of destination therapy utilizing first-generation LVAD technology [14]. In this series, the 1- and 2-year survival rates were 77 %. While these trials have shown a clear survival benefit, particularly in patients who are inotrope dependent [15], there still is a marked discrepancy between those that could potentially benefit from mechanical circulatory support as destination therapy and those that actually are offered and receive this therapy. Device-related adverse events and limitations in first-generation device durability have hindered device therapy from gaining widespread acceptance as destination therapy.

The emergence of second- and third-generation devices utilizing continuous-flow technology represents a significant advancement in addressing the limitations of pulsatile volume displacement devices. These devices offer the advantage of being smaller in size with smaller percutaneous leads, do not require valves, and have fewer moving parts with enhanced durability. A recent trial utilizing the HeartMate II axial flow device in a bridge-to-transplant population demonstrated improved durability and decreased infectious complications [16]. The need for chronic anticoagulation therapy with continuous-flow devices was reflected in the incidence of bleeding complications. Third-generation devices utilizing bearing-less configurations through magnetic or hydrodynamic levitation offer the potential for further enhanced durability with no contacting parts. Several third-generation devices are currently in clinical trials. Continued technological developments and improvements in device design, peripherals, and energy sources are necessary for mechanical circulatory support to become an effective means of long-term destination therapy.

Current Status of Destination Therapy

Following the results of the REMATCH trial, the use of LVADs as destination therapy was granted approval by the Food and Drug Administration (FDA) in November of 2002. Guidelines for approved destination therapy centers were outlined by the Centers for Medicare and Medicaid Services (CMS) [17]. In addition, a consensus statement regarding the requirements of centers performing destination therapy was released by the International Society of Heart and Lung Transplantation [18]. In an effort to facilitate data collection and further research efforts, the Interagency Registry for Mechanically Assisted Circulatory Support (INTERMACS) was created as a collaborative effort between the National Heart, Lung, and Blood Institute (NHLBI), CMS, the FDA, and the United Network for Organ Sharing (UNOS). As of August 2007, 68 centers have received CMS approval for destination therapy [19].

Despite these important regulatory advances, there remains a significant discrepancy between the number of patients that could benefit from mechanical circulatory support and those that actually are offered and receive LVADs. A recent analysis from the National Inpatient Sample identified approximately 300,000 patients admitted with a diagnosis of congestive heart failure or cardiogenic shock. Of these patients, only 291 underwent LVAD implantation. Factors identified as having a negative impact for device use included age greater than 65, female gender, race, geographic region, and admission to a nonacademic center [20].

Several barriers exist to the widespread acceptance of device therapy. The past several years have seen rapid progress in field of LVADs with regard to device development and patient management. Much of the contemporary data and outcomes, however, have not been disseminated to "gatekeeper" medical personnel who care for these patients. As a result, the use of mechanical support as part of the treatment armamentarium for advanced heart failure has not gained widespread acceptance, preventing in many cases the timely referral of these patients to specialized centers.

Economic and infrastructure barriers also exist. The effective care of advanced heart failure patients often requires significant resources in the form of specialized personnel, facility infrastructure, and ancillary services. As a result, the number of centers that are able to offer VAD therapy has been limited, making accessibility difficult for a significant portion of the heart failure population. Establishment of regional referral networks is necessary to make this care accessible to a greater number of patients. Greater emphasis and resources must be placed towards the development of such organized networks so that patients can be offered this potential lifesaving therapy.

The costs associated with device implantation and the perioperative care of device patients remain significant [21–23]. However, as experience has been gained in recent years, the cost for device therapy has declined. Miller and colleagues reported the hospital costs associated with patients receiving devices in the post-REMATCH era and found a 40 % reduction in cost from implantation to hospital discharge ($128,084 versus $210,187). In addition, there was a trend towards decreased length of stay and improved survival to discharge [24]. The cost associated with device therapy must also be evaluated in the context of the cost associated with medical therapy for patients suffering end-stage heart failure. A recent analysis of the expense associated with patients treated in the medical arm of the REMATCH trial demonstrated a mean cost of $156,169 expended in the last 2 years of life, with greater than 50 % of the cost incurred during the final 6 months of life [25]. A majority of the expense in the final 6 months of life was associated with inpatient costs. Thus, medical therapy in end-stage heart failure is also associated with significant expense but with inferior survival and quality-of-life outcomes when compared to LVAD therapy.

Patient Selection and Risk Stratification

Appropriate patient selection represents one the most critical determinants of successful outcomes with VAD therapy. The perioperative and long-term risks of device implantation must be weighed against the potential survival and quality-of-life benefit with mechanical support. Patient selection criteria must not be so stringent as to exclude ill patients that may benefit from device therapy, while at the same time avoiding high perioperative mortality rates by the inclusion of patients that have prohibitive risk. Complications associated with LVAD therapy that may limit its effectiveness include device failure, post-implant right ventricular failure, infection and sepsis, bleeding, and thromboembolism. Risk stratification systems such as the Heart Failure Survival Score and the Seattle Heart Failure Score are useful in identifying patients who may benefit from support with a VAD [26, 27]. VADs have been used to treat a wide variety of disease processes leading to both acute and chronic forms of heart failure including cardiogenic shock associated with myocardial infarction, postcardiotomy shock, myocarditis, and chronic ischemic and nonischemic cardiomyopathies.

Several reports have sought to identify significant preoperative variables that may predict risk and impact outcomes. The revised Columbia screening scale published in 2003 offers a way of stratifying the risk for LVAD therapy based on several clinical factors: mechanical ventilation, postcardiotomy, prior LVAD insertion, central venous pressure (CVP) >16 mmHg, and prothrombin time >16 s [28]. Each factor is given a weight, with a cumulative score of >5 predicting an operative mortality of 46 % versus a mortality rate of 12 % for a score ≤5. McCarthy and colleagues previously reported the results of 100 patients undergoing LVAD implantation [29]. In this group of patients, preoperative factors that increased the risk of death by univariate analysis included the need for mechanical ventilation or extracorporeal membrane oxygenation (ECMO), low pulmonary arterial pressures, and elevations in bilirubin, blood urea nitrogen, and creatinine. Deng et al. reported the results of 464 patients undergoing implantation of the Novacor left ventricular assist system (LVAS). Sepsis associated with respiratory failure, preoperative right heart failure, age >65 years, acute postcardiotomy state, and acute infarction were independent risk factors for death by multivariate analysis [30].

More contemporary risk models include those by Lietz et al. and by Matthews et al. [31, 32]. The risk model by Lietz and colleagues specifically looks at early survival in patients undergoing LVAD implantation for destination therapy. In this study, predictors of 90-day in-hospital mortality included the following: platelet count $\leq 148 \times 10^3/\mu L$, serum albumin ≤3.3 g/dl, INR >1.1, mean pulmonary pressure ≤25.3 mmHg, vasodilator therapy at time of implantation, AST >45 U/dl, hematocrit <34 %, BUN >51 U/dl, and lack of intravenous inotropic support. The Matthews risk score was developed to assess the risk of right ventricle (RV) failure but additionally describes the risk of early mortality following LVAD implantation. Patients identified to be at high risk for postoperative RV failure in this model were also found to be at increased risk for postoperative death following LVAD implantation.

The CMS established guidelines for destination therapy (DT) eligibility. Patient selection criteria are very similar to inclusion criteria established for the REMATCH trial, thus selecting for patients in class IV heart failure at the end stage of their disease. The timing of device therapy relative to the stage and severity of heart failure has a significant impact on long-term outcomes, with worsening survival seen as device therapy is instituted later in the progression of heart failure [33, 34]. Implementation of device therapy for destination therapy earlier in the progression of heart failure, before significant end-organ dysfunction, right ventricular failure, and cachexia have developed, will likely lead to improved outcomes.

Complications

In the early experience with LVADs for destination therapy there were frequent complications due to the severity of illness at the time of implantation and the durability of the first-generation pulsatile devices. The more common complications that contributed to death or a diminished quality of life included device failure, right ventricular failure, infection, bleeding, and thromboembolism.

Destination therapy by definition is an implantable LVAD used for lifelong support in patients with end-stage heart failure that are not transplant candidates. Thus, identifying patients at risk for postoperative RV failure is paramount and has important implications for selecting candidates for destination therapy. Approximately 20–30 % of patients undergoing left VAD placement will have postoperative right heart dysfunction [29, 35, 36]. Several studies have identified a variety of preoperative variables associated with postoperative RV failure. Ochiai et al., in an analysis of 245 patients undergoing LVAD placement, found preoperative circulatory support, female gender, and nonischemic etiology for heart failure as risks for postoperative RV failure requiring RVAD placement. In addition, hemodynamic parameters associated with RVAD use were low mean and diastolic pulmonary arterial pressures, low right ventricular stroke work (RVSW), and low RVSW index (RVSWI), most likely identifying patients with impaired RV contractility. Elevated pulmonary vascular resistance and pulmonary arterial pressures were not identified as risk factors [37]. Similar findings have been previously reported [38].

More recently, the right ventricular failure risk score (RVFRS), developed by Matthews and colleagues at the University of Michigan, provides a way of stratifying risk of postoperative RV failure [32]. Utilizing information from a prospectively collected database, 197 LVAD implants were examined. Right ventricular dysfunction was found in 35 % of cases. Independent predictors of RV failure were the preoperative requirement of a vasopressor, aspartate aminotransferase (AST) ≥80 IU/l, bilirubin ≥2.0 mg/dl, and serum creatinine of ≥2.3 mg/dl. Each clinical predictor was assigned a point score and a cumulative risk score was then derived. Survival to transplantation and overall survival declined as the RVFRS increased, again confirming the negative impact of postoperative RV failure on outcomes following LVAD implantation. Fitzpatrick and colleagues recently analyzed a series of 266 LVAD recipients looking for preoperative variables that would predict the need for biventricular mechanical circulatory support. These included low cardiac index, RV stroke work index, severe preoperative RV dysfunction, preoperative creatinine, previous cardiac surgery, and systolic blood pressure [39].

Infection remains a significant source of morbidity and mortality in patients receiving mechanical circulatory support. In the REMATCH trial, the leading cause of death in patients receiving devices was sepsis, accounting for 20 of 52 deaths in this group [7]. A subsequent analysis focusing on infection during the REMATCH trial showed that freedom from sepsis in patients with LVADs was 58 % at 1 year and 48 % at 2 years. The peak hazard for sepsis occurred early within 30 days from implantation [40]. In a recent trial reporting the use of the HeartMate II second-generation axial flow device (Thoratec Inc, Pleasanton, CA) in a bridge-to-transplant population, results are more encouraging. Device-related infection was seen in 14 % of patients. All device infections involved the percutaneous lead, with no infections seen in the pump pocket. Localized infection not related to device placement was seen in 28 % of recipients [16]. Nutritional optimization in the perioperative period is an important factor in preventing infectious complications. VAD patients are often malnourished and cachectic due to problems of anorexia, impaired gastrointestinal function due to low cardiac output, and a chronic catabolic state secondary to the neurohumoral changes associated with heart failure. As has been described, an interdisciplinary approach to nutritional assessment and management is highly effective [41]. Guidelines regarding the use of perioperative antibiotics have been previously reported [42]. In general, prophylaxis is directed toward common pathogens, such as staphylococci, as well as providing gram-negative coverage. Cooperation with infectious disease specialists is helpful in custom tailoring regiments based on sensitivities within a given institution.

Mediastinal bleeding following LVAD implantation is relatively common, occurring in some series in as many as 48 % of patients [29, 43]. In the recent continuous-flow LVAD trial, bleeding was the most common adverse event, seen once again primarily in the early postoperative period (0–30 days) [16]. Reoperation was required in 31 % of patients. This is likely a reflection of the severity of illness in this patient population and the need for postoperative anticoagulation with heparin and warfarin when using continuous-flow devices. Predisposing factors include passive hepatic congestion and impaired production of coagulation factors, compromised nutritional status, use of preoperative anticoagulation, extensive surgical dissection, and reoperative procedures. In addition, LVAD patients develop a coagulopathy secondary to interactions between circulating blood elements and the artificial device surfaces [44]. The development of acquired von Willebrand disease following device placement has also been described [45]. Preoperatively, every effort is made to normalize the coagulation profile. Diuresis with relief of hepatic congestion, administration of fresh frozen plasma, and vitamin K supplementation can all be utilized. If possible, anticoagulants such as warfarin and clopidogrel should be discontinued at least five days prior to surgery. A low threshold should be maintained for early re-exploration with excessive postoperative bleeding. Cardiac tamponade results in impaired right ventricular function, with subsequent decreased LVAD filling and reduced pump flows. Early reoperation also allows for evacuation of mediastinal and pump pocket hematoma which can serve as a nidus for infection.

Thromboembolic events can lead to devastating neurologic and end-organ injury and remain a concern in patients undergoing mechanical device placement. In the past, as many as one third of patients with an LVAD had a thromboembolic event [46]. There has been significant improvement since then due to improved technology and patient management. In the REMATCH trial, the rate of neurologic events was 4.35 times higher than in the medically treated group, with 47 % of such events being transient [7]. Difficulty in accurately comparing the incidence of thromboembolism among different devices is partly due to inconsistent definitions, as described by Pasque and Rogers [47]. The HeartMate XVE (Thoratec Inc., Pleasanton, CA), with its sintered titanium and textured polyurethane internal surfaces, has a relatively low incidence of thromboembolic events without the need for systemic anticoagulation with heparin or warfarin. Second- and third-generation rotary pumps usually require systemic anticoagulation to maintain an international normalized ratio (INR) between 2.0 and 3.0. In addition, depending on the system used, many patients are maintained on antiplatelet therapy with aspirin, dipyridamole, or clopidogrel. Pump thrombosis remains a potential mode of device failure with continuous-flow devices and can lead to thromboembolic complications. In the recent HeartMate II trial, the incidence of stroke was 8 % (6 % ischemic, 2 % hemorrhagic), and the incidence of transient ischemic attacks was 4 % [16]. Vigilant control of anticoagulation parameters is necessary to balance the risk of thrombus formation with the threat of late mediastinal bleeding.

Device Development

Efforts to improve device durability and maximize freedom from mechanical failure have been a major impetus for the evolution of device technology. Minimizing the risk of device failure is critical in establishing mechanical support as a feasible option for providing long-term support as destination therapy. First-generation LVADs such as the HeartMate XVE utilize pusher plate technology to generate pulsatile flow through displacement of blood volume. An extensive clinical experience has been accumulated worldwide with the use of pulsatile devices, particularly for bridge to cardiac transplantation. The design requires the devices to be somewhat large in size to accommodate the blood chamber, often precluding use in patients with a BSA of less than 1.5. Significant surgical dissection is usually required to create the device pocket. In addition, there are several moving and contacting parts, as well as inflow and outflow valves to maintain unidirectional flow. The percutaneous driveline is relatively large in size when compared to newer generation devices to accommodate both the electrical connections and the venting of air for the pumping chamber. Device failure can occur at any one of the components of the system. These include the inflow and outflow conduits, the pumping chamber, or the external peripherals. In the event of electrical failure of the device, the pusher plate can be driven pneumatically with either a hand pump or a pneumatic console. Due to the various sources of mechanical failure, durability is limited. In the REMATCH trial, device failure was the second most common cause of death behind sepsis [7]. While 1-year freedom from device failure and replacement was 87 %, this dropped off to 37 % by the second year [7, 48].

The development of continuous-flow LVADs represents a significant step towards addressing the shortcomings of first-generation technology. Many second-generation LVADs utilize an axial flow design with a rotating impeller to provide continuous non-pulsatile blood flow without the need for inflow or outflow valves. Although early concerns existed regarding the effects of non-physiologic continuous blood flow, studies have shown no adverse impact on end-organ function or ventricular unloading and remodeling [49–51]. Compared to pulsatile VADs, these devices offer the advantage of being smaller in size (Fig. 11.1).

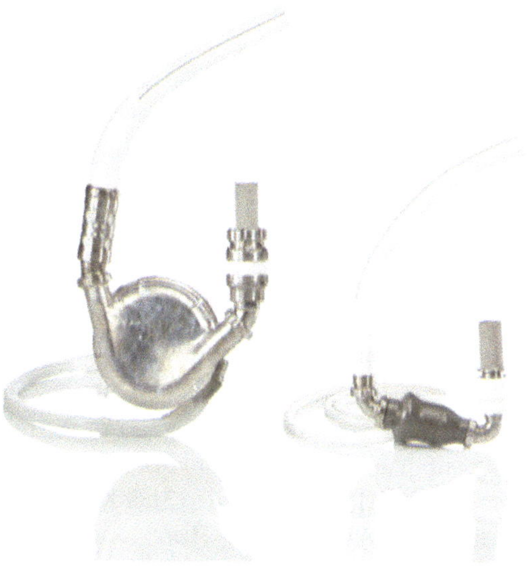

Fig. 11.1 The HeartMate XVE (Thoratec Inc., Pleasanton, CA) first-generation pulsatile LVAD and HeartMate II axial flow LVAD. (Courtesy of Thoratec Corp., used with permission.)

They also have fewer moving and contacting parts with potentially enhanced durability. In addition, there is no need for venting of the device, allowing for smaller percutaneous drivelines. Typically, such devices have a single moving component, the rotating impeller, which is suspended in place by contacting bearings. Early clinical experiences with devices such as the HeartMate II have been very promising with regard to device reliability and short- and mid-term outcomes [52, 53]. In the HeartMate II bridge-to-transplant trial, there were no primary pump failures [16].

Several LVADs with third-generation design have entered clinical trials. These include the HVAD (HeartWare Corp., Framingham, MA), the Duraheart (Terumo Heart Inc., Ann Arbor, MI), the Levacor VAD (World Heart Corp., Salt Lake City, Utah), and the VentrAssist device (Thoratec Corp., Pleasanton, CA) Figs. 11.2. In a recent review, third-generation devices were characterized by a noncontact bearing design, in contrast to second-generation axial flow devices which have a contact bearing configuration [54]. Noncontact design is achieved by suspension of the rotor using either magnetic or hydrodynamic levitation, or a combination of both. The theoretical advantage is the elimination of contacting parts and friction wear, with even greater potential for improved long-term durability. These devices also offer the advantages of small size and small percutaneous drivelines. The HeartWare HVAD is small enough in size to be implanted completely within the pericardial space, eliminating the need for a preperitoneal pocket. Third-generation design offers the promise of additional improvements in long-term device reliability, an important factor in achieving greater acceptance of LVADs for destination therapy.

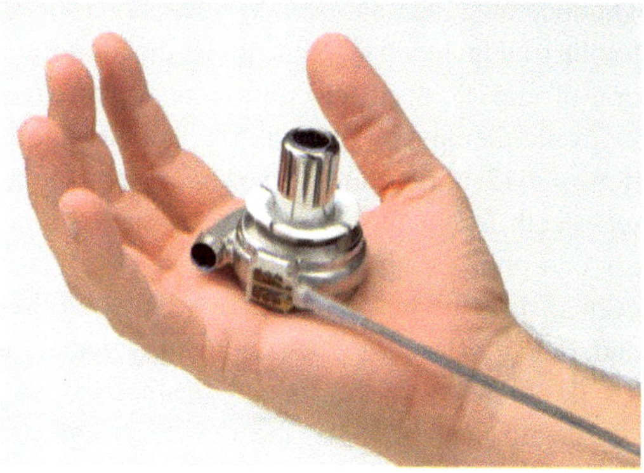

Fig. 11.2 The HeartWare HVAD (HeartWare Corp., Framingham, MA). (Courtesy of HeartWare Inc., used with permission.)

Current Outcomes

The REMATCH trial established definitively the survival and quality-of-life benefit with mechanical circulatory support for the treatment of end-stage heart failure [7]. The limitations of first-generation device therapy, however, were highlighted by the increased incidence of adverse events in LVAD patients. In this trial, 129 patients suffering from New York Heart Association (NYHA) class IV heart failure who were not candidates for cardiac transplantation were randomized to either optimal medical management or placement of a left VAD (HeartMate VE LVAD,

Thoratec Inc., Pleasanton, CA). Inclusion criteria for the trial included left ventricular ejection fraction of <25 %, need for continuous intravenous inotropic therapy, and a peak oxygen consumption of <12 ml/kg/min. The primary end point was death from any cause, with several secondary end points such as the incidence of adverse events, days of hospitalization, quality of life, and functional status. Device therapy led to a 48 % reduction in the risk of death from any cause. Survival rates for the device group and medically treated group at 1 year were 52 % and 25 %, respectively, and 23 % and 8 % at 2 years. In addition, assessments of quality of life and functional status were significantly better in the device group. The probability of device failure was 35 % at 2 years, with ten patients in the trial requiring device exchange.

During the course of the REMATCH trial, as clinical experience was gained and device enhancements made, outcomes improved. Park and colleagues analyzed the clinical results of patients undergoing device placement as stratified by era of the trial [10]. Patients receiving devices in the second half of the trial had 1- and 2-year survivals of 59 % and 38 %, as compared to 44 % and 21 % for patients undergoing LVAD placement in the first half of the trial. The overall rate of adverse events was also significantly lower in the late cohort of LVAD patients. This included decreased rates of sepsis, pump housing infection, renal failure, and perioperative bleeding.

Since the REMATCH trial, continued progress has been towards improving clinical results and decreasing the morbidity and mortality associated with device therapy. Lietz and coworkers reported the results of 280 patients undergoing LVAD placement for destination therapy following conclusion of the REMATCH trial [31]. The complete data of 222 of these patients was used to derive a preoperative risk score for 90-day in-hospital mortality. Using the risk score, patients were then stratified into four categories (low, medium, high, and very high risk). Overall survival in the group of post-REMATCH patients was 56 % and 31 % at 1 and 2 years, respectively. When stratified by risk categories, 1-year survival rates were 81.2 %, 62.4 %, 27.8 %, and 10.7 % for low-, medium-, high-, and very high-risk groups, respectively (Fig. 11.3). Survival to hospital discharge was 87.5 % in the low-risk group as compared to only 10.7 % in the very high-risk cohort. This analysis highlights the importance of patient selection as one of the critical determinants of successful outcomes with VAD therapy.

Long and colleagues reported their single-center experience with destination therapy [14]. When compared to the REMATCH trial, there were significantly improved survival rates of 77 % seen at 1- and 2-year follow-up (Fig. 11.4). In this group of patients, perioperative mortality was decreased to 8.1 %, compared to 31 % for patients in the REMATCH trial. There was also a significant reduction in the incidence of adverse events. Authors attributed the continuing improvement in destination therapy in the modern era to improvements in patient management, patient selection, and device design enhancements.

The development of second-generation axial flow pumps represents a significant advance in device therapy. Single-center experiences have shown reduced rates of morbidity and mortality with axial flow devices [55]. While the prediction, avoidance, and treatment of right ventricular dysfunction following LVAD placement remain a challenge, Patel and colleagues demonstrated a reduced need for RVAD implantation following LVAD placement with axial flow devices compared to pulsatile first-generation devices [56].

One of the largest clinical trials evaluating the use of mechanical circulatory support for destination therapy has recently completed enrollment. Patients in this trial were randomized to receive either the continuous-flow HeartMate II axial flow device or the pulsatile-flow HeartMate XVE LVAD in a 2:1 ratio. Preliminary results of the trial indicate significant advantages of the second-generation HeartMate II when compared to the HeartMate XVE, leading to the termination of randomization prior to completion of the trial. Several third-generation devices, as previously discussed, have entered clinical trials in the USA.

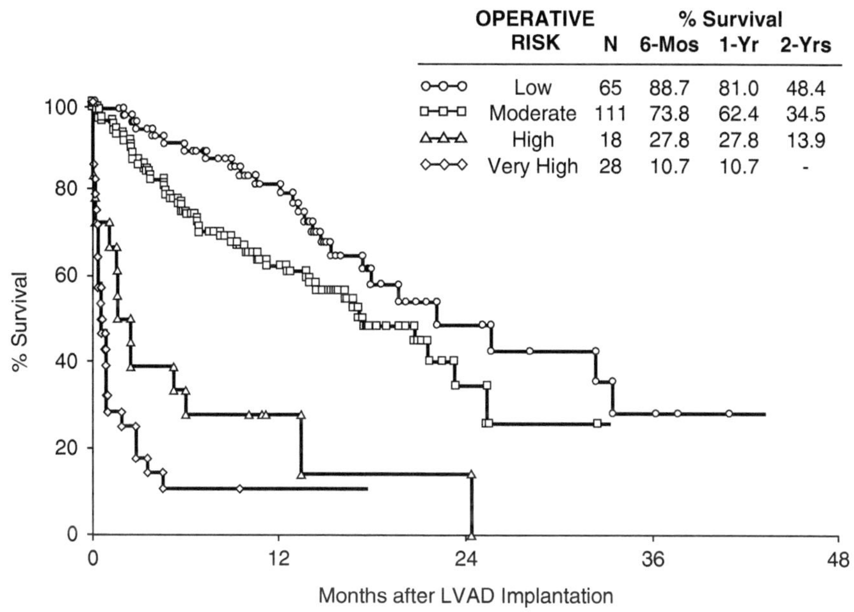

Fig. 11.3 LVAD survival stratified by DT risk score (adapted from Lietz K, Long JW, Kfoury AG, Slaughter MS, Silver MA, Milano CA, Rogers JG, Naka Y, Mancini D, Miller LW. Outcomes of left ventricular assist device implantation as destination therapy in the post-REMATCH era: implications for patient selection. Circulation. 2007; 116: 497–505.)

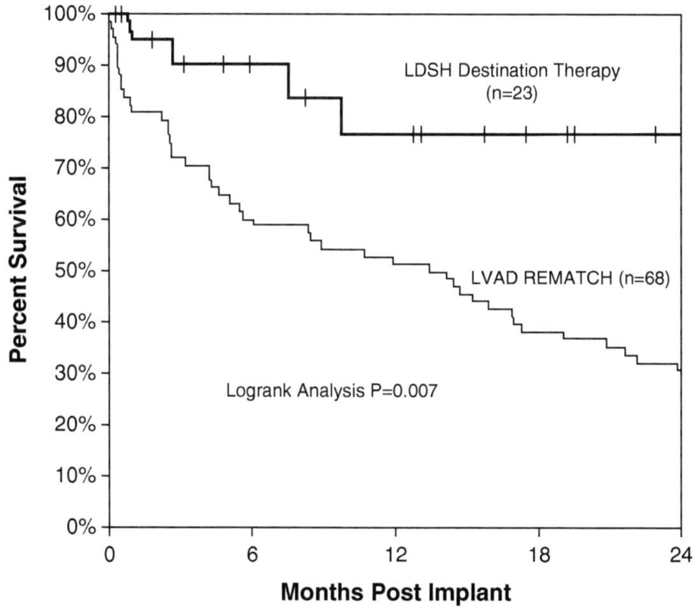

Fig. 11.4 Destination therapy survival at LDS Hospital, Salt Lake City, UT versus REMATCH trial (adapted from Long JW, Healy AH, Rasmusson BY, Cowley CG, Nelson KE, Kfoury AG, Clayson SE, Reid BB, Moore SA, Blank DU, Renlund DG. Improving outcomes with long-term "destination" therapy using left ventricular assist devices. J Thorac Cardiovasc Surg. 2008;135(6):1353–1361.)

Conclusions

VAD therapy has emerged as an important treatment option for patients suffering from end-stage heart failure. Since the results of the REMATCH trial, acceptance of LVADs as destination therapy has been slow. As experience with patient selection and management has grown and as device design has evolved, clinical outcomes with regard to survival and freedom from adverse events continue to improve. Efforts toward the development of smaller devices, transcutaneous energy sources, and minimally invasive implantation techniques are aimed at reducing complications associated with current device therapy. This will likely lead to an increase in the acceptance in the use of LVADs earlier in the progression of heart failure, potentially leading to further improvements in clinical outcomes. In addition, more widespread dissemination of the technology will improve access of therapy to the many patients who could benefit from LVAD support, likely leading to an increase in the use of devices for long-term destination therapy in patients not eligible for cardiac transplantation.

References

1. Hunt SA, Abraham WT, Chin MH, et al. ACC/AHA 2005 Guideline Update for the Diagnosis and Management of Chronic Heart Failure in the Adult-Summary Article. Circulation. 2005;112(12):1825–52.
2. Jessup M, Brozena S. Heart failure. N Engl J Med. 2003;348:2007–18.
3. Kannel WB. Incidence and epidemiology of heart failure. Heart Fail Rev. 2000;5(2):167–73.
4. Hershberger RE, Nauman D, Walker TL, et al. Care processes and clinical outcomes of continuous outpatient support with inotropes (COSI) in patients with refractory endstage heart failure. J Card Fail. 2003;9(3):180–7.
5. Gillum RF. Epidemiology of heart failure in the United States. Am Heart J. 1993;126:1042–7.
6. The International Society for Heart & Lung Transplantation. ISHLT Online. http://www.ishlt.org. Accessed 9 Jan 2013.
7. Rose EA, Gelijns AC, Moskowitz AJ, et al. Long-term use of left ventricular assist device for end-stage heart failure. N Engl J Med. 2001;345(20):1435–43.
8. Rogers JG, Butler J, Lansman SL, et al. Chronic mechanical circulatory support for inotrope-dependent heart failure patients who are not transplant candidates: results of the INTrEPID Trial. J Am Coll Cardiol. 2007;50:741–7.
9. Pae WE, Connell JM, Adelowo A, Clinical Utility Baseline Study (CUBS) Group, et al. Does total implantability reduce infection with the use of a left ventricular assist device? The LionHeart experience in Europe. J Heart Lung Transplant. 2007;26:219–29.
10. Park SJ, Tector A, Piccioni W, et al. Left ventricular assist devices as destination therapy: a new look at survival. J Thorac Cardiovasc Surg. 2005;129:9–17.
11. Dowling RD, Park SJ, Pagani FD, et al. Heartmate VE LVAS design enhancements and its impact on device reliability. Eur J Cardiothorac Surg. 2004;25:958–63.
12. Pagani FD, Long JW, Dembitsky WP, et al. Improved mechanical reliability of the Heartmate XVE left ventricular assist system. Ann Thorac Surg. 2006;82:1413–9.
13. Long JW, Kfoury AG, Slaughter MS, et al. Long-term destination therapy with the HeartMate XVE left ventricular assist device: improved outcomes since the REMATCH study. Congest Heart Fail. 2005;11:133–8.
14. Long JW, Healy AH, Rasmusson BY, et al. Improving outcomes with long-term "destination" therapy using left ventricular assist devices. J Thorac Cardiovasc Surg. 2008;135:1353–61.
15. Stevenson LW, Miller LW, Desvigne-Nickens P, et al. Left ventricular assist device as destination for patients undergoing intravenous inotropic therapy: a subset analysis from REMATCH (Randomized Evaluation of Mechanical Assistance in Treatment of Chronic Heart Failure. Circulation. 2004;110:975–81.
16. Miller LW, Pagani FD, Russell SD, et al. Use of a continuous-flow device in patients awaiting heart transplantation. N Engl J Med. 2007;357:885–96.
17. Centers for Medicare & Medicaid Services. Centers for Medicare & Medicaid Services website. http://www.cms.hhs.gov. Accessed 9 Jan 2013.
18. Deng MC, Young JB, Stevenson LW, Board of Directors of the International Society for Heart and Lung Transplantation, et al. Destination mechanical circulatory support: proposal for clinical standards. J Heart Lung Transplant. 2003;22:365–9.
19. Centers for Medicare & Medicaid Services. Medicare approved facilities/trials/registries. http://www.cms.hhs.gov/MedicareApprovedFacilitie/VAD/list.asp. Accessed 9 Jan 2013.
20. Joyce DL, Conte JV, Russell SD, et al. Disparities in access to left ventricular assist device therapy. J Surg Res. 2009;152:111–7.
21. Dembitsky WP. REMATCH and beyond: the cost of treating heart failure using an implantable left ventricular assist device. Semin Cardiothorac Vasc Anesth. 2006;10:253–5.
22. Clegg AJ, Scott DA, Loveman E, et al. The clinical and cost-effectiveness of left ventricular assist devices

for end-stage heart failure: a systematic review and economic evaluation. Health Technol Assess. 2005;9: 1–148.
23. Oz MC, Gelijns AC, Miller LW, et al. Left ventricular assist device as permanent heart failure therapy: the price of progress. Ann Surg. 2003;238:577–85.
24. Miller LW, Nelson KE, Bostic RR, et al. Hospital costs for left ventricular assist devices for destination therapy: lower costs for implantation in the post-REMATCH era. J Heart Lung Transplant. 2006;25: 778–84.
25. Russo MJ, Gelijns AC, Stevenson LW, et al. The cost of medical management in advanced heart failure during the final two years of life. J Cardiac Fail. 2008;14:651–8.
26. Levy WC, Mozaffarian D, Linker DT, et al. The Seattle Heart Failure Model: prediction of survival in heart failure. Circulation. 2006;113:1424–33.
27. Aaronson KD, Schwartz JS, Chen TM, et al. Development and prospective validation of a clinical index to predict survival in ambulatory patients referred for cardiac transplant evaluation. Circulation. 1997;95:2597–9.
28. Rao V, Oz MC, Flannery MA, et al. Revised screening scale to predict survival after insertion of a left ventricular assist device. J Thorac Cardiovasc Surg. 2003;125(4):855–62.
29. McCarthy PM, Smedira NO, Vargo RL, et al. One hundred patients with the Heartmate left ventricular assist device: evolving concepts and technology. J Thorac Cardiovasc Surg. 1998;115(4):904–12.
30. Deng MC, Loebe M, El-Banayosy A, et al. Mechanical circulatory support for advanced heart failure: effect of patient selection on outcome. Circulation. 2001;103:231–7.
31. Lietz K, Long JW, Kfoury AG, et al. Outcomes of left ventricular assist device implantation as destination therapy in the post-REMATCH era: implications for patient selection. Circulation. 2007;116:497–505.
32. Matthews JC, Koelling TM, Pagani FD, et al. The right ventricular failure risk score: a pre-operative tool for assessing the risk of right ventricular failure in left ventricular assist device candidates. J Am Coll Cardiol. 2008;51:2163–72.
33. UAB School of Medicine. Interagency Registry for Mechanically Assisted Circulatory Support. http://www.intermacs.org. Accessed 9 Jan 2013.
34. Lietz K, Miller LW. Destination therapy: current results and future promise. Semin Thorac Cardiovasc Surg. 2008;20:225–33.
35. Goldstein DJ, Oz MC, Rose EA, et al. Implantable left ventricular assist devices. N Engl J Med. 1998;339: 1522–33.
36. Kavarana MN, Pessin-Minsley MS, Urtecho J, et al. Right ventricular dysfunction and organ failure in left ventricular assist device recipients: a continuing problem. Ann Thorac Surg. 2002;73:745–50.
37. Ochiai Y, McCarthy PM, Smedira NG, et al. Predictors of severe right ventricular failure after implantable left ventricular assist device insertion: analysis of 245 patients. Circulation. 2002;106(Suppl I):I198–202.
38. Fukamachi K, McCarthy PM, Smedira NG, et al. Preoperative risk factors for right ventricular failure after implantable left ventricular assist device insertion. Ann Thorac Surg. 1999;68:2181–4.
39. Fitzpatrick JR, Frederick JR, Hsu VM, et al. Risk score derived from pre-operative data analysis predicts the need for biventricular mechanical circulatory support. J Heart Lung Transplant. 2008;27:1286–92.
40. Holman WL, Park SJ, Long JW, et al. Infection in permanent circulatory support: experience from the REMATCH trial. J Heart Lung Transplant. 2004;23: 1359–65.
41. Holdy K, Dembitsky W, Eaton LL, et al. Nutrition assessment and management of left ventricular assist device patients. J Heart Lung Transplant. 2005;24: 1690–6.
42. Chinn R, Dembitsky W, Eaton L, et al. Multicenter experience: prevention and management of left ventricular assist device infections. ASAIO J. 2005;51: 461–70.
43. Frazier OH, Rose EA, Oz MC, et al. Multicenter clinical evaluation of the HeartMate vented electrical left ventricular assist system in patients awaiting heart transplantation. J Thorac Cardiovasc Surg. 2001;122: 1186–95.
44. Spanier T, Oz MC, Levin H, et al. Activation of coagulation and fibrinolytic pathways in patients with left ventricular assist devices. J Thorac Cardiovasc Surg. 1996;112:1090–7.
45. Geisen U, Heilmann C, Beyersdorf F, et al. Non-surgical bleeding in patients with ventricular assist devices could be explained by acquired von Willebrand disease. Eur J Cardiothorac Surg. 2008;33:679–84.
46. Pagani FD, Aaronson KD. Mechanical devices for temporary support. In: Franco KL, Verrier ED, editors. Advanced therapy in cardiac surgery. 2nd ed. Hamilton: BC Decker; 2003. p. 460–83.
47. Pasque MK, Rogers JG. Adverse events in the use of HeartMate vented electric and Novacor left ventricular assist devices: comparing apples and oranges. J Thorac Cardiovasc Surg. 2002;124(6):1063–7.
48. Dembitsky WP, Tector AJ, Park S, et al. Left ventricular assist device performance with long-term circulatory support: lessons for the REMATCH trial. Ann Thorac Surg. 2004;78:2123–30.
49. Thalmann M, Schima H, Wiesenthaler G, et al. Physiology of continuous blood flow in recipients of rotary cardiac assist devices. J Heart Lung Transplant. 2005;24:237–45.
50. Sezai A, Shiono M, Orime Y, et al. Major organ function under mechanical support: comparative studies of pulsatile and nonpulsatile circulation. Artif Organs. 1999;23(3):280–5.
51. Garcia S, Kandar F, Boyle A, et al. Effects of pulsatile- and continuous-flow left ventricular assist devices on left ventricular unloading. J Heart Lung Transplant. 2008;27:261–7.

52. Frazier OH, Gemmato C, Myers TJ, et al. Initial clinical experience with the Heartmate II axial-flow left ventricular assist device. Tex Heart Inst J. 2007;34: 275–81.
53. Griffith BP, Kormos RL, Borovetz HS, et al. Heartmate II left ventricular assist system: from concept to first clinical use. Ann Thorac Surg. 2001;71:S116–20.
54. Pagani FD. Continuous-flow left ventricular assist devices with "3rd generation" design. Semin Thorac Cardiovasc Surg. 2008;20:255–63.
55. John R, Kamdar F, Liao K, et al. Improved survival and decreasing incidence of adverse events with the Heartmate II left ventricular assist device as bridge-to-transplant therapy. Ann Thorac Surg. 2008;86: 1227–35.
56. Patel ND, Weiss ES, Schaffer J, et al. Right heart dysfunction after left ventricular assist device implantation: a comparison of the pulsatile Heartmate I and axial-flow Heartmate II devices. Ann Thorac Surg. 2008;86:832–40.

Newer-Generation Rotary Blood Pumps

12

Steven M. Parnis, Mehmet Hakan Akay, and O.H. Frazier

In 1812, LeGallois first proposed the concept of supporting or replacing the failing heart and circulation [1]. The foundation for mechanical circulatory support was laid by research into organ perfusion and preservation by many investigators, including DeBakey, Lindbergh, and Gibbon [2–4]. In the first reported use of a rotary blood pump to support the failing left ventricle, Dennis and colleagues utilized a transseptal technique in the 1950s to cannulate the left atrium, bypass the left ventricle, and return blood to the femoral artery with a roller pump [5]. In 1963, Hall and colleagues reported the first clinical implantation of a left ventricular assist device (LVAD) [6]. This pulsatile device was implanted within the chest and was connected between the left atrium and the descending thoracic aorta. The first successful use of an LVAD occurred in 1967, when DeBakey used a paracorporeal pulsatile device in a patient in cardiogenic shock. The pump was connected to the left atrium and right subclavian artery (Fig. 12.1). After 4 days, the device was removed under local anesthesia, and the patient was discharged home.

Throughout the 1960s and 1970s, several programs were initiated by the National Heart Institute (which later became the National Heart, Lung, and Blood Institute or NHLBI) to develop cardiac assist devices that could assist or replace the failing heart [7]. These programs produced several of the first-generation implantable pulsatile LVADs, including the HeartMate XVE (Thoratec Corporation, Pleasanton, CA), the Novacor Left Ventricular Assist System (World Heart, Inc., Oakland, CA), and the LionHeart Left Ventricular Assist System (Arrow International, Reading, PA). Altogether, these devices were implanted as bridges to transplantation or as destination therapy in several thousand patients worldwide who were not transplant candidates [8–10]. Currently, the Novacor and LionHeart devices are no longer being used clinically, although the HeartMate XVE is still available and used at many institutions.

In the mid-1980s, a miniature axial-flow blood pump (Fig. 12.2), the Hemopump—developed by Richard Wampler, MD, and the Nimbus Corporation [11]—underwent preclinical testing and first clinical use at the Texas Heart Institute in Houston [12]. This experience confirmed that a miniature rotary blood pump could unload the compromised left ventricle and provide adequate

S.M. Parnis, B.S.
Center for Cardiac Support, Texas Heart Institute at St. Luke's Episcopal Hospital, 6770 Bertner Ave., MC 1-268, Houston, TX 77030, USA
e-mail: sparnis@texasheart.org

M.H. Akay, M.D.
Department of Mechanical Circulatory Support, Heart Transplantation, Texas Heart Institute at St. Luke's Episcopal Hospital, 6770 Bertner Avenue, MC 2-114A, Houston, TX 77030, USA
e-mail: mhakay@hotmail.com

O.H. Frazier, M.D. (✉)
Department of Transplant/Mechanical Circulatory Support, Texas Heart Institute at St. Luke's Episcopal Hospital, 6770 Bertner Ave., C 355, Houston, TX 77030, USA
e-mail: lschwenke@heart.thi.tmc.edu

J.A. Morgan and Y. Naka (eds.), *Surgical Treatment for Advanced Heart Failure*,
DOI 10.1007/978-1-4614-6919-3_12,

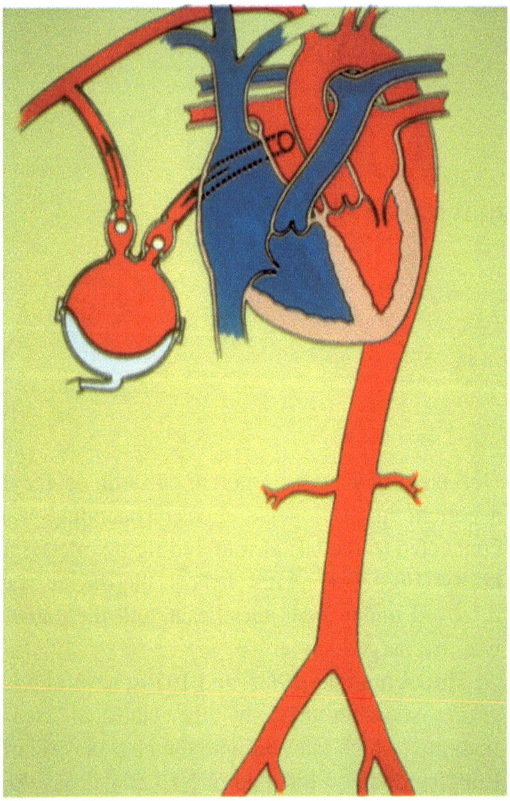

Fig. 12.1 The paracorporeal pulsatile left ventricular assist device used by Dr. Michael E. DeBakey in the 1960s (image property of Texas Heart Institute)

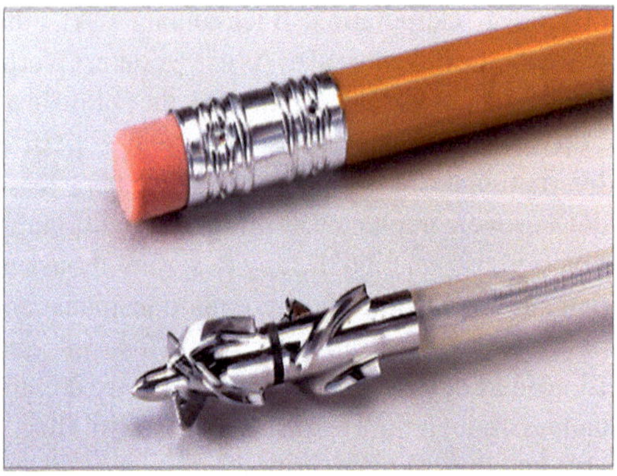

Fig. 12.2 The Hemopump miniature axial-flow blood pump is about the size of the eraser on an ordinary pencil. The successful clinical use of this device encouraged further development of implantable rotary blood pumps (image property of Texas Heart Institute)

systemic support while improving the potential for myocardial recovery. In 1994, NHLBI initiated the innovative ventricular assist systems program to encourage the development of a totally implantable ventricular assist system [13]. This program resulted in the next generation of smaller, implantable continuous-flow blood pumps [14–17].

Today, numerous rotary blood pumps are undergoing clinical trials designed to test their safety and effectiveness so that they may be used as bridges to transplantation, bridges to recovery, or destination therapy. Rotary pumps in current clinical use can be classified as to whether they have axial or centrifugal flow, have magnetically suspended or attached bearings, or are suitable for short- or long-term use. Axial-flow and centrifugal pumps typically have a central rotor containing permanent magnets. Electrically controlled coils, embedded in the housing of the blood pump, couple with magnets located in the impellers, thereby controlling rotational speed. Centrifugal pumps typically contain rotors shaped to accelerate blood flow towards the outer wall of the pump. In contrast, axial-flow pumps typically contain rotors that are more cylindrical. Helical blades on these cylindrical rotors cause blood flow to accelerate along the spinning axis of the rotor.

Another feature of continuous-flow pumps is the method used to suspend the rotor or impeller. Early continuous-flow pumps used solid fixed bearings, which are vulnerable to friction-related bearing wear, do not allow for washout of tight gaps, and sometimes allow thrombus to build up. Today, many continuous-flow pumps utilize electromagnetic and hydrodynamic suspension, which can virtually eliminate pump wear and also reduce damage to blood cells. Compared to earlier LVADs, these devices are much smaller and simpler, having only one moving part; as a result, they are less susceptible to infection and failure. They require a less invasive implant procedure and fit a wider size range of patients. Today's continuous-flow pumps are not only more efficient than previous models but are also much more comfortable for patients, allowing them to return to a relatively normal lifestyle.

This chapter focuses on the current use of continuous-flow pumps for both temporary and long-term support of patients with acute and chronic heart failure.

Short-Term Support

Continuous-flow pumps designed for temporary use may be appropriate in several clinical settings involving cardiogenic shock (e.g., acute myocardial infarction or postcardiotomy heart failure) and to provide cardiac support during coronary revascularization procedures. Although these devices may be inserted by cardiovascular surgeons in the operating room, they are usually and most effectively applied by cardiologists in the catheterization laboratory. Short-term pumps may also be used for bridging to a long-term cardiac assist device. The systems described in this section have been approved by the United States Food and Drug Administration (FDA) and been used for cardiac support in thousands of cases, for either left ventricular, right ventricular, or biventricular support.

Impella

The Impella System (Abiomed, Inc., Danvers, MA) consists of a small axial-flow blood pump that is similar to the earlier Hemopump. Three Impella models are used for left-sided cardiac support: the Impella LP 2.5, Impella LP 5.0, and Impella LD. All three models are catheter-mounted axial-flow pumps and have a distal cannula that is placed across the aortic valve in retrograde fashion to directly unload the left ventricle. The pump and pump outlet are located in the ascending aorta, into which blood is ejected for systemic support. The Impella RD is used for right-sided cardiac assistance and is connected to the right atrium and pulmonary artery. This device has CE mark approval and is undergoing clinical trials in the United States. Currently, the Impella 2.0 and 5.0 have both FDA and CE mark approvals.

The Impella pumps are connected to an external drive unit by a 2.8-mm flexible drive cable and a purge system (using a heparinized 40 % glucose solution), which continuously flushes the pump and motor housing.

The Impella LP 2.5 consists of a 4-mm (12F) microaxial blood pump mounted on a 9F pigtail catheter (Fig. 12.3). It is inserted percutaneously, with the aid of fluoroscopic guidance, in either the catheterization laboratory or the operating room. The device is inserted through the femoral artery via a 13F sheath over a guidewire.

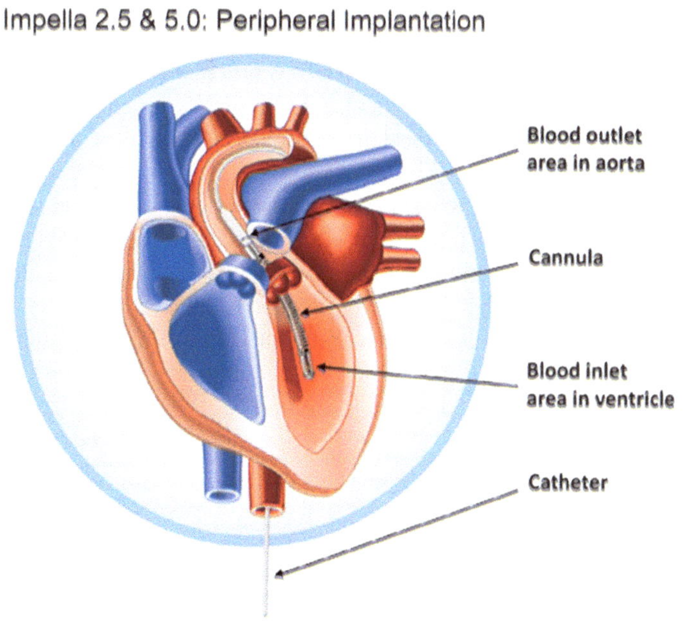

Fig. 12.3 The Impella 2.5 and 5.0 axial-flow pumps (Abiomed, Inc., Danvers, MA) are inserted via the femoral artery and advanced across the aortic valve for short-term cardiac support. The two pumps are exactly alike, except that the 5.0 model is larger

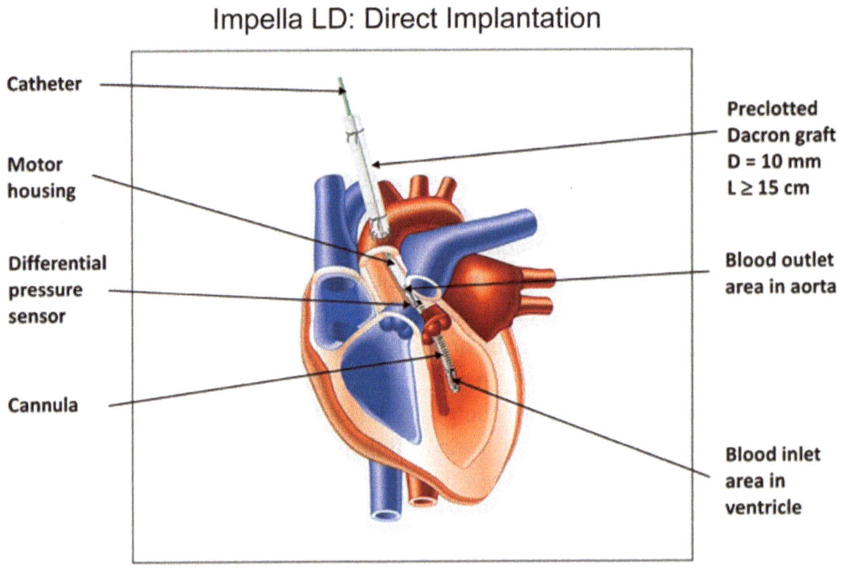

Fig. 12.4 The Impella LD (Abiomed, Inc., Danvers, MA) has a shorter cannula than the Impella 2.5 or 5.0. The LD is inserted surgically via the ascending aorta and advanced across the aortic valve

The system can provide up to 2.5 L/min of support against a normal physiologic afterload.

The Impella LP 5.0—a larger version of the Impella LP 2.5 device—consists of a 6.4-mm microaxial pump and a 7.3-mm-diameter (21F) cannula. The device is inserted into the femoral artery via a prosthetic graft and is advanced into the left ventricle with the aid of fluoroscopic guidance. It can provide up to 5.0 L/min of blood flow.

The Impella LD is the same as the Impella LP 5.0 but has a shorter (55-mm) left ventricular cannula (Fig. 12.4). The device is surgically implanted directly into the left ventricle via the ascending aorta.

The Impella RD is used for right-sided support alone and can only be inserted surgically. This small microaxial-flow blood pump has a short caged inlet that is inserted directly into the right atrium and a ringed outlet graft that is anastomosed to the pulmonary artery. It can deliver blood flows of up to 5 L/min.

TandemHeart

The TandemHeart (Cardiac Assist, Inc., Pittsburgh, PA) is a percutaneously inserted left ventricular assist system for temporary use during high-risk percutaneous coronary interventions (PCIs) or off-pump coronary bypass; it is also used for bridging to transplantation and for treating acute myocardial infarction and postcardiotomy shock. The two-stage catheter system dilates the puncture site in the atrial septum and provides transseptal access by means of a transseptal cannula that drains blood from the left atrium (Fig. 12.5). An extracorporeal centrifugal blood pump returns blood to an arterial femoral cannula, which is positioned at the level of the femoral bifurcation.

Use of this technique to support the failing left ventricle dates back to the 1950s, when Dennis and colleagues [5] used a transseptal approach to cannulate the left atrium, bypass the left ventricle, and return blood to the femoral artery with a roller pump. Seven of their eight patients survived for a short period, but there were no long-term survivors because revascularization procedures had not yet been developed.

The FDA-approved TandemHeart percutaneous ventricular assist device represents a clinically meaningful application of Dennis's concept [18–21]. The external centrifugal pump weighs 227 g, operates at 3,000–7,500 rpm, and supplies

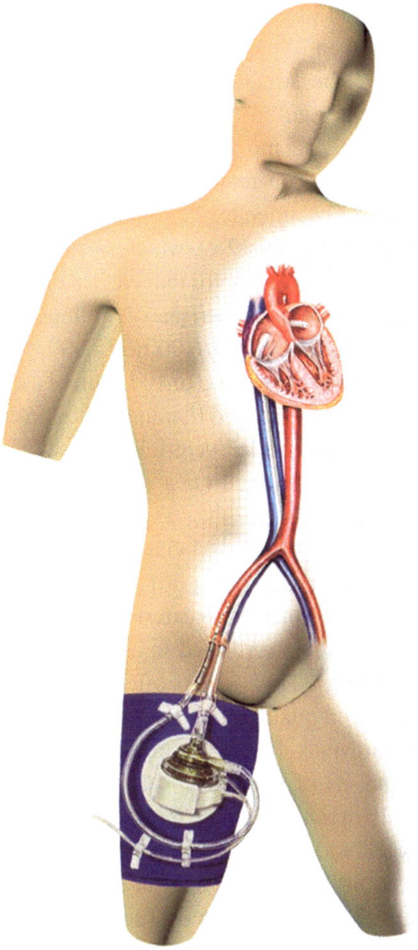

Fig. 12.5 The cannulas of the TandemHeart (CardiacAssist, Inc., Pittsburgh, PA) are inserted via the femoral artery and vein. The inflow cannula is placed within the left atrium by means of a transseptal technique

up to 4 L/min of continuous flow [22]. Pump inflow is achieved through a 21F cannula that is placed in the left atrium through an atrial transseptal puncture via the femoral vein. The cannula draws oxygenated blood from the left atrium into the external centrifugal pump. A 15F or 17F outflow cannula is placed in the femoral artery. The pump controller, which rotates and controls the impeller of the centrifugal pump, as well as an anticoagulant infusion line, protects the hydrodynamic bearing by cooling it and providing an anticoagulation agent.

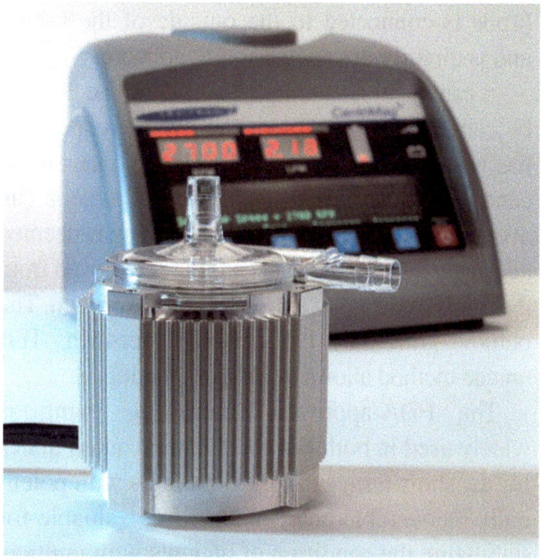

Fig. 12.6 The CentriMag Ventricular Assist System (Levitronix LLC, Waltham, MA) (image property of Texas Heart Institute)

CentriMag

The CentriMag ventricular assist system (Levitronix LLC, Waltham, MA) is used for short-term left, right, or biventricular support (Fig. 12.6). The extracorporeal centrifugal blood pump contains a rotor that is magnetically levitated and spins friction free. The rotor is encased in a polycarbonate housing. The inlet to the blood pump is concentric with the axis of the rotor, and the pump outlet is perpendicular to the inlet. Blood enters via the inlet and contacts the spinning rotor; energy in the form of pressure and velocity is then transferred from the rotor to the blood, which exits the outlet port at flows of up to 10 L/min. The blood pump is attached to a motor which, when magnetically coupled, powers the pump. A cable connects the motor to a console that controls pump speed and monitors pump function.

The cannulas are inserted into either the right or left atrium (for venous drainage) or into the pulmonary artery or aorta, depending on the type of support required. The cannulas are attached to standard 3/8-inch tubing, which is connected to the pump's inflow and outflow ports. For continuous pump-flow monitoring, an ultrasonic flow probe is connected to the outside of the tubing and is directly connected to the console.

A cannulation technique that allows the chest to be completely closed and that avoids reoperation has been revived from the 1960s. By placing the cannula through a graft [23, 24], the surgeon can avoid reopening the chest when weaning is deemed adequate. Instead, the inlet cannula is removed from the inside of the graft, and the graft is oversewn. The outflow graft may be similarly oversewn. This unique method allows quick explantation.

The FDA-approved CentriMag pump is widely used in both Europe and the United States for the short-term support of patients with potentially recoverable heart failure. It is valuable for stabilizing the condition of patients with multiorgan system failure and an uncertain neurologic status. It is also used for supporting patients after an acute myocardial infarction, for bridging to recovery, for postcardiotomy shock, and for short-term right ventricular assistance in combination with implantable LVADs.

Long-Term Support

Experience gained with implantable pulsatile blood pumps for long-term support helped pave the way for the widespread use of continuous-flow rotary blood pumps for this purpose. Typically, these pumps are smaller and require less power than their pulsatile predecessors. Although continuous-flow devices have no flexing or moving diaphragms, no membranes, and no valves to ensure unidirectional flow, they generally do necessitate chronic anticoagulation therapy (i.e., warfarin). Percutaneous drivelines are also smaller than those of first-generation pumps, and improved management techniques have decreased the incidence of infection. Nevertheless, complications (e.g., percutaneous driveline site infections or external pump cable fractures) still do exist.

HeartMate II

The HeartMate II LVAD (Thoratec Corporation, Pleasanton, CA) consists of an implantable axial-flow blood pump, a controller module, an alternating-current power-based unit, and external batteries. The small blood pump measures 4 cm in diameter and 6 cm in length; it weighs 375 g and has one moving part, a high-speed impeller that spins on inlet and outlet ball-and-cup bearings. The impeller is contained within the pump housing (Fig. 12.7), which surrounds a brushless direct-current motor that creates a spinning magnetic field to activate the impeller. Rotational speeds range from 6,000 to 15,000 rpm, and the device can provide up to 10 L/min of continuous output. The sintered titanium inflow cannula is inserted into the left ventricle via a sewing ring, and blood is returned via a 12-mm outflow graft anastomosed to the ascending aorta (Fig. 12.8). Power is delivered via a percutaneous lead that exits the right upper portion of the abdomen; the lead is connected to external controllers and either an AC-power-based unit or wearable portable batteries. This system offers patients a greatly improved quality of life.

The HeartMate II has received CE mark approval and, as of September 2010, also FDA approval. It has supported more than 5,000 patients worldwide for up to 6 years as a bridge to transplantation, a bridge to recovery, or destination therapy. In clinical bridge-to-transplant trials performed at 35 centers from March 2005 to April 2008, 469 patients received a HeartMate II; 250 of these patients underwent cardiac transplantation, 12 underwent ventricular recovery and had the device explanted, 106 had died during the support period, and 100 remained on LVAD support. The 250 transplant recipients had a survival rate of 97 % at 30 days and 87 % at 1 year. With regard to reliability, the HeartMate II is greatly improved over its predecessor, the first-generation HeartMate XVE pulsatile device. In the Randomized Evaluation of Mechanical Assistance for the Treatment of Congestive Heart Failure (REMATCH), which assessed the HeartMate XVE LVAD [25], nearly 50 % of the support group required a device exchange by 18 months due to mechanical malfunction or infection. In contrast, no mechanical failures of the device pumping mechanism were observed in a clinical trial of the HeartMate II as a bridge to transplantation [26]. Because of its improved

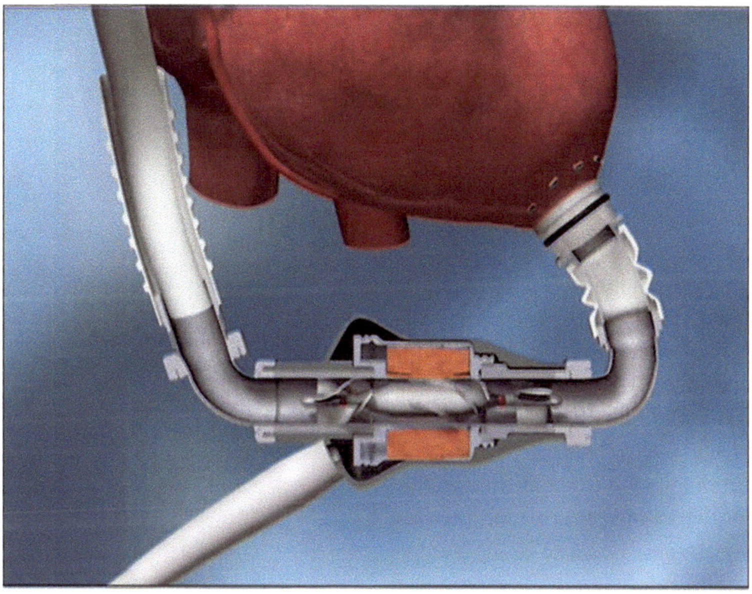

Fig. 12.7 The HeartMate II (Thoratec Corporation, Pleasanton, CA) has one moving part—a high-speed impeller that is contained in the pump housing

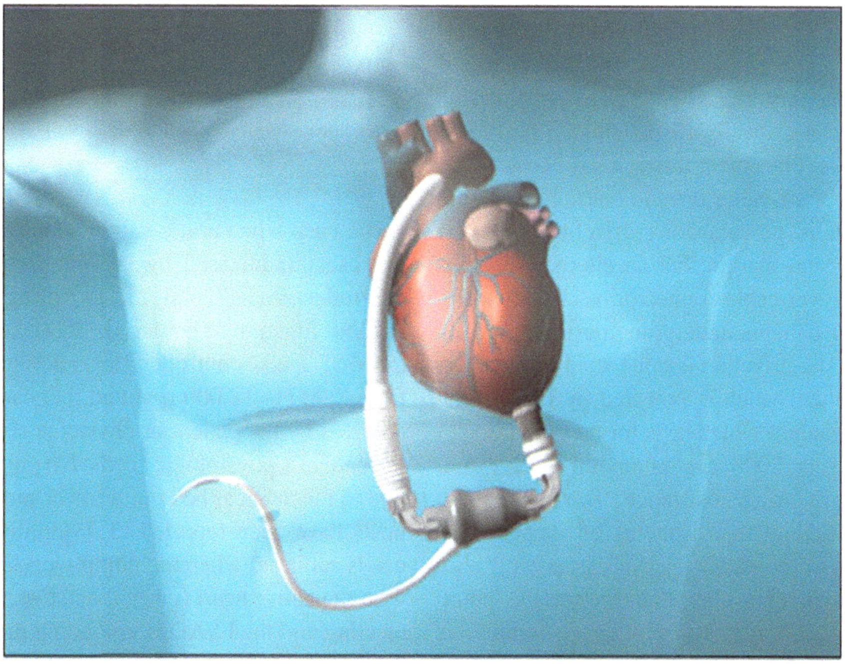

Fig. 12.8 The HeartMate II left ventricular assist device with the inflow cannula inserted in the left ventricle and the outflow graft anastomosed to the ascending aorta. The pump is placed in a subdiaphragmatic pocket

features, the HeartMate II is the first implantable rotary blood pump to have widespread use.

Jarvik 2000

In 1989, in collaboration with Dr. Robert Jarvik, the Texas Heart Institute began initial development of the Jarvik 2000, a long-term, implantable pump with nonlubricated bearings (Jarvik Heart, Inc., New York, NY). The titanium blood pump is about the size of a C-cell battery. It weighs 90 g, measures 2.5 cm in diameter, and displaces 25 mL. Within the pump housing is a sealed, brushless, electromagnetic, direct-current motor. The rotor, the only moving part, is held in place by two ceramic bearings. Because of the pump's small size, the senior author (OHF) recommended placing the pump directly into the intraventricular cavity [27, 28]. The device is connected to the arterial circulation by a 16-mm Hemashield outflow graft to the descending thoracic aorta (Fig. 12.9), but the outflow graft could also be attached to the supraceliac aorta, ascending aorta, or first part of the descending aorta [29]. In most cases, the pump can be placed without the use of cardiopulmonary bypass [30]. This enhances its usefulness in critically ill patients with chronic heart failure. Placement through a subcostal incision may be of value in redo sternotomy situations [31]. A percutaneous driveline exits the right subcostal margin, but an alternative skull-pedestal power-cable connector has been used in Europe for patients undergoing destination therapy [32]. The driveline is connected to an external controller, which is powered by lithium ion batteries, each of which lasts for up to 8 h.

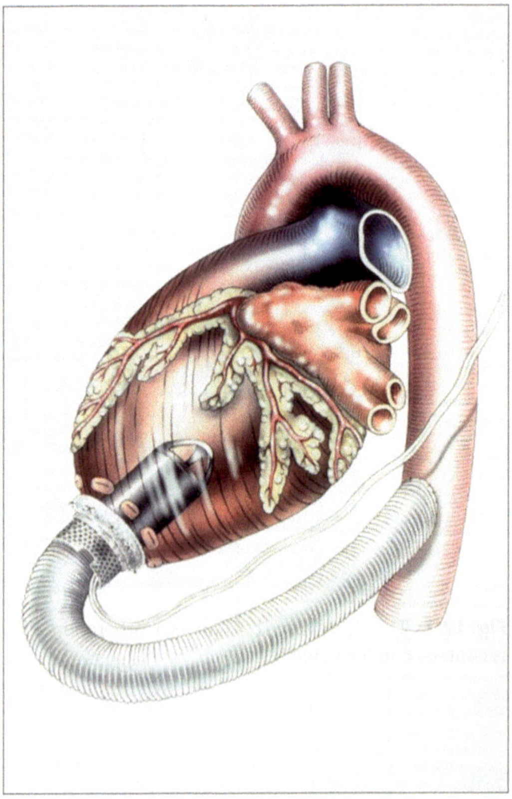

Fig. 12.9 The Jarvik 2000 blood pump (Jarvik Heart, Inc., New York, NY) is inserted into the left ventricle with the outflow graft attached to the descending thoracic aorta (image property of Texas Heart Institute)

The Jarvik 2000 can pump up to 7 L/min against physiologic resistance. The addition of sintered titanium microspheres on its intraventricular blood-contacting surfaces, as well as a phased speed controller that lowers the pump speed to 7,000 rpm for 6 s every minute, is designed to decrease the risk of thrombus formation in the ventricle around the base of the pump (addressed by the sintered titanium microspheres), thrombus formation in the noncoronary aortic cusp when aortic valve opening is limited or absent (addressed by the intermittent speed controller), and a septal shift impairing right ventricular function. The Jarvik 2000 also has an external speed controller that allows variations from 8,000 to 12,000 rpm and that can easily be adjusted by the patient or physician according to the patient's physiologic needs. No pump failures due to mechanical bearing wear or pump thrombosis have been reported [33]. Optimal clinical use is achieved when the pump works in parallel with the native heart (when the native ventricle is ejecting and the LVAD is unloading the ventricle throughout the cardiac cycle) [34]. This pump has provided more than 7 years of continuous destination therapy for a patient who received it in June 2000 in Oxford, England [35].

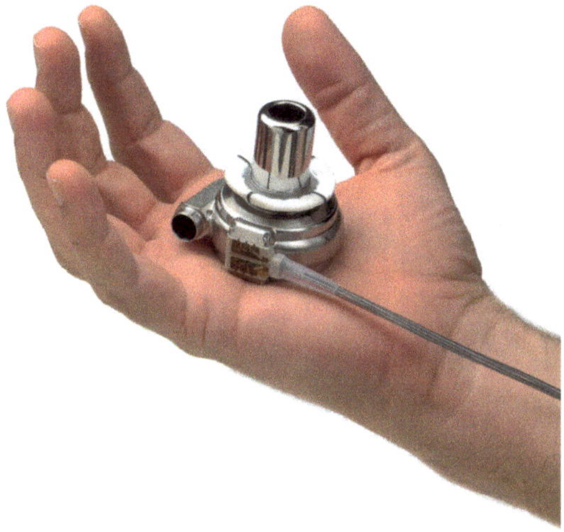

Fig. 12.10 The HeartWare ventricular assist device (HeartWare, Inc., Miami Lakes, FL) is a small centrifugal pump (image courtesy of HeartWare, Inc. Caution: Investigational device. Limited by Federal Law to investigational use in the USA)

Magnetically Suspended Centrifugal Pumps

With first-generation implantable rotary blood pumps, or axial-flow pumps, a major concern was the use of mechanical bearings, which could potentially become worn and impair performance and durability. To address this concern, engineers began to develop implantable, magnetically suspended pumps, which have the potential for longer durability. Most of these pumps have a magnetically levitated (maglev) impeller that eliminates the need for mechanical bearings and physical contact between moving parts. By generating higher torque at a lower speed, these pumps should minimize wear, heat generation, and hemolysis. Several maglev designs are being developed and should soon see widespread use.

HeartWare HVAD

The HeartWare HVAD (HeartWare, Inc., Miami Lakes, FL) is a small (displacement volume, 50 mL; weight, 145 g), continuous-flow, centrifugal pump (Fig. 12.10) that uses a hybrid system—a combination of passive magnetic and hydrodynamic thrust bearings—to create contact-free rotation of a wide-blade impeller, the only moving part within the pump. The front and rear housing are titanium-ceramic hybrid assemblies. Both housings contain sealed motor stators, which rotate the wide-blade impeller and allow power redundancy. Radial and axial support is provided by a magnetic center post in the rear housing and three stacks of magnets in the impeller. When the pump is turned on, the impeller is pushed away from the front housing and begins to rotate. A very thin cushion of blood maintains the gap between the impeller and the front housing. Once power is applied to the device, there are no points of mechanical contact within the pump. This is expected to improve device reliability and reduce the risk of blood trauma as blood cells pass through the pump.

The HVAD pump is implanted within the pericardial sac (Fig. 12.11). The titanium inflow cannula is inserted into the ventricular cavity via a sewing ring that contains a metallic C-clamp to allow secure attachment to the base of the pump. Blood is returned via a 10-mm outflow graft attached to the ascending aorta. A percutaneous driveline exits the right subcostal margin and is connected to an external microprocessor controller, which is powered by lithium ion batteries. A tablet computer monitor displays system information and allows for alternating-current power options. The HVAD can generate up to 10 L/min of forward flow. It has been awarded a CE mark in Europe. It has been approved as a bridge to heart transplantation by the FDA and is undergoing a clinical trial for use as destination therapy in the United States.

DuraHeart

The DuraHeart (Terumo Heart, Inc., Ann Arbor, MI) is an implantable centrifugal blood pump that uses magnetic levitation to suspend a rotating impeller within a titanium housing (Fig. 12.12). The pump is 72 mm in diameter, is 45 mm thick, weighs 540 g, and has a displacement volume of 180 mL. It can provide up to 8 L/min of blood flow at a head pressure of 120 mmHg and pump speeds of 1,200–2,600 rpm. The impeller is suspended magnetically by three electromagnets mounted in the upper housing and on the motor side of the impeller; it is rotated by means

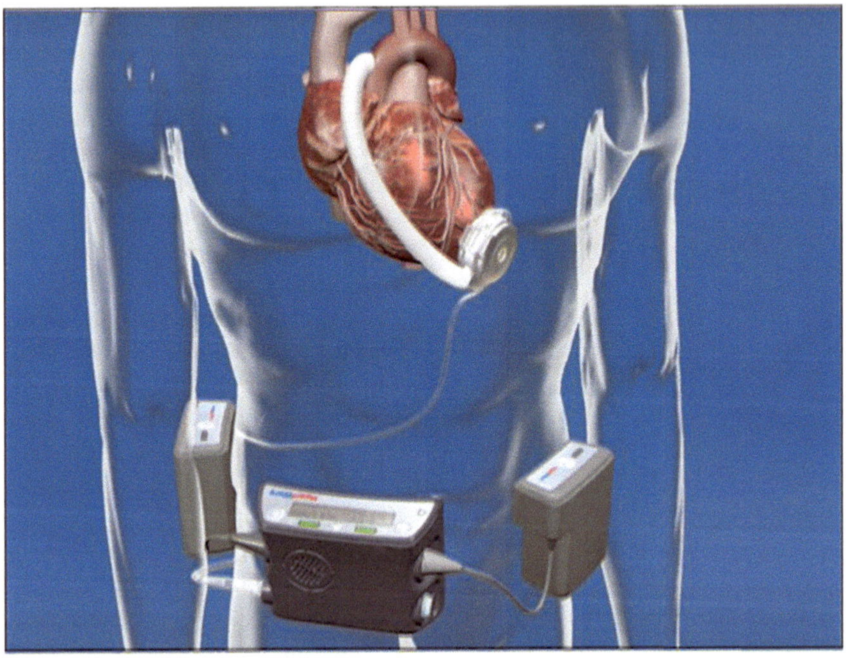

Fig. 12.11 The HeartWare pump is placed within the pericardial sac. The outflow graft is attached to the ascending aorta. The percutaneous driveline exits the right subcostal margin and is connected to the external controller and batteries (image courtesy of HeartWare, Inc. Caution: Investigational device. Limited by Federal Law to investigational use in the USA)

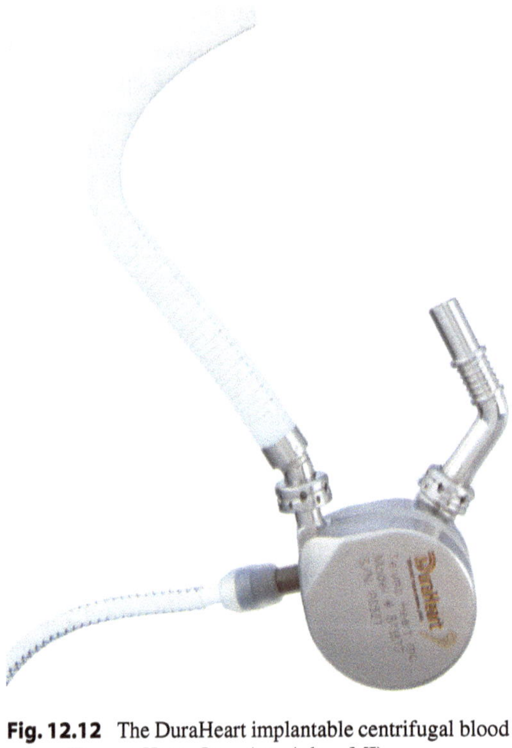

Fig. 12.12 The DuraHeart implantable centrifugal blood pump (Terumo Heart, Inc., Ann Arbor, MI)

of magnetic coupling between the impeller and a brushless direct-current motor. Tilting and axial placement of the impeller are monitored by three position sensors to ensure that the impeller is free floating at the center of the pump housing. This also maintains consistent washout of the blood path within the pump. A titanium inflow conduit connects the pump to the heart, and blood is retuned via a 12-mm Gelweave graft (Terumo Heart, Inc.) to the ascending aorta. The pump is placed in an abdominal pocket and is connected to an external controller via a percutaneous lead that exits the abdominal wall. The controller can be powered by wearable external batteries or by a console and charger system.

The DuraHeart was awarded a CE Mark in 2007 and is currently undergoing clinical trials in the United States. In 6 US patients and 68 European patients with support durations of more than 3 years, the DuraHeart has yielded results similar to those of other rotary blood pumps [36]. No pump mechanical failure or pump thrombosis has been reported.

Summary

Small, continuous-flow, rotary blood pumps have greatly expanded the options for treating both acute and chronic heart failure. Because of their increased reliability and effectiveness, these pumps provide clinicians with an "off-the-shelf" circulatory support device for the treatment of heart failure. Continuous-flow pumps are easier to implant than their predecessors and can be explanted if ventricular recovery occurs. These advances in design, engineering, and clinical implementation have ushered in a new era for the support and management of end-stage heart failure. The next challenge is to make mechanical circulatory support the gold standard for the treatment of patients with advanced heart failure.

References

1. LeGallois CJJ. Experiences on the principle of life. Philadelphia: Thomas; 1812 [Translation of LeGallois CJJ, Experiences sur la Principe de la Vie. Paris, 1812].
2. DeBakey ME. A simple continuous flow blood transfusion instrument. New Orleans Med Surg J. 1934;87: 386–9.
3. Lindbergh CA. An apparatus for the culture of whole organs. J Exp Med. 1935;62:409–32.
4. Gibbon JH. Application of a mechanical heart and lung apparatus to cardiac surgery. Minn Med. 1957;37:171–85.
5. Dennis C, Carlens E, Senning A, Hall DP, Moreno JR, Cappelletti RR, et al. Clinical use of a cannula for left heart bypass without thoracotomy. Ann Surg. 1962;156:623–37.
6. DeBakey ME, Liotta D, Hall CW. Left ventricular bypass pump for cardiac assistance. Clinical experience. Am J Cardiol. 1971;27:3–11.
7. National Heart, Lung, and Blood Institute. Report of the workshop on the artificial heart: planning for evolving technologies. Bethesda: U.S. Department of Commerce, National Information Service; 1944.
8. UAB School of Medicine. Interagency Registry for Mechanically Assisted Circulatory Support. http://www.intermacs.org. Accessed 8 Oct 2010.
9. WorldHeart Corporation. Novacor-LVAS. http://www.worldheart.com/about/novacor-lvas.cfm. Accessed 8 Oct 2010.
10. Thoratec Corporation. HeartMate® XVE LVAD. http://www.thoratec.com/vad-trials-outcomes/clinical-outcomes/heartmate-xve-lvad.aspx. Accessed 8 Oct 2010.
11. Wampler RK, Moise JC, Frazier OH, Olsen DB. In vivo evaluation of a peripheral vascular access axial flow blood pump. ASAIO Trans. 1988;34:450–4.
12. Frazier OH, Wampler RK, Duncan JM, Dear WE, Macris MP, Parnis SM, et al. First human use of the Hemopump, a catheter-mounted ventricular assist device. Ann Thorac Surg. 1990;49: 299–304.
13. Watson JT. AS Innovative ventricular assist systems. ASAIO J. 1994;40:M902.
14. Griffith BP, Kormos RL, Borovetz HS, Litwak K, Antaki JF, Poirier VL, et al. HeartMate II Left Ventricular Assist System: from concept to first clinical use. Ann Thorac Surg. 2001;71:S116–20.
15. Burke DJ, Burke E, Parsaie F, Poirier V, Butler K, Thomas D, et al. The Heartmate II: design and development of a fully sealed axial flow left ventricular assist system. Artif Organs. 2001;25: 380–5.
16. Parnis SM, Conger JL, Fuqua Jr JM, Inman RW, Tamez D, Macris MP, et al. Progress in the development of a transcutaneously powered axial flow blood pump ventricular assist system. ASAIO J. 1997;43:M576–80.
17. Fukamachi K, Ochiai Y, Doi K, Massiello AL, Medvedev AL, Horvath DJ, et al. Chronic evaluation of the Cleveland Clinic CorAide left ventricular assist system in calves. Artif Organs. 2002;26:529–33.
18. Satoh H, Kobayashi T, Nakano S, Shimazaki Y, Kaneko M, Matsuda H. Clinical application of percutaneous left ventricular support with a centrifugal pump. ASAIO J. 1993;39:153–5.
19. Edmunds Jr LH, Herrmann HC, DiSesa VJ, Ratcliffe MB, Bavaria JE, McCarthy DM. Left ventricular assist without thoracotomy: clinical experience with the Dennis method. Ann Thorac Surg. 1994;57:880–5.
20. Fonger JD, Zhou Y, Matsuura H, Aldea GS, Shemin RJ. Enhanced preservation of acutely ischemic myocardium with transseptal left ventricular assist. Ann Thorac Surg. 1994;57:570–5.
21. Pavie A, Leger P, Nzomvuama A, Szefner J, Regan M, Vaissier E, et al. Left centrifugal pump cardiac assist with transseptal percutaneous left atrial cannula. Artif Organs. 1998;22:502–7.
22. Kar B, Adkins LE, Civitello AB, Loyalka P, Palanichamy N, Gemmato CJ, et al. Clinical experience with the TandemHeart percutaneous ventricular assist device. Tex Heart Inst J. 2006;33:111–5.
23. John R, Liao K, Lietz K, Kamdar F, Colvin-Adams M, Boyle A, et al. Experience with the Levitronix CentriMag circulatory support system as a bridge to decision in patients with refractory acute cardiogenic shock and multisystem organ failure. J Thorac Cardiovasc Surg. 2007;134:351–8.
24. De Robertis F, Birks EJ, Rogers P, Dreyfus G, Pepper JR, Khaghani A. Clinical performance with the Levitronix Centrimag short-term ventricular assist device. J Heart Lung Transplant. 2006;25:181–6.
25. Rose EA, Gelijns AC, Moskowitz AJ, Heitjan DF, Stevenson LW, Dembitsky W, et al. Long-term use of a left ventricular assist device for end-stage heart failure. N Engl J Med. 2001;345:1435–43.

26. Miller LW, Pagani FD, Russell SD, John R, Boyle AJ, Aaronson KD, et al. Use of a continuous-flow device in patients awaiting heart transplantation. N Engl J Med. 2007;357:885–96.
27. Frank CM, Palanichamy N, Kar B, Wilson JM, Gregoric ID, Loyalka P, et al. Use of a percutaneous ventricular assist device for treatment of cardiogenic shock due to critical aortic stenosis. Tex Heart Inst J. 2006;33:487–9.
28. Frazier OH, Myers TJ, Westaby S, Gregoric ID. Use of the Jarvik 2000 left ventricular assist system as a bridge to heart transplantation or as destination therapy for patients with chronic heart failure. Ann Surg. 2003;237:631–7.
29. Myers T, Frazier OH, Delgado R. Use of mechanical devices in treating heart failure. In: Hosenpud J, Greenberg B, editors. Congestive heart failure. 3rd ed. Philadelphia: Lippincott Williams & Wilkins; 2006. p. 776–81.
30. Frazier OH. Implantation of the Jarvik 2000 left ventricular assist device without the use of cardiopulmonary bypass. Ann Thorac Surg. 2003;75: 1028–30.
31. Westaby S, Frazier OH, Pigott DW, Saito S, Jarvik RK. Implant technique for the Jarvik 2000 Heart. Ann Thorac Surg. 2002;73:1337–40.
32. Frazier OH, Myers TJ, Jarvik RK, Westaby S, Pigott DW, Gregoric ID, et al. Research and development of an implantable, axial-flow left ventricular assist device: the Jarvik 2000 Heart. Ann Thorac Surg. 2001;71:S125–32.
33. Siegenthaler MP, Frazier OH, Beyersdorf F, Martin J, Laks H, Elefteriades J, et al. Mechanical reliability of the Jarvik 2000 heart. Ann Thorac Surg. 2006;81:1752–8.
34. Frazier OH, Myers TJ, Westaby S, Gregoric ID. Clinical experience with an implantable, intracardiac, continuous flow circulatory support device: physiologic implications and their relationship to patient selection. Ann Thorac Surg. 2004;77:133–42.
35. Westaby S, Frazier OH, Banning A. Six years of continuous mechanical circulatory support. N Engl J Med. 2006;355:325–7.
36. Morshuis M, El-Banayosy A, Arusoglu L, Koerfer R, Hetzer R, Wieselthaler G, et al. European experience of DuraHeart magnetically levitated centrifugal left ventricular assist system. Eur J Cardiothorac Surg. 2009;35:1020–8.

Total Artificial Heart

13

Hannah Copeland, Jack G. Copeland, and Richard G. Smith

History

Heart disease continues to be the leading cause of death in the United States with almost 700,000 people, or 29 % of deaths, per year. Medical management of advanced heart failure remains the primary therapy for most patients, but surgery offers a large number of patients more curative approaches including a host of conventional operations, mechanical circulatory support with a family of devices for short and long duration, and cardiac transplantation. The use of the total artificial heart (TAH) is one such intervention that has grown exponentially in the past 10 years.

Initially, VADs were used as a bridge-to-transplantation, and TAHs were used for long-term support. The first TAH was implanted in a dog at the Cleveland Clinic in 1957. Calves later became the better experimental model due to the calves' ability to tolerate the cardiopulmonary bypass and have less thrombogenicity. These preliminary experiments led to the development of a "permanent" TAH. In 1964, the United States Government National Heart Initiative instituted an order to produce a TAH.

In 1969, Dr. Denton Cooley was the first to implant a TAH, also known as the Liotta TAH, in a human as bridge-to-transplant [1]. That patient lived for 64 h on the device and later died of pneumonia and sepsis 32 h after transplantation. The next TAH was not implanted for another 12 years. In 1981, Dr. Cooley implanted a TAH in a 36-year-old male who had suffered cardiac failure after a coronary artery bypass graft. He was implanted with an Akutsu TAH for 53 h until transplantation. The gentleman later died 8 days after transplantation, also from sepsis. The same year, the US Food and Drug Administration (FDA) granted approval to permanently implant the Jarvik-7 TAH at the University of Utah. The first recipient of that device was Barney Clark; he lived for 112 days on the device [2].

In 1985, Dr. Jack Copeland at the University of Arizona implanted the unapproved Phoenix TAH in order to save a man who had cardiac graft failure [3]. The device was placed as a bridge-to-transplant. The implantation created a great deal of controversy, though, resulted in the FDA acceptance of the one-time use of any device in a true emergency. The patient died secondary to sepsis after a second transplant. The first successful

H. Copeland, M.D.
Division of Cardiovascular and Thoracic Surgery, Loma Linda University Medical Center, Loma Linda, CA 92354, USA
e-mail: hannahcopeland411@gmail.com

J.G. Copeland, M.D. (✉)
Division of Cardiovascular and Thoracic Surgery, University of California, San Diego, 9300 Campus Point Drive #7892, La Jolla, CA 92037-7892, USA
e-mail: jackcope3@gmail.com

R.G. Smith, MSEE
Artificial Heart Program, University of Arizona Medical Center, 1501 North Campbell Avenue, Tucson, AZ 85724, USA
e-mail: richard.smith@uahealth.com

J.A. Morgan and Y. Naka (eds.), *Surgical Treatment for Advanced Heart Failure*,
DOI 10.1007/978-1-4614-6919-3_13, © Springer Science+Business Media New York 2013

bridge-to-transplant was on August 29, 1985 [4]. A young man on a TAH, a Jarvik-7 100, for 9 days was successfully bridged to transplant by Copeland and his team. This patient lived for 5 years posttransplant and eventually died of posttransplantation lymphoproliferative disease. This initial device had a stroke volume of 100 mL. A year later, a smaller device with a stroke volume of 70 mL, the Jarvik7-70, (Symbion, Inc., Salt Lake City, UT) was developed; this device fits most patients and with minimal changes has evolved into the SynCardia TAH-t (SynCardia Systems Inc., Tucson, AZ).

Shortly afterward, to better understand the use of the Jarvik-7, patient selection, and prevention of two of the major complications, thromboembolism and infection, an investigational device exemption (IDE) study was started. Unfortunately, that study failed to provide critical information necessary to answer these questions and was stopped by the FDA in the USA in early 1991. Though, simultaneously in Paris, La Pitié Hospital, reported no neurological complications in 60 consecutive Jarvik-7 patients who were treated with a multidrug anticoagulation protocol [5].

In late 1991, the Jarvik-7 was transferred from Symbion to a company called CardioWest, formed by the University Medical Center in Tucson, AZ, and Medforte in Salt Lake City, Utah. Subsequently the device was renamed the CardioWest TAH. A new IDE study was established and implemented in five centers in the USA in January of 1993. The trial was conducted over 9 years, including 95 implant patients and 35 control patients. The manufacturing of the device was transferred from Vancouver to Tucson. A new company was created in 2002, SynCardia Systems, Inc., in order to finish the IDE study and assist in the application for commercial use of the device.

Later in 2004, the CardioWest TAH-t was approved as the first and only TAH by the FDA for use as a bridge-to-transplant as reported the same year in the New England Journal of Medicine [6]. The SynCardia TAH-t is a sound surgical option for patients awaiting a heart transplant who are failing maximal medical and inotropic support. It is currently used in 60 centers in the USA and over 40 in Europe. The FDA study documented a 79 % survival to transplantation and a posttransplantation survival equal to first time primary cardiac recipients over a period of 5 years.

Description of the Device

The official FDA mandated the name of this device is the SynCardia TAH-t; the "t" refers to the fact that the device is temporary. Although it was originally intended and designed as a long-term cardiac replacement and might be a long-term device in the future, the SynCardia TAH-t is currently used as a temporary measure to bridge patients to transplantation. It is driven by 3 different consoles; a large pneumatic console with a complete duplicate backup driver nicknamed "Big Blue" (Fig. 13.1). The large console is being replaced by a 55 lb in house console called Companion 2 and a much smaller outpatient driver, the Freedom Driver. Over 1,000 SynCardia TAH-ts (TAH) have been implanted for over 150 patient-years. Over 75 patient-years on device have been in outpatients.

The TAH replaces both native ventricles with separate right and left prosthetic ventricles that are lined with smooth segmented polyurethane. The polyurethane diaphragm is four layered, a safety feature. Both artificial ventricles together weigh 160 g and displace 400 mL. This orthotopic biventricular pneumatic pump can pump a maximum in vivo output of 9–10 L/min at a central venous pressure (CVP) of <10 mm Hg. The maximal stroke volume is 70 mL, but 99 % of the time the device is run using a fill volume of about 50–60 mL per stroke, and it fully ejects with each beat (Fig. 13.2a, b).

The blood flow path is the same as the native heart with an inflow distance from atrium to device of less than 5 mm and a blood path from left atrium to aorta or right atrium to pulmonary artery of less than 20 cm. The implantable ventricles contain Medtronic Hall (Medtronic, Inc., Minneapolis, MN) valves that are 27 cm on the inflow side and 25 cm on the outflow side. The outflow conduits are made of Dacron (Maquet, Chicago, IL) and measure 3 cm from the ventricular outflow valve to the aorta and 6 cm from right ventricular outflow to the pulmonary artery (Fig. 13.3).

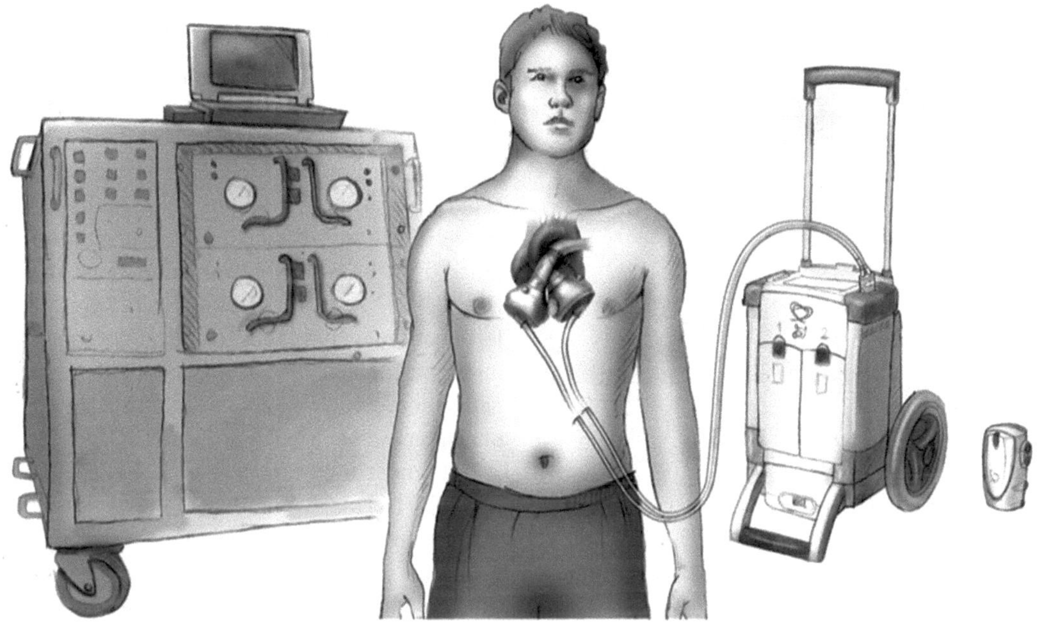

Fig. 13.1 Current driver for CardioWest TAH-t on left shown with new drivers drawn to scale: Companion Driver attached to patient weighs 18 kg, the much smaller Freedom Driver, further to the left weighs 2 kg (this article was published in Sabiston & Spencer's Surgery of the Chest, 8th edition, Zimmerman H, Copeland JG, Aquila Allen LA, Smith RG, "Total artificial heart," pp. 1525–1532, copyright Elsevier 2010)

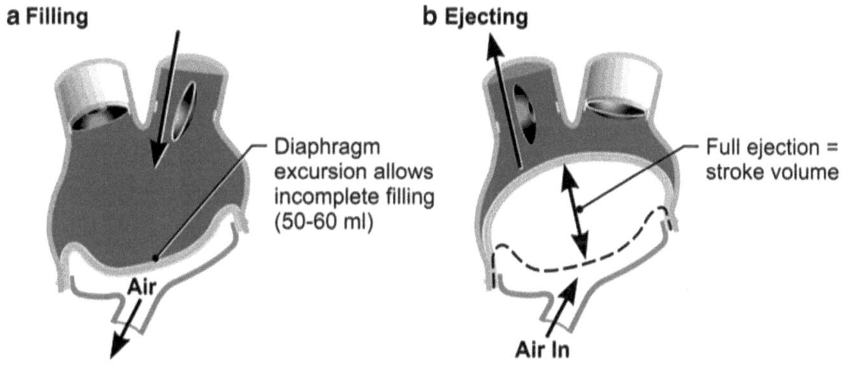

Fig. 13.2 (**a**) This shows pump diastole or filling. Partial filling allows for increased venous return scenarios (exercise, right left imbalance, Valsalva maneuver, etc.). The driver console beat rate % systole and vacuum are set to allow filling with about 50–60 mL/beat with the patient at rest. (**b**) Ejection pressures are set to always cause a maximal diaphragm excursion ("full eject"). For the left ventricle, the ejection pressure is set at 60 mm Hg greater than the anticipated systolic pressure. For the right ventricle, the ejection pressure is set at 30 mm Hg higher than the anticipated pulmonary artery pressure

The principles of cardiac physiology and the Starling curve are clearly evident with the TAH. Since the ventricles are set to fill to about 50–60 mL per beat, the patient can have an increased venous return of 10–20 mL per beat (for a total of 70 mL) for such circumstances as exercise, when the patient would have an increased venous return and in turn increased stroke volume and increased cardiac output by 1.5–2.5 L/min. The drivers are set to allow filling the ventricles to 70–85 % of full capacity with an ejection of 100 %. The decreased filling

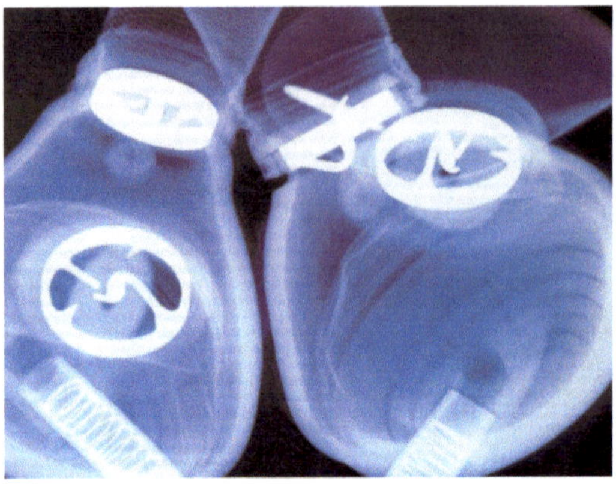

Fig. 13.3 Radiograph of the CardioWest TAH-t ventricles showing the 27 mm diameter inflow and 25 mm diameter outflow valves, the four-layered diaphragm, the plastic cases, and the spiral wound drive lines

allows the pneumatic ventricles to accommodate for differences in left and right ventricular volumes that occur with such conditions as bronchial flow, coughing, Valsalva maneuvers, exercise, and transfusion. Also, this characteristic of the device prevents "overpumping" of the right to left ventricle, which, therefore, prevents pulmonary edema. In the non-pneumatic, electromechanical, and hydroelectric experimental TAHs, no such forgiving pneumatic "cushion" exists and balancing the ventricles continues to be a major challenge.

Patient Selection

In 2004, the results of the FDA IDE study for the SynCardia TAH-t in bridge-to-transplantation were published in the New England Journal of Medicine. The prospective study was conducted from January 1993 to September 2002 with a total of 130 patients: 81 patients in the protocol group, 35 retrospective control group, and 14 did not meet the criteria for the study though were implanted for the purpose of compassionate care. In that study, the indication for implantation was severe end-stage biventricular failure in patients who were considered reasonable candidates for cardiac transplantation. Thus, most patients had been listed for cardiac transplantation then decompensated and were felt to be too sick to be treated with a left ventricular assist device (LVAD). When we examined risk factors in this study [7], we concluded that the indications for implantation of the TAH are "(1) irreversible biventricular heart failure, (2) acute decompensation after cardiotomy, (3) cardiogenic shock after acute myocardial infarction, (4) stone heart, (5) irreversible cardiac rejection or graft failure, (6) failed LVAD and/or biventricular assist device (BiVAD), (7) decompensating heart failure with left ventricular thrombus, (8) acquired ventricular septal defect, (9) prosthetic or incompetent native aortic valve in cardiogenic shock, or (10) unresponsive ventricular arrhythmia."

The most important criterion for implantation of a TAH is availability of the device at the institution as well as the surgeon's experience. The patients must be candidates for a cardiac transplantation. Destination therapy as an indication for this device is likely to be covered in the near future, since it has been approved by the FDA and awaits final funding approval.

In the FDA study the selection inclusion criteria for the patients were fairly rigid. However, nearly 20 % of patients could not be weaned from cardiopulmonary bypass prior to device implant, and nearly 40 % were on intra-aortic balloon pump support, and 40 % had a history of prior cardiac surgery, and the mean creatinine was 1.7 mg/dL and bilirubin 2.0 mg/dL preimplantation (see Table 13.1).

Thus, patients that qualify for implantation of the TAH have severe biventricular disease, typically have multiple-system organ failure, and are at imminent risk of death. Copeland et al. compared the use of the LVAD, BiVAD, and TAH [8]. In this retrospective study, 75 % of TAH patients survived to transplantation as compared with 56 % of those on Novacor LVADs (Novacor, WorldHeart Inc., Ottawa, Ontario, Canada) and 38 % of those on Thoratec BiVADs (Thoratec Inc. Pleasanton, CA). A multivariate analysis that reported risk factors for the CardioWest TAH and compared them with similar studies of LVADs and BiVADs [7], concluded that the TAH was preferred for patients who had been diagnosed with renal and hepatic dysfunction, had elevated venous pressure, right heart failure, required

Table 13.1 Inclusion and exclusion criteria for the CardioWest TAH-t investigational device exemption (IDE) study

Inclusion criteria
Eligible for transplant (institutional criteria)
NYHA class IV
BSA 1.7–2.5 m^2, or T10 ≥ 10 cm (distance on CT scan from anterior vertebral body to sternum inner table at level of tenth thoracic vertebra)
Hemodynamic insufficiency demonstrated by A or B below:
A. CI ≤ 2.0 L/min/m^2 and one of the following:
SAP ≤ 90 mm Hg
CVP ≥ 18 mm Hg
B. Two of the following:
65
Dopamine ≥ 10 μg/kg/min
Dobutamine ≥ 10 μg/kg/min
Epinephrine ≥ 2 μg/kg/min
Other drugs at maximum levels
Intra-aortic balloon pump (IAPB)
Cardiopulmonary bypass (CPB)
Exclusion criteria
Use of any VAD
Pulmonary vascular resistance ≥ 8 Wood (640 dynes-s/cm^5)
Dialysis in previous 7 days
Serum creatinine ≥ 5 mg/dL
Cirrhosis with total bilirubin ≥ 5 mg/dL
Cytotoxic antibody ≥ 10 %

mechanical ventilation, and had a previous cardiac operation. The TAH significantly decreased the CVP and increased the systemic pressure, which, in turn, lead to increase in the organ perfusion pressure reversing multiple-system end-organ failure. The TAH is an excellent alternative for patients who are refractory to medical therapy and at high risk for an LVAD or BiVAD.

At La Pitie, LePrince et al. evaluated the use of the CardioWest TAH over a 15-year experience [9], from 1986 to 2001 in 127 patients. The study concluded that CardioWest TAH was the device of choice for those patients who are truly sick with biventricular failure as a bridge-to-transplantation. They reported a low incidence of neurological events. This success can be attributed to the anticoagulation protocol. This will be further discussed in detail later in this chapter. Furthermore, LePrince et al. noted that a small body size correlated with a higher rate of death for these patients.

In addition, at Bad Oeynhausen, Morshuis et al. [10] reported a 5-case series that showed that the CardioWest TAH could also be used successfully for an acute myocardial infarction for a patient in cardiogenic shock. They noticed that approximately 7 % who are diagnosed with a myocardial infarction develop cardiogenic shock. In this case study, Morshuis et al. noted a hospital mortality of 60–100 % with medical therapy. By the time the patient develops cardiogenic shock, it is too late to save the infarcted myocardium with medical therapy or stenting. Thus, mechanical circulatory support systems are excellent options, especially the TAH. The SynCardia TAH-t was shown to have higher pump flows than other BiVADs. In comparison, patients with cardiogenic shock are not accustomed to the severely decreased perfusion systemically and thus, the TAH with higher pump flows prevented the systemic decreased perfusion to multiple organ systems. The Bad Oeynhausen team was also able to stop the use of catecholamines which also further damage multiple organ systems. There is a risk of failure of recovery with VADs and in turn thrombosis of the ventricle which is easily prevented with the use of the TAH because the native ventricles are completely removed. Morshuis et al. concluded that the TAH "represents the only life-saving therapeutic option in patients with irreversible cardiogenic shock."

Along with the indications for patient selection, a surgeon must evaluate other factors prior to implantation. The following size factors that significantly improve the outcome for patients prior to implantation of TAH are body surface area (BSA) ≥2 m^2, left ventricular end-diastolic dimension of ≥70 mm, anterior posterior diameter of the heart at the level of T10 on computed tomography (CT) scan of ≥10 cm from the inner table of the sternum to the anterior edge of the T10 vertebra, and a calculated native heart volume by CT scan of ≥1500 mL; these are factors that give assurance that the SynCardia TAH-t will fit into the recipient and function normally. A risk factor analysis taken from the FDA study of the SynCardia TAH-t found several factors that increased the risk of death [7] (see Tables 13.2 and 13.3).

The patients in that study had an average cardiac index of 1.9 L/min/m^2, a pulmonary capillary wedge pressure (PCWP) ranged from 11 to 43 mm Hg, and average CVP of 20 mm Hg. The laboratory values were consistent with multisystem organ failure with average values such as sodium of 132 mmol/L, creatinine of 1.7 mg/dL, total bilirubin of 2.0 mg/dL, and an INR of 2.0. Comparison of multivariate risk factors found in this study with those reported for other devices suggested that the CardioWest TAH could be used in sicker patients with less concern for factors that increase risk with LVADs and BiVADs.

Postoperative Care: Anticoagulation and Nutrition

Post-implantation of the CardioWest TAH, the patient must be placed on strict anticoagulation therapy that is adjusted based on the patient's laboratory values. The risks for thrombus formation after the implantation of the device are from the patient's condition: pre-bypass, post-bypass, and post-implant combined with blood reactivity as a result activation of platelets, coagulation proteins, fibrinolysis, leukocytes, and proinflammatory cytokines. In addition, biomaterials of the device increase the risks of thrombus as well the flow dynamics of the device such as turbulence and stagnation of blood. Furthermore, the patients must be monitored closely in order to provide him/her with adequate anticoagulation and simultaneously minimize or, better yet, prevent bleeding. This is a fine line the physician must walk. Postoperatively, the patient is placed on heparin at starting dose of 2–5 units/kg/h, aspirin at 41–81 mg/day for each increment of platelet count of 50,000 per mL above 150,000, dipyridamole at 75–100 mg for 6–8 h if the platelet count is >50,000/mL, and pentoxifylline at a dose of 200–400 mg PO for 8 h. Patients are transitioned from heparin to warfarin at a starting dose of 2–7.5 mg/day typically on postoperative day 7 to maintain an INR of 2 to 3 [11].

To maintain the balance between adequate anticoagulation and prevention of bleeding, a multisystem monitoring is helpful. The following tests are followed: thromboelastography, platelet aggregation, CBC (especially the platelet count), PFA-100, PT/INR, PTT, fibrinogen, D-dimer, liver function tests, total protein, albumin, prealbumin, cholesterol, CRP, and BUN. For patients treated with continuous infusion heparin, thromboelastography is an excellent method of monitoring coagulability. Thromboelastography measures the interaction between platelets and clotting factors and thus provides information about fibrin formation, clot rate, clot strengthening, and stability of the clot. A physician can determine if a patient is hypo-, normo-, or hypercoaguable. The goal of anticoagulation of TAH recipients is to maintain them in the normocoagulable range by thromboelastography.

This anticoagulation regimen has reduced the total incidence of stroke to 2.7 %, the lowest of all devices when compared to the Thoratec Heartmate II, Novacor, and Thoratec. Based on the University Medical Center CardioWest study, there was a stroke rate of 0.12 per patient per year.

In addition to anticoagulation, these patients are anemic and require supplements such as iron, vitamin C, folic acid, and vitamin B-12. Some patients are also prescribed Epogen (epoetin alfa). This may make patients more hypercoagulable and necessitate adjustment of the postoperative anticoagulation therapy regimen.

The key to a successful anticoagulation is to individualize the therapy to the patient. In addition, having a designated individual that monitors patients' anticoagulation specifically while on the CardioWest TAH ensures that the balance between adequate anticoagulation and bleeding prevention can be achieved.

In addition to anticoagulation therapy, nutrition is an extremely important part of the postoperative care. It is important to place these patients on gastrointestinal prophylaxis with either H2 blockers or proton pump inhibitors. While on the CardioWest TAH, these patients will have a high calorie need and may require high protein shake supplements throughout the day to ensure that they meet their new caloric intake demands.

Table 13.2 Univariate analysis of risk factors for death in CardioWest bridge-to-transplantation with three end points

Pre-op prognostic factor	Risk of death from implant to transplant odds ratio (p-value)	Risk of death to 30 days posttransplant odds ratio (p-value)	Risk of death to 1 year posttransplant odds ratio (p-value)
Ischemic cardiomyopathy	ns	3.45 (0.02)	2.70 (0.05)
Male gender	ns	ns	ns
History of smoking	3.45 (0.05)	3.23 (0.03)	ns
Heavy alcohol intake	ns	ns	ns
History of hypertension	ns	ns	ns
Cardiac arrest within 24 h	ns	ns	ns
Anticoagulated	ns	ns	ns
On heart-lung machine	3.33 (0.05)	ns	ns
On IABP	ns	ns	ns
On ventilator	ns	ns	ns
Obtunded	ns	ns	ns
Prior mediastinal operation	4.00 (0.02)	3.70 (0.01)	3.33 (0.02)
Prior percutaneous angioplasty	ns	ns	ns
Pacemaker	ns	ns	ns
Automatic internal defibrillator	ns	ns	2.70 (0.05)
Diabetes	ns	ns	ns
Age ≥ 55	ns	ns	2.56 (0.05)
Body surface area ≥ 2 m^2	ns	ns	ns
Cardiac index ≥ 2 L/min/m^2	ns	ns	ns
Syst vasc resistance ≥ 1,200	ns	ns	ns
Pulm vasc resistance ≥ 250	ns	ns	ns
Heart rate ≥ 100 beats/min	ns	ns	ns
Systolic arterial pressure ≥ 90	ns	ns	ns
Pulmonary art syst press ≥ 50	0.25 (0.02)	0.32 (0.04)	0.37 (0.06)
Pulmonary art mean press ≥ 25	ns	ns	ns
PCWP mean ≥ 25 mm Hg	ns	ns	ns
Central venous pr ≥ 16 mm Hg	ns	ns	ns
Central venous pr ≥ 20 mm Hg	ns	ns	ns
Serum sodium ≥ 130 mEq/L	ns	ns	ns
BUN ≥ 40 mg/dL	ns	ns	ns
Serum creatinine ≥ 2 mg/dL	ns	ns	ns
Total bilirubin ≥ 2 mg/dL	ns	ns	ns
Total bilirubin ≥ 4 mg/dL	ns	ns	ns
SGOT ≥ 50 IU/L	ns	ns	ns
WBC ≥ 12,000/mL	ns	ns	ns
Platelet count ≥ 150,000/mL	0.19 (0.01)	0.30 (0.03)	ns
Fibrinogen ≥ 400 mg/dL	ns	ns	ns
Prothrombin time ≥ 16 s	ns	3.03 (0.03)	2.81 (0.04)
INR ≥ 2	ns	ns	ns
PTT ≥ 35 s	ns	ns	ns
pH ≥ 7.4	ns	ns	ns
$PaCO_2$ ≥ 30 Torr	ns	ns	ns
HCO_3 ≥ 20 mEq/L	ns	ns	ns

Table 13.3 Multivariate risk factor analysis for death in bridge-to-transplantation using the CardioWest TAH-t at three end points

End point	*N*	Variable	Odds ratio for death	95 % confidence interval	*p*-Value
Survival to transplant	69	History of smoking	34	2.19–500	0.01
Survival to 30-days post transplant	69	History of smoking	9.70	1.42–66	0.02
Survival to 30-days post transplant	69	Prothrombin time ≥ 16 s	4.74	1.04–21	0.04
Survival to 1-year post transplant	69	Prothrombin time ≥ 16 s	3.80	1.01–14	0.05

Small frequent meals are best tolerated on the TAH-t. While on the TAH, patients will increase their appetite and achieve an adequate nutritional status that will better prepare them for transplantation.

Good nutrition in combination with physical therapy will also provide for a healthy body ready for transplantation while on the TAH. Emphasis should be placed on physical rehabilitation to prevent muscular atrophy, respiratory compromise, and risk of infection. At the University of Arizona, the patients on the CardioWest TAH attended cardiac rehabilitation in the hospital gymnasium at least three times per week with the assistance of the nursing staff, engineers of the TAH, and the device nurse practitioner.

Implantation and Explantation of the CardioWest TAH-t

Prior to surgery, patients are prepped with an arterial line, central line, and standard mechanical ventilation. Care in the position of the tip of the central line is mandatory. It should not pass beyond the superior vena cava (SVC)–right atrial junction. Central lines of all types that are used during the duration of the implantation should also respect this limit. Any line that passes into the right atrium is a threat to jam the tricuspid valve, a fatal and preventable complication. With the proliferation of personnel capable of placing central lines, it is important to educate everyone and to have the radiology staff mark the position of the tips of such lines on all radiographs. A transesophageal echocardiogram is required for the evaluation of deairing, adequate device fit, and the absence of compression of the inferior vena cava (IVC) (most commonly seen in tight fit situations) and the left pulmonary veins (occasionally seen when the A–P diameter is limited). The atrial inflow connectors are trimmed to appropriate size, and the outflow conduits are sprayed with a thin layer of CoSeal (Baxter Inc., Deerfield, Illinois) then trimmed: aortic to 3 cm stretched length distal to the quick connector, pulmonic 6 cm stretched length distal to the quick connector.

The aorta, superior and IVC are cannulated. Umbilical tape is placed around the cavae as chokers. There is limited dissection around the aorta and pulmonary artery, which allows for minimal adhesions at time of transplantation. Then, cardiopulmonary bypass is instituted and the heart fibrillated. Total bypass is completed by pulling on chokers around the cavae. Next, the surgeon removes the native ventricles. While excising the ventricles, the surgeon must be sure to preserve the annulus of both the tricuspid and mitral valves. The incision is made on the ventricular side of the atrioventricular (AV) groove of the right ventricle then extended laterally to the acute margin and anteriorly across the right ventricular outflow tract and just proximal to the pulmonary valve. Then posteriorly, the incision is extended across the interventricular septum to the left side and then anteriorly about 1 cm on the ventricular side of the AV groove. The remaining muscle is trimmed to within 1–1.5 cm of the AV valves; the chordae are trimmed leaving 2 mm edge of valve tissue along the annulus. The great vessels are separated from each other only enough to give modest mobility thus leaving undissected tissue for explant (Figs. 13.4, 13.5 and 13.6)

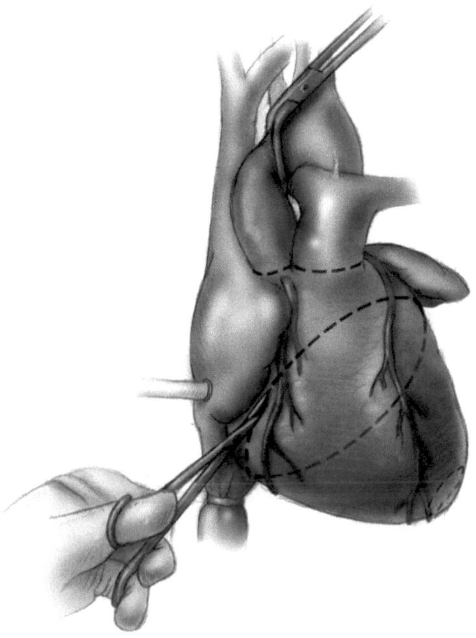

Fig. 13.4 The lines of cardiectomy are shown

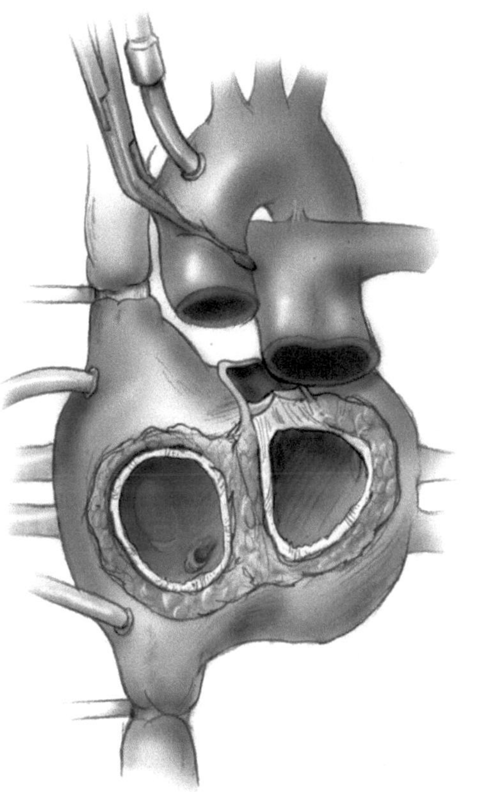

Fig. 13.6 On the "atrial cuffs" ventricular myocardium has been trimmed down to about 1 cm from the 2 mm circumferential AV valve remnant. The great vessels have been transected at the level of the sinotubular junctions

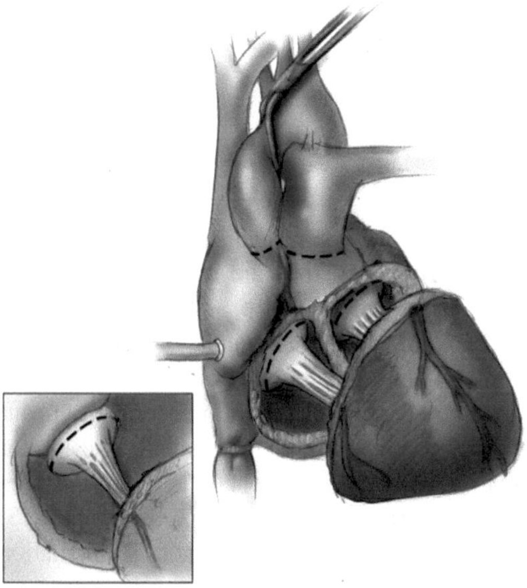

Fig. 13.5 The lines of resection are shown. Note that about 1 cm of ventricular tissue is retained and a 2 mm length of AV valve is also retained. Both of these strengthen the attachment of the atrial quick connectors (this article was published in Sabiston & Spencer's Surgery of the Chest, 8th edition, Zimmerman H, Copeland JG, Aquila Allen LA, Smith RG, "Total artificial heart," pp. 1525–1532, copyright Elsevier 2010)

The atria are now prepared with Teflon felt buttresses that encircle them. The buttresses have a twofold purpose—it can tamponade and control bleeding from the AV groove and strengthen the anastomosis to the inflow connector. The buttresses are approximately 10 mm in width and 10 cm in length. These buttresses, usually 2½ or 3, are placed on the outer edge of the atrial cuff and sewn in place with a running 3-0 polypropylene suture on an MH needle (Fig. 13.7). Next, the coronary sinus is oversewn with a 3-0 polypropylene suture (Fig. 13.8).

The atrial inflow connector is inverted and placed inside the left atrial cuff on the lateral wall and sewn in circumferentially with a 3-0 polypropylene on an MH needle in a running fashion (Fig. 13.9). The right quick connector is inverted and similarly sewn in place.

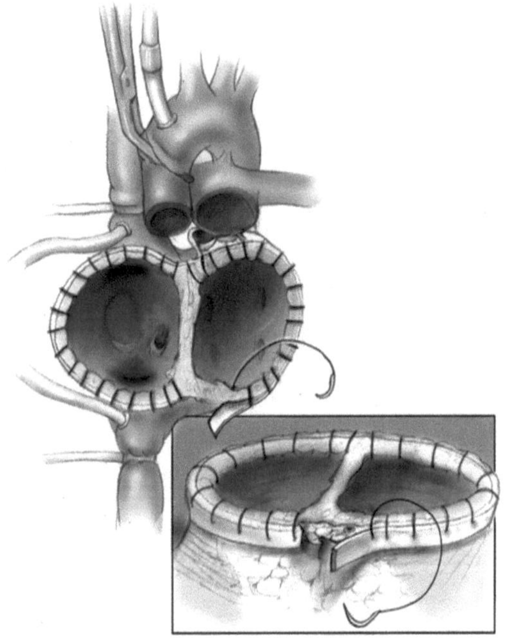

Fig. 13.7 A circumferential 10 mm strip of Teflon felt is sewn to the outside (not the septum) of the combined atrial cuffs. This strengthens the cuff for the quick connect anastomosis, and the epicardial to endocardial whipstitch occludes the many cut vessels in the AV groove fat (this article was published in Sabiston & Spencer's Surgery of the Chest, 8th edition, Zimmerman H, Copeland JG, Aquila Allen LA, Smith RG, "Total artificial heart," pp. 1525–1532, copyright Elsevier 2010)

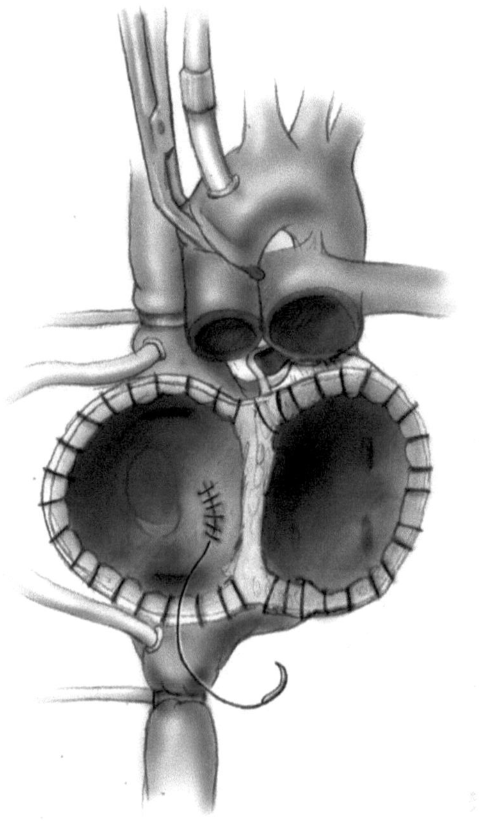

Fig. 13.8 Over sewing the coronary sinus

After finishing, the inflow connectors are returned to normal everted positions. Hemostasis is now checked with a plastic leak tester that fits in the inflow connector. A syringe with 60–100 cc in volume is injected into a three-way stopcock connected to the tester to test the atrial suture line. For example, the surgeon's hand is posterior to the left atrium and compresses the right and left pulmonary veins, and an assistant injects the saline and an observation for leaks is made. Next, using Freer elevator, the seal between the tester and connector is broken. This is repeated for the right side with the exception that the superior and IVC are already obstructed by the previously placed umbilical tapes. Sutures are placed if there are any identified leaks with a 3-0 MH polypropylene (Fig. 13.10).

Then, great vessel anastomoses are made with 4-0 polypropylene suture. The CoSeal preclotted aortic outflow conduit is 3 cm stretched length beyond the quick connector, and the pulmonic conduit is 6 cm stretched length. After making the anastomoses, they are tested for leaks (see Figs. 13.11 and 13.12).

Next a "neopericardium" is constructed of three 0.1 mm polytetrafluoroethylene (PTFE) of 15 cm × 20 cm sheets. The neopericardium has been shown to decrease mediastinal adhesion formation by decreasing contact between the prosthetic ventricles and mediastinal tissues [12, 13]. This markedly facilitates eventual explantation. One sheet is sutured on the right side of the heart just lateral to the cavae and at the posterior angle where the pericardium reflects onto the cavae. On the left side another sheet is sutured to the pericardial reflection anterior to the left pulmonary veins. The third sheet covers the diaphragm and is sutured near the left inferior pulmonary vein and near the IVC. The sheets are folded onto

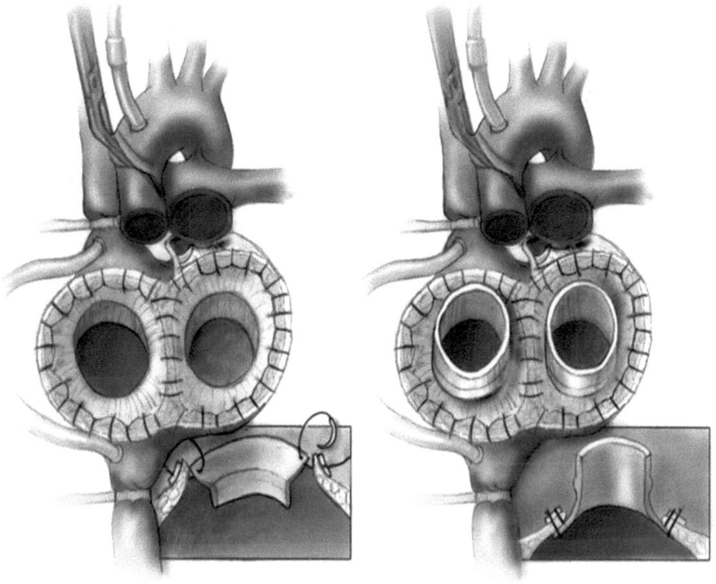

Fig. 13.9 Inverted (*left side* of diagram) cuffs are sewn in place then everted (*right side* of diagram)

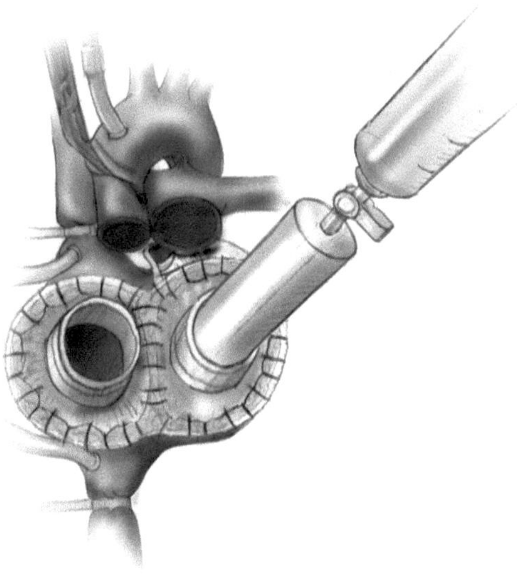

Fig. 13.10 Testing the left atrial cuff suture line for leaks

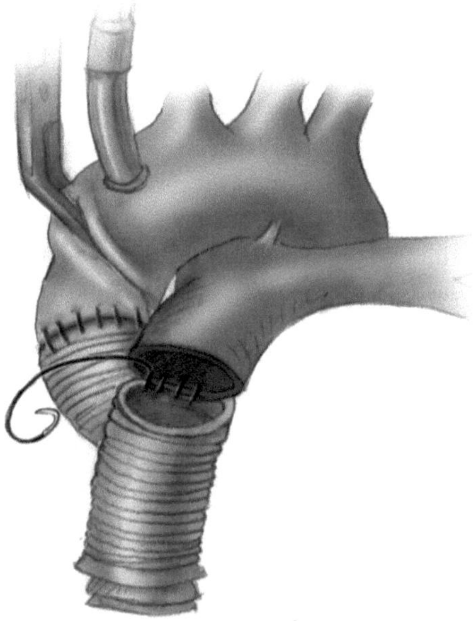

Fig. 13.11 Great vessel anastomoses

themselves until the CardioWest TAH is implanted. Once the ventricles are in place, the sheets are pulled up to completely cover both ventricles and are held in place with sutures or clips. We also place ribbons of PTFE about 5 mm wide around the SVC, IVC, and aorta. These loops are very loose and are left in place to facilitate placement of umbilical tapes around the cavae and aorta at device explantation. This construction of neopericardium and vessel looping has significantly shortened the skin incision to

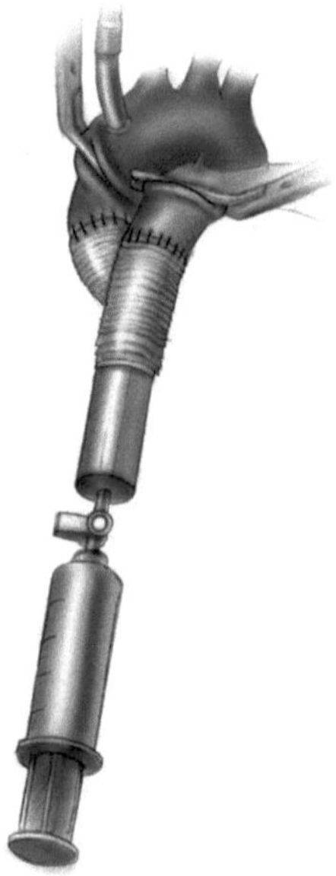

Fig. 13.12 Testing the pulmonary artery anastomosis. Note the clamp on the pulmonary artery

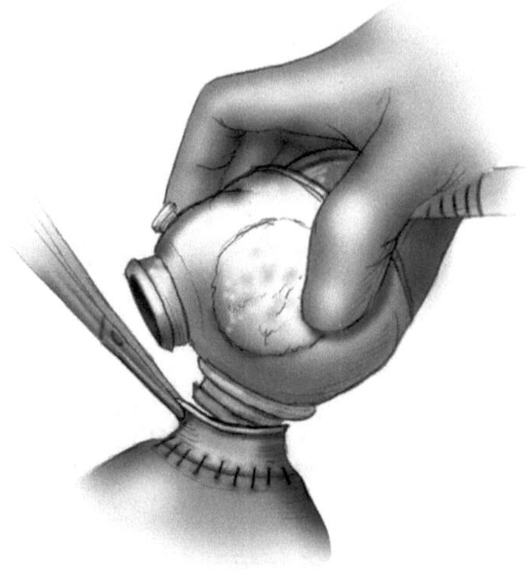

Fig. 13.13 Making the atrial connection. On the one side, we place side by side two medium heavy needle holders. The rigid atrial connector is "backed in" as if buttoning a button. It pops into the elastic quick connector with a snapping sound. The surgeon must check to be sure that the rigid connector is circumferentially fully engaged with the atrial quick connect (this article was published in Sabiston & Spencer's Surgery of the Chest, 8th edition, Zimmerman H, Copeland JG, Aquila Allen LA, Smith RG, "Total artificial heart," pp. 1525–1532, copyright Elsevier 2010)

start of cardiopulmonary bypass time [12], and it has diminished the thickening of the pericardium that was seen previously.

The driveline conduits that connect to the ventricles are positioned in subcutaneous pathways. The left-sided ventricle conduit is placed in the epigastrium at approximately the level of the midclavicular line and about 2 in. below the costal margin. The line is pulled through from the mediastinum to a 1 inch transverse skin incision using a 40 French straight chest tube. The driveline conveniently fits into the chest tube; thus, only one pass per driveline is necessary. The same approach is used to place the right-sided driveline conduit, just 4–5 cm medial to the left driveline, assuring the prevention of necrosis between the two sites. The driveline conduits are immediately connected to the 6 ft long PVC drivelines. This prevents fluid and particles from entering the drivelines. Then the console ends of these large lines are passed off and connected to the driver.

Now, the artificial ventricles can be placed, first the left. The atrial connection is made keeping the aortic quick connector as close to the native aorta as possible (Fig. 13.13).

Next the ventricle is filled with saline and it is wise to wait for the left atrium to fill from bronchial collateral flow before proceeding to the aortic connection. Maximal attempts at deairing are encouraged at this point before making the aortic connection. Once the aortic connection is done, we go on to the right ventricle connections. First the right atrial connection is made keeping the pulmonary artery rigid connecter as close to the pulmonary artery as possible. Just before making the pulmonary artery connection, the IVC tape is released for enough time to fill the prosthetic right ventricle with blood. Once this connection is completed, we place the patient in steep Trendelenburg position and release the aortic cross-clamp just after making a good size needle hole in the ascending aorta. The final appearance of the device is shown in Fig. 13.14.

We then remove caval tapes and start pumping at the low rate of 40 beats per minute. Using

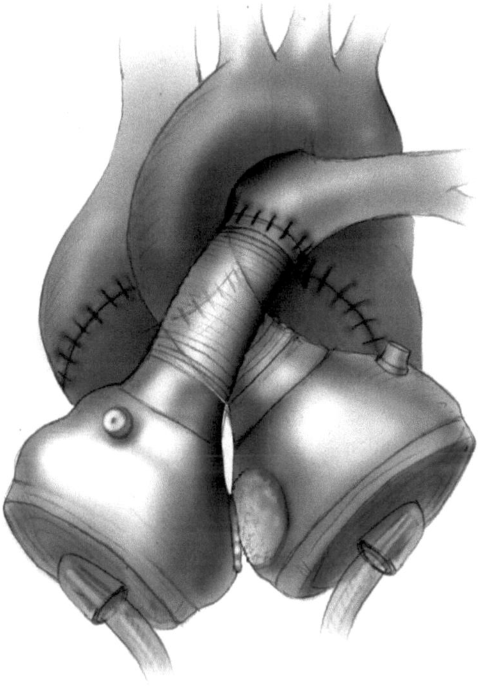

Fig. 13.14 Final appearance of the implanted ventricles (this article was published in Sabiston & Spencer's Surgery of the Chest, 8th edition, Zimmerman H, Copeland JG, Aquila Allen LA, Smith RG, "Total artificial heart," pp. 1525–1532, copyright Elsevier 2010)

transesophageal echo and with pulmonary ventilation, we gradually increase the beat rate as we separate from cardiopulmonary bypass. We attempt to completely deair prior to going to beat rates above 100. Once we verify that there is no more air in the heart, we discontinue cardiopulmonary bypass, close our vent site, and administer protamine.

At this point the pump output should be about 7 L/min and the CVP 10–15 mm Hg with a physiologic systemic pressure. Alpha agent support may be necessary if the systemic vascular resistance is low. Hemostasis is the next priority. The most complete hemostasis possible should be present before attempts at closing. Multiple chest tubes should be placed. We usually make small openings in the mediastinal pleura and insert tubes into both thoracic cavities as well as leaving 2–3 tubes in the mediastinum. Prior to closing the chest, the PTFE sheets are placed around the entire device.

Transesophageal echo is used to ensure the absence of compression of the IVC and the left pulmonary veins as the chest is being closed. Also, careful attention should be directed to the systemic and CVPs and the pump output. It is normal for the CVP to rise and the output and systemic pressure to fall with initial chest closure, but there should be a fairly prompt rebound to "normal" after a few minutes and some additional volume replacement.

Explantation

Explantation of the CardioWest TAH-t at the time of transplantation is much easier now that we use the neopericardium. Still we start 1.5–2 h before the anticipated arrival time of the donor heart. Our shortest time to establishing cardiopulmonary bypass through the chest in this setting was 14 min, though it usually takes about 45 min. Some groups start by heparinizing and cannulating the groin. We have in most cases kept all cannulation within the mediastinum. Once the chest is reopened, removal of the right-sided PTFE sheet exposes the right atrium for placement of caval cannulas. Using the PTFE ribbons around the cavae and the aorta, we tie one end of an umbilical tape to the divided PTFE and pull on the other end to pass the tape. With the aorta exposed and controlled with an umbilical tape and snares around the cavae, we then place purse string sutures, heparinize, cannulate, and begin bypass before doing any further dissection. Once we are on bypass, the CardioWest driver is turned off, the aorta cross-clamped, and total bypass instituted by tightening the caval snares. We then remove the ventricles at the quick connect levels and divide the drivelines near the exit site from the mediastinum. Once the device has been removed, there is more room for further dissection. The great vessels are cut fresh just distal to the conduit anastomoses. The atrial quick connectors are undercut just posterior to their anastomoses and taken together. Care is exercised to keep particulate debris away from the left atrial cuff in particular as well as the other three cuffs. If the left side of the pericardium is abnormally stiff or thickened, we remove it down to near the left phrenic nerve. This eliminates the possibility of constriction of the transplanted heart.

Because the recipient has been chronically anticoagulated, we anticipate a coagulopathy at this time. We do not recommend preemptive use of activated clotting factors [14]. Rather, we prime the pump with 4–6 units of fresh frozen plasma, give 2–4 units of platelets after the protamine, and give some additional fresh frozen plasma. We wait for hemostasis, sometimes up to several hours, rather than give activated factors. During that time, we use copious topical vancomycin solution for irrigation. A sense of restraint in blood and component replacement is advised to avoid right ventricular distention.

Table 13.4 Specific indications for the TAH

1. Incessant arrhythmias
2. Biventricular dysfunction
3. Prosthetic aortic valve
4. Thrombus in ventricle
5. Ventricular septal defects
6. Massive acute myocardial infarction
7. Stone heart, or failure to wean from cardiopulmonary bypass or ECMO, or unresponsive cardiac arrest in a potential transplant candidate
8. Graft failure posttransplantation

Table 13.5 Algorithm for patient and device selection

Patient condition	CardioWest TAH-t	BiVAD	LVAD
Unstable	Yes	Yes	No
Biventricular failure	Yes	Yes	No
Stable	No	No	Yes
BSA $\geq$ 1.7 m^2	Yes	No	No
BSA < 1.7 m^2	No	Yes	Yes
Bridge to recovery	No	Probably not	Yes

Summary

We implanted 108 CardioWest TAH-ts and found that this device has been used in about one-third of our cases alongside LVADs and BiVADs, each also used one-third of the time. There have been some situations that necessitate TAH use (Table 13.4).

In Table 13.5, our algorithm for device and patient selection is shown. This has developed over the past 23 years and reflects the availability of the three types of devices at our institution for most of that time. It summarizes in a few words sets of complex concepts. For instance, "unstable" is a term that is loosely used in our literature, but here means severe instability to the point of carrying significantly increased risk if an LVAD were used. Much of this, sorting out of risk factors has been done by those who have specialized in LVAD implants [15]. "Unstable" in this setting refers to renal and hepatic dysfunction, previous cardiac surgery, elevated CVP, etc. "Biventricular failure" refers to patients who are anticipated to have right heart failure after LVAD implantation. We know the mortality for such patients on LVAD support approaches 50 %. "Stable" in this algorithm means that the patient is stable on one or two inotropic infusions, having good end-organ function, and not requiring intensive hemodynamic monitoring and minute-to-minute therapy changes to maintain life. "BSA" or body surface area in this algorithm is used as a marker of adequate size for implantation of a TAH. In large patients with large hearts, there is never a sizing problem, and seldom is there a problem in large patients with normal size hearts for their body size, also seldom is there a problem with normal size patients who have very large hearts, i.e., left ventricular end-diastolic diameter (LVEDD) of >70 mm on echo. Judgment must be learned in this area, and surgical innovation may be necessary in smaller patients. Finally, bridge to recovery is a definite contraindication to the use of a TAH, and in our experience, it has been rare to see anyone sick enough for a BiVAD to have cardiac recovery.

The CardioWest TAH-t is a simple and powerful tool for surgeons and cardiologists treating unstable end-stage heart failure. It has been shown to salvage a high percentage of patients with relatively few adverse events. It was designed as a "permanent" device to last 4 years or more. This limit has not been tested in humans, but durability has not been an issue with implant times that often exceed 1 year. The device has been approved by the FDA as a temporary bridge-to-transplantation and by CMS (Centers for Medicare and Medicaid Services) for the highest-paying DRG (diagnosis-related group). No other TAH has achieved such approval status. We believe that it has an important place in rescuing sick patients. Acceptance by nearly all major transplant centers in the world has been gratifying. As the portable divers become more available, out-of-hospital care will be possible, costs for hospital length of stay will be dramatically cut, and use of the device is anticipated to increase rapidly in Europe, North America, and Australia.

References

1. Cooley DA, Liotta D, Hallman GL, Bloodwell RD, Leachman RD, Milam JD. First human implantation of cardiac prosthesis for staged total replacement of the heart. Trans Am Soc Artif Intern Organs. 1969;15:252–66.
2. Devries WC, Anderson J, Joyce L, Anderson F, Hammond EH, Jarvik RK, Kolff WJ. Clinical use of the total artificial heart. N Engl J Med. 1984;310:273–8.
3. Vaughn CC, Copeland JG, Cheng K, Austin J, Levinson MM. Interim heart replacement with a mechanical device: an adjunct to management of allograft rejection. J Heart Transplant. 1985;4:502–5.
4. Copeland JG, Levinson MM, Smith RG, Icenogle TB, Vaughn C, Cheng K, Ott R, Emery RW. The total artificial heart as a bridge to transplantation. A report of two cases. JAMA. 1986;256:2991–5.
5. Szefner J, Cabrol C. Control and treatment of hemostasis in patients with a total artificial heart: the experience at La Pitie. In: Piffare R, editor. Anticoagulation, hemostasis, and blood preservation in cardiovascular surgery. Philadelphia: Hanley and Belfus; 1993. p. 237–64.
6. Copeland JG, Smith RG, Arabia FA, Nolan PE, McClellan D, Tsau PH, Sethi GK, Bose RK, Banchy ME, Covington. Cardiac replacement with a total artificial heart as a bridge-to-transplantation. N Engl J Med. 2004;351:859–67.
7. Copeland JG, Smith RG, Bose RK, Tsau PH, Nolan PE, Slepian MJ. Risk factor analysis for bridge to transplantation with the CardioWest total artificial heart. Ann Thorac Surg. 2008;85:1639–44.
8. Copeland JG, Smith RG, Arabia FA, Nolan PE, Mehta VK, McCarthy MS, Chisholm KA. Comparison of the CardioWest total artificial heart, the Novacor left ventricular assist system and the Thoratec ventricular assist system in bridge to transplantation. Ann Thorac Surg. 2001;71(3 Suppl):S92–7.
9. Leprince P, Bonnet N, Rama A, Leger P, Borsier X, Levasseur JP, Szefner J, Vassier E, Pavie A, Gandjbakhch. Bridge to transplantation with the Jarvik-7 (CardioWest) total artificial heart: a single center 15-year experience. J Heart Lung Transplant. 2003;22:1296–303.
10. Morshuis M, Reiss N, Arsoglu L, Tenderich G, Korfer R, El-Banayosy A. Implantation of CardioWest total artificial heart for irreversible acute myocardial infarction shock. Heart Surg Forum. 2007;10:E251–6.
11. Copeland JG, Arabia FA, Tsau PH, McClellan D, Smith RG, Slepian MJ. Total artificial hearts: bridge to transplantation. Cardiol Clin. 2003;21:110–3.
12. Copeland JG, Arabia FA, Smith RG, Covington D. Synthetic membrane neo-pericardium facilitates total artificial heart explantation. J Heart Lung Transplant. 2001;20:654–6.
13. Leprince P, Rhamati M, Bonnet N, Bors V, Rama A, Lege P, Gandjbakhch I, Pavie A. Expanded polytetrafluoroethylene membranes become more wrap surfaces of circulatory support devices in become more undergoing bridge to heart transplantation. Eur J Cardiothorac Surg. 2001;19:302–6.
14. Wegner JA, DiNardo JA, Arabia FA, Copeland JG. Blood loss and transfusion requirements in patients implanted with a mechanical circulatory support device undergoing cardiac transplantation. J Heart Lung Transplant. 2000;19:504–6.
15. Rao V, Oz MC, Flannery MA, Catanese KA, Argenziano M, Naka Y. Revised screening scale to predict survival after insertion of a left ventricular assist device. J Thorac Cardiovasc Surg. 2003;125:855–62.

14 Right Ventricular Dysfunction in Patients Undergoing Left Ventricular Assist Device Implantation: Predictors, Management, and Device Utilization

Abeel A. Mangi

Background

Right ventricular dysfunction occurs fairly frequently during the conduct of standard cardiac operations, but is largely a reversible and transient phenomenon. It is generally thought to be caused by embolization of air down the right coronary artery, incomplete or inadequate revascularization, or inadequate myocardial protection. Conventional and widely used strategies such as reperfusing the heart at higher blood pressure, revascularization, or "resting" the empty beating heart on bypass are known to ameliorate the severity of this condition.

For the purposes of this chapter, we define nonreversible failure of the right ventricle as the need for postoperative inotropic support for greater than 14 days, inhaled nitric oxide for greater than 48 h, right-sided circulatory support, or hospital discharge on an inotrope. Nonreversible failure of the right ventricle represents the more malignant form of this syndrome and is seen in 0.04–0.1 % of postcardiotomy cases. Unfortunately, the incidence of right ventricular dysfunction after left ventricular assist device (LVAD) implantation that fails to resolve in the operating room is reported to range from 20 % to 50 % and imposes a considerable burden in terms of postoperative morbidity and mortality. Should this syndrome supervene, the mortality of an LVAD operation increases from 19 % to 43 % [1]. Although most patients can be maintained with prolonged inotropic support, 10–15 % may require implantation of a separate right ventricular support device (RVAD).

A.A. Mangi, M.D. (✉)
Department of Cardiac Surgery, Yale New Haven Hospital/Yale University School of Medicine, Boardman 204, 333 Cedar Street, New Haven, CT 06510, USA
e-mail: abeel.mangi@gmail.com

The Implications of Right Ventricular Dysfunction

Persistent right ventricular dysfunction after LVAD implantation has been shown to independently predict higher incidences of end-organ dysfunction, longer intensive care unit and hospital lengths of stay, and increased morbidity and increased mortality in patients awaiting transplantation [2–4]. Right ventricular (RV) dysfunction severe enough to require RVAD implantation is independently predictive of death.

Impaired Hepatic Perfusion

Patients who require LVAD implantation have tenuous end-organ function, usually because of both right and left ventricular failure. It is well recognized that blood flow is distributed away from splanchnic organs in the setting of systemic hypotension such as that may occur in patients with severe left-sided heart failure. This diversion

J.A. Morgan and Y. Naka (eds.), *Surgical Treatment for Advanced Heart Failure*,
DOI 10.1007/978-1-4614-6919-3_14,

of flow is accomplished by mesenteric vasoconstriction, which, in turn, leads to decrease in portal venous return to the liver. Since the majority of oxygen flow to the liver comes from the portal circulation, this can result in centrilobular necrosis and a resultant release of hepatic enzymes. The need to place such a patient on cardiopulmonary bypass (CPB) with attendant hypotension and hemodilution exacerbates mesenteric vasoconstriction, furthering liver injury by the mechanisms discussed earlier [5].

When right-sided heart failure occurs in addition to left-sided heart failure, the addition of "passive hepatic congestion," which might more accurately be termed venous hypertension of the liver, serves to exacerbate hepatic hypoxia. This is because the column of low pressure portal venous blood cannot negotiate the high pressure column of venous blood and can no longer perfuse the hepatocytes. The addition of right-sided failure therefore serves to exacerbate hepatic hypoxia already present because of left-sided heart failure. This is one explanation for why even after correcting left ventricular performance with cardiac replacement therapies, the overwhelming majority of patients, in some estimate, as high as 94 % demonstrate persistent hepatic dysfunction [6].

Systemic Inflammatory Response Due to Splanchnic Hypoperfusion

More troubling is the systemic inflammatory response that hepatic dysfunction can engender. Rossi and associates studied 11 randomly selected patients with normal cardiac chamber size and function, who were undergoing elective isolated coronary artery bypass graft surgery with the use of CPB [7]. In the absence of significant macrocirculatory changes and postoperative complications, a correlation existed between the damage to the gastrointestinal mucosa, subsequent increased permeability, *Escherichia coli* bacteremia, and the activation of a self-limited inflammatory response. In the liver sinusoid, free intravascular lipopolysaccharide (LPS) produced from degradation of the bacterial cell wall binds to LPS-binding protein (LBP). This complex has a high affinity for the CD14 cell surface receptor on the Kupffer cell, causing activation and secretion of inflammatory cytokines including, but not limited to, TNF-α, IL-1β, and IL-6; eicosanoids; intercellular adhesion molecules; platelet-activating factor; oxygen-free radicals; and nitric oxide. Simultaneously, soluble CD14 binds with the LPS/LBP complex and activates endothelial cells, which then release a similar inflammatory cascade. The secretion of TNF-α sets in motion the cellular, metabolic, and vascular responses of systemic inflammatory response syndromes, septic shock, and multiple-system organ failure syndromes [8]. Although transient splanchnic ischemia may be self-limiting and clinically irrelevant in relatively healthy patients with normal hepatic function, one would hypothesize that this cannot hold true for patients with end-stage heart disease who already have severely compromised liver function. In fact, such a hypothesis holds true. Studying a group of 16 patients undergoing LVAD implantation, Masai and co-workers demonstrated that patients with hyperbilirubinemia and inflammatory reactions before LVAD support showed worsening of hyperbilirubinemia, inflammatory cytokine, and hyaluronan levels despite adequate hemodynamics achieved under LVAD support. These results suggest that inflammatory response contributes to subsequent aggravation of hepatic dysfunction, with cholestasis and fibrosis and with ongoing derangement in hepatic sinusoidal microcirculation even under adequate systemic circulatory support [9]. Whether such a syndrome can be ameliorated by the use of antibodies to TNF-alpha or by empiric use of drugs known to blunt the systemic inflammatory response syndrome, such as Xigris, is speculative and needs to be considered in light of the specific complications that these drugs carry.

Prolonged Hospital Stay and Greater Mortality Awaiting Transplant

Irrespective of what the causes of right-sided failure after LVAD implantation are, it is indisputable that a prolonged requirement for inotropic support translates into a longer intensive care unit stay, a longer overall hospital stay, as well as into a greater mortality rate. Masai et al. [9] have demonstrated that patients who suffer RV dysfunction after LVAD implantation have higher postoperative creatinine (2.2 mg/dL versus 1.5 mg/dL), greater need for postoperative continuous venovenous hemodialysis (73 % versus 26 %), greater transfusion requirement (43.2 units versus 24.7 units of packed red blood cells), greater requirement for platelet transfusion (58 units versus 30 units), longer intensive care unit stays (33 days versus 9 days), and higher mortality (42.8 % versus 14.5 %).

Of most interest, the higher mortality rate persists even after inotropes have been successfully weaned off and is directly correlated with the duration of inotropic support [2]. When Schenk et al. examined 176 patients who underwent isolated LVAD implantation, they noted that although 100 % of patients were on inotropes on the day of operation, when they could be discontinued, this was most often accomplished between postoperative days 3 and 5. By postoperative day 7, 57 % of patients were still inotrope dependent; by postoperative day 14, 33 % of patients were still inotrope dependent; and by postoperative day 21, 22 % of patients were still inotrope dependent. Patients with nonischemic etiologies of heart failure and those with right ventricular stroke work indices less than 500 mmHg mL/m^2 were most likely to be on inotropes for greater than 14 days. Most striking, however, was the finding that duration of inotropic support impacted 6-month survival. Specifically, patients who tolerated discontinuation of inotropic support on the first postoperative day had a 6-month survival of 72 %, but those who required inotropic support until postoperative days 10, 30, and 60 had a 6-month survival of 64 %, 57 %, and 46 %, respectively.

Morgan et al. [4] suggest that timing of RVAD implantation influences survival to transplantation, likely reflecting a selection bias in candidates for LVAD support, and heightened vigilance in the immediate postoperative course. They demonstrate that survival to transplant in patients who underwent early RVAD implantation (i.e., within 24 h) was 70 % versus a survival rate of 57 % in those who underwent RVAD implantation greater than 24 h after LVAD implantation. This finding is statistically significant ($p<0.001$).

In addition, these authors [4] demonstrated that the diminishment in survival when right ventricular support is needed *persists after transplantation.* Patients who require RVAD in addition to LVAD have a 1-, 5-, and 10-year posttransplant actuarial survival rate of 71.4 %, 71.4 %, and 71.4 %, respectively, whereas patients requiring LVAD only have a posttransplant actuarial survival rate of 90.5 %, 80.4 %, and 78.5 % at 1, 5, and 10 years. While this discussion of right ventricular failure is therefore germane to patients being bridged to transplantation, it is of even more importance in destination therapy patients, in whom transplantation is not an option, and in whom appropriate selection is critically important.

Mortality After RVAD Implantation

RV failure of a magnitude that requires RVAD implantation emerges as an independent predictor of death in every series on the subject. In the series from Frazier et al. [10], 4 out of 34 patients undergoing LVAD implantation as bridge to transplant required RVAD placement, and none survived to transplantation. In the analysis, RV failure was the only variable that correlated with a negative outcome. Echoing these results, Goldstein et al. [11] report that 21 of 22 patients requiring RVAD died awaiting transplantation, and Kormos et al. report that 40 % of patients requiring RV support succumbed prior to transplantation [12]. In the Cleveland Clinic series, 16 patients required RVAD implantation within 2 days of LVAD implantation, and the remaining two required RVAD implantation on postoperative days 3 and 12 because of respiratory failure followed by severe RV dysfunction. High dose inotropic support preceded RVAD implantation in 17 of 18 patients. Survival to transplantation decreased dramatically with time in this cohort and was 47 % at postoperative day 10, 29 % at postoperative day 20, and only 22 % at postoperative day 30. Overall, survival to transplant was 27 % versus 83 % in patients who did not require RVAD implantation [2].

Predictors of RV Dysfunction After LVAD Implantation

Right ventricular dysfunction after LVAD implantation is common, is difficult to control, and may have disastrous clinical and programmatic implications. It is intuitive, therefore, that by identifying patients at risk for RV dysfunction, preoperative maneuvers may be undertaken to reduce the likelihood of postoperative RV dysfunction, and that in patients deemed prohibitive risks, that alternative means of biventricular support such as the total artificial heart be considered. Consensus is starting to emerge in the literature on what preoperative symptom complex constitutes high risk for postoperative RV dysfunction.

In general, two schools of thought dominate the discussion of, and approach to, preoperative risk factors for right ventricular failure after LVAD implantation. The first emphasizes patient characteristics and features, and the other emphasizes analysis of hemodynamic parameters. From a practical perspective, both factors probably carry equal weight and should be considered while evaluating a patient for mechanical circulatory support.

Clinical Predictors of Right Ventricular Failure

Kormos et al. [13] have argued that non-hemodynamic preoperative clinical factors are more predictive of RV failure because "patients who are more clinically compromised and have more marginal end-organ function tend to require more extensive right ventricular support after LVAS implantation." Studying 32 patients, Kormos et al. demonstrated that patients with borderline multiorgan failure, elevation of bilirubin or creatinine, with a fever around the time of implantation, those demonstrating a requirement for pure pressors, adult respiratory distress syndrome, or right ventricular infarction are at exceedingly high risk for perioperative right ventricular failure requiring prolonged inotropic support or right-sided circulatory support.

This view has been echoed by Pagani et al. who in a study of 32 patients suggested that there was a higher tendency to develop right ventricular failure necessitating mechanical assistance after LVAD implant in patients who came to medical attention in cardiac arrest, with severe hemodynamic instability (systolic blood pressure ≤ 75 mm Hg) requiring short-term circulatory support with ECMO and with evidence of multiorgan failure (defined as serum creatinine level >3 mg/dL or oliguria; international normalized ratio >1.5 or transaminases >five times normal or total bilirubin >3 mg/dL; and needing mechanical ventilation) [14].

Recently Fukumachi et al. [15] analyzed 100 patients, Ochiai et al. [16] studied 245 patients, and Matthews et al. [17] have looked at 197 patients undergoing LVAD implantation. Using univariate analyses, all three authors have suggested that patient-specific factors do indeed predict the need for prolonged right ventricular inotropic support and/or right ventricular assist device. Common factors identified by all three authors include small body surface area, female sex (which may be a surrogate for smaller body surface area or BSA), younger patient age, the presence of myocarditis, and higher preoperative levels of serum aspartate transaminase levels (AST 637 versus 146, $p=0.0059$).

Additional factors identified separately by the three authors using univariate analysis include the following. Fukamachi et al. identified the need for preoperative use of intra-aortic balloon counter-pulsation, extracorporeal membrane oxygenation, short-term mechanical support, positive pressure ventilation, body temperature, and renal function as assayed by BUN or creatinine as predictive of the need for right-sided mechanical support [15]. Ochiai et al. identified the need for preoperative mechanical ventilation (83 % versus 56 % $p=0.015$) and preoperative circulatory assistance (48 % versus 18 %

$p = 0.003$) predicted the need for prolonged postoperative inotropic support [16]. Matthews et al. identified the presence of renal replacement therapy (odds ratio 9.93), dependence upon vasopressin (odds ratio 7.24), serum creatinine greater than 2.3 (odds ratio 5.56), dependence on Neo-Synephrine (odds ratio 3.59), serum bilirubin greater than 2 (odds ratio 3.59), serum AST >80 (odds ratio 3.2), a white blood cell count greater than 12,200 (odds ratio 3.36), dependence on ventilator (odds ratio 3.18), need for preoperative mechanical circulatory support ECMO/Tandem (Cardiac Assist Inc., Pittsburgh, PA, USA)/Abiomed (Danvers, MA, USA) (odds ratio 3.17), prior cerebrovascular event (odds ratio 2.99), cardiopulmonary arrest within 24 h of operation (odds ratio 2.61), and dependence upon intravenous antiarrhythmic therapy (OR 2.56) as predictive of RV failure [17].

Upon multivariate analysis, Fukumachi et al. [15] and Ochiai et al. [16] demonstrated that the need for preoperative circulatory support (odds ratio 5.3), female gender (odds ratio 4.5), and nonischemic etiology of cardiogenic shock (odds ratio 3.3) were strongly predictive of the need for postoperative right-sided circulatory support.

Upon multivariate analysis, Matthews et al. demonstrated that the need for a pressor requirement (weighted to receive 4 points), elevation in creatinine (weighted to receive 3 points), elevation in bilirubin (weighted to receive 2.5 points), and elevation in AST (weighted to receive 2 points) strongly predicted postoperative RV failure. The scoring system developed by Matthews et al. predicts that patients with a score greater than 5.5 have a 15-fold greater chance of developing right ventricular failure when compared to patients with a score less than 3 [17].

Although very sophisticated, for practical purposes, however, it is not very different from the earlier descriptions of preoperative predictions of RV failure after LVAD implantation that we described earlier in this section—that is, patients in hemodynamic extremis with evidence of hepatic or renal dysfunction are at prohibitively high odds for right ventricular failure after LVAD implantation and are probably best served with institution of biventricular support at initial operation.

Hemodynamic Predictors of Right Ventricular Failure

Right heart catheterization prior to LVAD implantation has been used to ascertain what, if any, hemodynamic factors are predictive of RV failure. Ochiai et al. [16] demonstrated, by univariate analysis, that patients requiring RVAD had lower mean pulmonary artery pressure (PAP) (33 mmHg versus 37 mmHg, $p = 0.04$), lower diastolic PAP (25 mmHg versus 29 mmHg, $p = 0.03$), and lower RVSW (543 mmHg mL versus 780 mmHg mL, $p = 0.037$). These results were verified by Fukamachi et al. [15] who, using univariate analyses, demonstrated that lower cardiac output (2.8 L/min versus 3.5 L/min, $p = 0.019$), lower mean PAP (31 mmHg versus 38 mmHg, $p = 0.015$), and lower right ventricular stroke work index (RV-SWI) (151 mmHg/mL/m^2 versus 368 mmHg/mL/m^2, $p = 0.011$) were all predictive of postoperative RVAD support. RV SWI in particular emerged as a highly specific predictor, with a specificity of 100 %, sensitivity of 54 %, positive predictive value of 100 %, and a negative predictive value of 20 %. This is also borne out by Matthews et al. [18], who demonstrate that RVSWI <450 has an odds ratio of 2.32 in predicting postoperative failure of the RV and that PA systolic pressure >50 is protective against postoperative RV failure, with an odds ratio of 0.49. Similarly, Morgan et al. [4] suggest that a high central venous pressure (CVP) coupled with low pulmonary artery (PA) pressure and a low RVSWI are predictive of right ventricular failure after LVAD implantation. In fact it has been demonstrated that patients *without* pulmonary hypertension were more likely to develop RV failure and die [18, 19] after LVAD implantation.

Farrar et al. [20] reported that only 46 % of patients with ischemic cardiomyopathy required RVAD whereas 63 % of patients with nonischemic cardiomyopathy required RVAD. Alternatively, 46 % of biventricular assist devices (biVADs) had nonischemic etiology as opposed to 40 % of those with ischemic cardiomyopathy. In addition, RVAD patients had higher incidence of reop for bleeding (57 % versus 27 % $p = 0.003$). They had poorer survival to transplantation (17 % versus

74 % $p < 0.001$) and required LVAD support for 94 days as opposed to 27 days in the no-RVAD group ($p = 0.002$). The low PAP and low RVSWI are referred to again, implying that depressed RV contractility before LVAD insertion was not strong enough to elevate PAP in the presence of high pulmonary vascular resistance (PVR) [19].

The implications of these findings are that when RV contractility is inadequate to generate a high PAP, the right ventricle is incapable of coping with the changes imposed by LVAD implantation. However, irreversibility of pulmonary hypertension, particularly when associated with high right atrial pressure, may suggest concomitant pulmonary disease or irreversible injury to the right ventricle. In such cases, a 4- to 8-week-long trial of selective pulmonary vasodilators (milrinone, sildenafil, prostaglandins) with serial right heart catheterization may be warranted in an attempt to lower PVR and improve cardiac index.

In summary, therefore, patients with nonischemic cardiomyopathy; with a hemodynamic profile suggesting elevation in CVP and diminution of PA pressures, and a low RVSWI; and a clinical profile that suggests the need for vasopressors, mechanical support, renal, respiratory, or hepatic dysfunction are at extremely high risk for post-LVAD right-sided heart failure and should be considered for a priori biventricular support.

Assessment of Right Ventricular Geometry, Function, and Tricuspid Valve Regurgitation

Pre-implant echocardiographic assessment of the right ventricle offers an important guide to preoperative and intraoperative management of right ventricular function. A dilated right ventricle that has lost its triangular "wedge-shaped" configuration on a zero-degree four-chamber view and assumes a globular shape is of concern. Contribution by the basal, free wall, and apical segments of the right ventricle are important to assess. Position of the interatrial septum and interventricular septum is important to assess when actuating a continuous-flow LVAD. Excessive unloading of the left ventricle causes the interventricular septum to shift leftward. This, in turn, induces a series of disadvantageous geometrical changes in the right ventricle that eliminate the septal contribution to RV stroke volume. In addition, the annulus of the tricuspid valve that corresponds to the septal leaflet is distorted, perhaps resulting in worsening tricuspid regurgitation.

The presence of severe functional tricuspid regurgitation is often an indicator of severe right ventricular dysfunction due to long-standing volume and pressure overload. Therefore, a reluctance to repair the tricuspid valve often exists, owing to concern over exacerbating right ventricular dysfunction. It is, however, being realized that severe preoperative tricuspid insufficiency is a risk factor for early right ventricular failure. The mechanism behind this may be acute and overwhelming volume and pressure overload of the right ventricle. Because of the low pressure sink in the systemic venous chambers, blood would preferentially stream into the systemic venous chambers instead of into the pressurized pulmonary circuit. Accordingly, left-sided chambers (and therefore the LVAD) would remain underfilled, which would potentiate the inability of the device to unload the pulmonary circuit, resulting in a tight spiral of early and overwhelming right ventricular failure. Accordingly, the presence of severe tricuspid regurgitation should be repaired or treated with rigid annuloplasty. Destruction of tricuspid leaflets may require valvular replacement, but this is unusual.

Mild to moderate tricuspid regurgitation and a functional valve would probably improve with a reduction in RV afterload that typically occurs during LVAD support.

If the right ventricle is ischemic, consideration should be given to surgical revascularization at the time of LVAD implantation.

Pathophysiology of Right Ventricular Dysfunction

There are four fundamental causes by which the right ventricle fails after implantation of an LVAD. These are ischemia, alterations in interventricular balance, position of the interventricular septum, and the need to simultaneously perform volume and pressure work.

Ischemia of the right ventricle, or the interventricular septum, can occur in a patient with unrevascularized ischemic cardiomyopathy or when the intracavitary pressure of a distended and overloaded right ventricle exceeds coronary perfusion pressure. Ways in which this situation can be avoided is by revascularizing the right coronary artery at the time of LVAD implantation, or by separating from bypass with a volume underloaded right ventricle, and at a high systemic blood pressure.

In general, under conditions that assume a balanced circulation, left ventricular output must by necessity be equal to right ventricular output. When an LVAD is implanted, it introduces an imbalance in interventricular balance such that the right ventricle must now match LVAD output. In patients who have suffered an isolated massive left ventricular infarction, this is generally not difficult for what is essentially a normal right ventricle. However, in patients who suffer nonischemic diffuse biventricular cardiomyopathy, the augmentation of preload returning to the right ventricle after implantation of an LVAD may unmask right ventricular dysfunction. In addition, under ideal circumstances, right ventricular afterload should decrease, with a drop in passive pulmonary hypertension. This however as we will see is not always the case.

Bleeding requiring massive blood product resuscitation, hypercarbia or acidemia, mechanical pulmonary problems, and pulmonary endothelial dysfunction after CPB can increase PVR acutely after LVAD implantation. In a situation where a diseased right ventricle is already being asked to perform volume work, the imposition of pressure work in addition can be simply overwhelming. The right ventricle can perform volume work or can perform pressure work. But it is very rare that a right ventricle can perform both pressure and volume work simultaneously.

Finally, right ventricular developed pressure is determined by performance of the free wall of the right ventricle as well as by position and function of the interventricular septum. As continuous-flow devices become more commonplace, an understanding of the role of the position of the interventricular septum is very important. As a continuous-flow LVAD is actuated, and as the left ventricle is unloaded, the septum is "sucked" towards the left. This results in an immediate increase in the diastolic compliance of the right ventricle. As capacitance of this chamber increases, and septal contribution to right ventricular performance is taken away by suctioning it into the left ventricle, fatigue of the right ventricular free wall can occur over the next few hours resulting in right ventricular failure. An analogy that is somewhat applicable here is that of a "hammer on an anvil," with the free wall serving as a hammer and the septum as the anvil. Increasing the distance between the hammer and the anvil requires expenditure of greater energy to deliver the blow of the hammer into the anvil. Eventually, in a diseased right ventricle, that energy requirement proves prohibitively high. The other, and more dangerous, circumstance is one in which the left ventricle is allowed to distend by having pump speeds that are too low. This can cause immediate failure of the right ventricle by causing septal shift into the right ventricle and immediate distension of the right ventricle.

Management of Right Ventricular Dysfunction

Meticulous attention to the conduct of the operation can enable even a patient with marginal right ventricular function to tolerate LVAD implantation, whereas sloppy technique can endanger even a well prepared and relatively healthy right ventricle.

Patients with ischemic cardiomyopathy who have flow-limiting lesions in the right coronary artery, posterior descending coronary, or left anterior descending coronary should be revascularized at the time of LVAD implantation in order to salvage hibernating myocardium and in order to perfuse the right ventricle and interventricular septum.

Bleeding needs to be avoided or minimized. In patients with long-standing right ventricular dysfunction and passive hepatic congestion, the synthetic function or the liver is often compromised. Accordingly, we pretreat patients with vitamin K the day prior to operation, the day of the operation, and postoperatively if possible. The CPB circuit is primed with fresh frozen plasma instead of crystalloid. Operative technique needs to be meticulous, with compulsive attention to hemostasis "on the way in," with particular attention to drying up the pump pocket and any sites of adhesions within the mediastinum prior to heparinization. Internalization of the LVAD is performed prior to heparinization in order to avoid drive line hematomas that can go on to get infected. We use Bovie electrocautery, the argon beam coagulator, adjunctive hemostatic agents liberally.

In the rare event that the patient develops a profound coagulopathy during a particularly long, difficult, or tedious re-operative dissection, we will pack the mediastinum with sponges and return the patient to the intensive care unit, where a blood product resuscitation will be undertaken in an attempt to reverse the coagulopathy. Once corrected, we will return to the operating room in order to proceed with LVAD implantation. If a severe coagulopathy occurs after implantation of the LVAD, a balance has to be struck between correction of the coagulopathy by blood product resuscitation and overwhelming the right ventricle by aggressively volume loading it. In select cases, we may choose to pack to mediastinum and leave the chest open for 24–48 h, permitting a gradual resuscitation, and then return to the operating room for a washout and chest closure. In addition, massive transfusions can result in transfusion-associated lung injury with attendant increases in PVR, which can then, in turn, impose pressure work on an already volume overloaded right ventricle. We avoid the use of recombinant factor 7 because of its prohibitive cost as well as unpredictability and fear of thrombotic events in the setting of a freshly implanted blood-artificial surface interface.

We pay assiduous attention to ventilation and maintenance of the acid–base balance. Hypercarbia and acidemia can cause an increase in PVR which can be detrimental to the performance of the right ventricle. After separating from CPB, we will maintain patients on an intensive care unit ventilator both in the operating room as well as on transport to the intensive care unit, in an attempt to avoid perturbations in ventilatory parameters.

Although there are centers that use inhaled nitric oxide (iNO) liberally, our institutional bias has been to use iNO more selectively, primarily because of its prohibitive cost. Generally, iNO will be employed in the setting of recalcitrant right ventricular dysfunction in patients for whom right ventricular mechanical support is not an option, destination therapy patients, for example. Alternatively, if PVR cannot be decreased by augmenting LVAD support (in the case of severe right ventricular dysfunction), the temporary addition of iNO may be used to decrease RV afterload, thereby enabling more efficient use of the LVAD in the immediate postoperative period.

We avoid the extended use of CPB and will attempt to perform the aortic anastomosis off pump, if possible limiting the use of CPB to opening the apex of the heart. In selective cases, particularly with access to the axial flow pumps and centrifugal pumps, we will attempt to perform the entire implantation off pump or at the very least to continue ventilating at low tidal volumes.

Several authors have demonstrated, over the course of the past decade, that interrupting pulmonary blood flow during CPB impairs endothelial cell signal transduction in the pulmonary arteries and branch vessels [21] and impedes the ability of the pulmonary vasculature to relax normally, which then adversely impacts right ventricular performance by imposing the requirement to do both pressure and volume work. Therefore, we routinely maintain ventilation despite the initiation of full CPB.

Finally, the conduct by which the patient is separated from CPB is a critically important phase of the operation. De-airing maneuvers are of critical importance. We routinely flood the operative field with carbon dioxide and do not initiate LVAD support until the systemic chambers are completely and thoroughly de-aired, using intraoperative transesophageal echocardiography as a guide.

After actuation of the device at low flow, separation from CPB is performed very gradually, keeping a very close eye on right ventricular performance. Any hemodynamic or visual sign of impeding failure (such as inability to fill the reservoir of a displacement-style pulsatile device, elevation in CVP, or sudden distension) should be met by immediate return to full CPB, reevaluation, and optimization of medical therapy. Most authors will gradually come up to flow that can partially support the left-sided systemic circulation (i.e., 3 L/min) while maintaining low flow on full CPB (i.e., 2 L/min). This strategy will provide 5 L of systemic flow while forcing the right ventricle to perform only 3 L of work (while 2 L are provided by the heart lung machine). This can gradually be weaned, allowing the right ventricle to slowly assume its full workload.

Other authors [22] have advocated cannulating the main PA with a "Y" connector from the aortic line and separating from bypass by coming up to full flow on the LVAD and simultaneously clamping the aortic line and diverting 5 L of flow from the right atrium (RA) to the PA, thereby providing full right heart bypass. This can then also be gradually weaned, allowing the right ventricle to assume its full workload. With the advent of continuous-flow devices, in which septal position is of critical importance in enabling right ventricular performance, such a strategy may hold limited appeal.

We pay particular attention to separating from CPB in sinus rhythm or attempt to maintain atrioventricular synchrony with the use of temporary epicardial pacing leads. If the patient has biventricular pacing systems in place, we attempt to separate with these devices.

Separation from CPB is done at high or above normal blood pressure in order to maintain adequate coronary perfusion pressure. In a patient with coronary artery disease or a graft-dependent coronary circulation, particularly with volume-related distension of the right ventricle, hypotension can result in a very rapid and tight downward spiral that is very difficult to break without institution of right-sided ventricular support.

As referred to above, we make every effort to decrease RV afterload with the use of intravenous phosphodiesterase inhibitors such as milrinone and low dose epinephrine to promote bronchodilatation and vasodilatation of the pulmonary vasculature. In addition, as referred to above, assiduous maintenance of the acid–base balance, prevention of hypercarbia and acidemia is very important. We also make every effort to drain pleural effusions, treat mucus plugging or lobar collapse aggressively, and, if pulmonary compliance is low, have a very low threshold to leave the chest open.

Mechanical Circulatory Support Utilization: Indications for Biventricular Support, Isolated Right Ventricular Support, and Types of Devices

The following serves as a general series of recommendations for appropriate triage for patients in end-stage heart failure being considered for mechanical circulatory support.

A hemodynamically stable patient (Interagency Registry for Mechanically Assisted Circulatory Support [INTERMACS] profile 2, 3 or 4) with CVP < 15, pulmonary capillary wedge pressure [PCWP] > 25 on stable doses of inotropes and without pressors may be considered for LVAD implantation.

A hemodynamically stable patient (Intermacs profile 2, 3, or 4) with CVP > 15, PCWP > 25 may be considered for a "challenge" to the right ventricle by augmenting left-sided perfusion and venous return with implantation of an intra-aortic balloon pump. If the patient is able to mobilize fluid and diurese, if PA pressures remain high and do not fall, and if CVP does not climb further, consideration may be given to proceeding to isolated LVAD implantation. If implantation of a right ventricular assist device is required, implantation should not be delayed. Leaving the operating room with borderline LVAD flows, marginal hemodynamics, low LA pressure, high RA pressures, and high doses of inotropes and/or pressors in the anticipation of recovery usually results in a suboptimal clinical outcome. Interval return to the operating room for placement of an RVAD in such a setting is usually associated with a high mortality.

A hemodynamically unstable patient (Intermacs profile 1), any patient who is dependent on pressors, who requires ECMO or mechanical ventilation, who has an unexplained fever, adult respiratory distress syndrome, hepatic or renal dysfunction, intractable ventricular arrhythmias, or an overwhelming right ventricular infarction should be considered for implantation of temporary biventricular assist device implantation. Over time, and after having been stabilized with appropriate management, some of these patients may become eligible for implantation of a permanent implantable LVAD. Others may require permanent biventricular assist device implantation or total artificial heart implantation. Certain patients with specific and unusual presentations—such as giant cell myocarditis, failed cardiac allograft, pulmonary edema despite maximal medical therapy, and ischemic cardiomyopathy where surgery threatens the right ventricle—may be candidates for a priori permanent biventricular support.

Isolated right ventricular support may be required in the setting of a hemodynamically significant right ventricular myocardial infarction, in the postcardiotomy condition, or in patients with end-stage cor pulmonale due to primary pulmonary disease, or after heart transplantation with allograft dysfunction. In these circumstances, consideration should be given to pulmonary support with concomitant extracorporeal membrane oxygenation.

References

1. Dang NC, Topkara VK, Mercando M, Kay J, Kruger KH, Aboodi MS, et al. Right heart failure after left ventricular assist device implantation in patients with chronic congestive heart failure. J Heart Lung Transplant. 2006;25:1–6.
2. Schenk S, McCarthy PM, Blackstone EH, Feng J, Starling RC, Navia JL, et al. Duration of inotropic support after left ventricular assist device implantation: risk factors and impact on outcome. J Thorac Cardiovasc Surg. 2006;131:447–54.
3. Kavarana MN, Pessin-Minsley MS, Urtecho J, Catanese KA, Flannery M, Oz MC, et al. Right ventricular dysfunction and organ failure in left ventricular assist device recipients: a continuing problem. Ann Thorac Surg. 2002;73:745–50.
4. Morgan JA, John R, Lee BJ, Oz MC, Naka Y. Is severe right ventricular failure in left ventricular assist device recipients a risk factor for unsuccessful bridging to transplant and post-transplant mortality. Ann Thorac Surg. 2004;77:859–63.
5. Ba ZF, Wang P, Koo DJ, Cioffi WG, Bland KI, Chaudry IH. Alterations in tissue oxygen consumption and extraction after trauma and hemorrhagic shock. Crit Care Med. 2000;28:2837–42.
6. Frazier OH, Rose EA, Oz MC, Dembitsky W, McCarthy P, Radovancevic B, et al. Multicenter clinical evaluation of the HeartMate vented electric left ventricular assist system in patients awaiting heart transplantation. J Thorac Cardiovasc Surg. 2001;122:1186–95.
7. Rossi M, Sganga G, Mazzone M, Valenza V, Guarneri S, Portale G, et al. Cardiopulmonary bypass in man: role of the intestine in a self-limiting inflammatory response with demonstrable bacterial translocation. Ann Thorac Surg. 2004;77:612–8.
8. Rietschel ET, Brade H, Holst O, Brade L, Müller-Loennies S, Mamat U, et al. Bacterial endotoxin: chemical constitution, biological recognition, host response, and immunological detoxification. Curr Top Microbiol Immunol. 1996;216:39–81.
9. Masai T, Sawa Y, Ohtake S, Nishida T, Nishimura M, Fukushima N, et al. Hepatic dysfunction after left ventricular mechanical assist in patients with end-stage heart failure: role of inflammatory response and hepatic microcirculation. Ann Thorac Surg. 2002;73(2):549–55.
10. Frazier OH, Rose EA, Macmanus Q, Burton NA, Lefrak EA, Poirier VL, et al. Multicenter clinical evaluation of the HeartMate 1000 IP left ventricular assist device. Ann Thorac Surg. 1992;53:1080–90.
11. Goldstein DJ, Seldomridge JA, Chen JM, Catanese KA, DeRosa CM, Weinberg AD, et al. Use of aprotinin in LVAD recipients reduces blood loss, blood use, and perioperative mortality. Ann Thorac Surg. 1995;59:1063–8.
12. Kormos RL, Borovetz HS, Armitage JM, Hardesty RL, Marrone GC, Griffith BP. Evolving experience with mechanical circulatory support. Ann Surg. 1991; 214:471–7.
13. Kormos RL, Gasior TA, Kawai A, Pham SM, Murali S, Hattler BG, et al. Transplant candidate's clinical status rather than right ventricular function defines need for univentricular versus biventricular support. J Thorac Cardiovasc Surg. 1996;111:773–83.
14. Pagani FD, Lynch W, Swaniker F, Dyke DB, Bartlett R, Koelling T, et al. Extracorporeal life support to left ventricular assist device bridge to heart transplant: a strategy to optimize survival and resource utilization. Circulation. 1999;100(19 Suppl):II206–10.
15. Fukamachi K, McCarthy PM, Smedira NG, Vargo RL, Starling RC, Young JB. Preoperative demographic risk factors for right ventricular failure after

implantable left ventricular assist device insertion. Ann Thorac Surg. 1999;68:2181–4.
16. Ochiai Y, McCarthy PM, Smedira NG, Banbury MK, Navia JL, Feng J, et al. Predictors of severe right ventricular failure after implantable left ventricular assist device insertion: analysis of 245 patients. Circulation. 2002;106(12 Suppl 1):I198–202.
17. Matthews JC, Koelling TM, Pagani FD, Aaronson KD. The right ventricular failure risk score a pre-operative tool for assessing the risk of right ventricular failure in left ventricular assist device candidates. J Am Coll Cardiol. 2008;51(22):2163–72.
18. Smedira NG, Massad MG, Navia J, Vargo RL, Patel AN, Cook DJ, et al. Pulmonary hypertension is not a risk factor for RVAD use and death after left ventricular assist system support. ASAIO J. 1996;42: M733–5.
19. Levin HR, Burkoff D, Chen J, Oz MC, Packer M, Rose EA. Right ventricular performance (but dot outflow resistance) is a major pre-operative determinant of right heart failure in patients with chronic heart failure who receive a left ventricular assist device. J Am Coll Cardiol. 1994;23(2 Suppl 1):838A.
20. Farrar DJ, Hill JD, Pennington DG, McBride LR, Holman WL, Kormos RL, et al. Preoperative and post-operative comparison of patients with univentricular and biventricular support with the Thoratec ventricular assist device as a bridge to cardiac transplantation. J Thorac Cardiovasc Surg. 1997;113:202–9.
21. Carvalho EM, Gabriel EA, Salerno TA. Pulmonary protection during cardiac surgery: systematic literature review. Asian Cardiovasc Thorac Ann. 2008;16: 503–7.
22. Loebe M, Potapov E, Sodian R, Kopitz M, Noon GP. A safe and simple method of preserving right ventricular function during implantation of a left ventricular assist device. J Thorac Cardiovasc Surg. 2001; 122(5):1043.

15 Ventricular Assist Devices and Transplantation for Adults with Congenital Heart Disease

Jonathan M. Chen and Robert A. Sorabella

While corrective surgery for congenital heart lesions generally obviates the need for further operative repairs, concurrent cardiomyopathy, acquired ischemic damage, and progressive failure of the systemic ventricle can all too often lead to end-stage heart failure in this complex cohort. While the principles of ventricular assist device (VAD) support or transplantation in these settings are no different than for those patients with dilated cardiomyopathy, prior palliative procedures, the presence of progressive aortopulmonary collaterals, and the existence of multiple prior operations significantly complicate later mechanical ventricular assistance and transplantation. In this setting, surgical flexibility and creativity are essential to adjust to the challenges of anatomy and physiology that the adult with congenital heart disease presents.

J.M. Chen, M.D. (✉)
Department of Pediatrics and Cardiothoracic Surgery, New York Presbyterian Hospital, Cornell Campus, 525 E. 68th Street, Suite M404, New York, NY 10023, USA
e-mail: jmc23@columbia.edu

R.A. Sorabella, M.D.
Division of Cardiothoracic Surgery, Department of Surgery, New York Presbyterian Hospital, Columbia Campus, 177 Fort Washington Ave., Milstein Hospital Building, Room 7GN-435, New York, NY 10023, USA
e-mail: ras2112@columbia.edu

Ventricular Assistance

The most common indications for mechanical ventricular assistance in adults with congenital heart disease are progressive concurrent cardiomyopathy, the failing systemic right ventricle, and the failing Fontan. While most adult patients with congenital disease are closely followed throughout their lifetime, "acquired" cardiomyopathy and heart failure may represent the cumulative insult of several prior operative repairs, progressive ischemic damage, or ongoing volume overload from aortopulmonary collaterals on myocardium that is inherently abnormal (e.g., noncompaction). In patients with corrected transposition of the great vessels (ccTGA), an additional sustained risk of complete heart block may contribute substantially to this progression. The failed Fontan candidates, incomplete volume unloading, significant atrioventricular valve regurgitation, malignant atrial tachyarrhythmias, and significant cyanosis or ascites in aggregate contribute significant risk to any such procedure.

The tenets of mechanical support in this setting, then, must address several key questions. First, is the indication for support short or long term—is this supportive therapy for the patient with ccTGA until they can be properly paced (with uni- or biventricular pacing), or is this an adult with a Mustard or Senning whose right ventricle has finally decompensated and is unsalvageable? Second, will the mechanical assistance address the problem? Single ventricular support of the failing

J.A. Morgan and Y. Naka (eds.), *Surgical Treatment for Advanced Heart Failure*, DOI 10.1007/978-1-4614-6919-3_15, © Springer Science+Business Media New York 2013

Fontan will not necessarily improve oxygenation, in particular because of the ongoing need for passive pulmonary blood flow. In such a situation, extracorporeal membrane oxygenation (ECMO) therapy may be most appropriate. Creative solutions for assistance of pulmonary arterial flow may also actually be what is required if the ventricular function is reasonable.

Third, in the presence of prior repairs, is the proposed assistance feasible? A patient with a Mustard/Senning who requires biventricular support will present unique challenges to obtain right ventricular assist device (RVAD) inflow, given the location and orientation of the systemic venous baffle. The extensive trabeculations within a systemic right ventricle may increase the risk of obstruction of the inflow cannula if not properly resected. Creative solutions to single ventricular support through a previously unused approach (e.g., thoracotomy) must take into account ventricular looping and apical directionality (e.g., dextrocardia). Additionally, those with right ventricular to pulmonary artery conduits generally have such severe calcification of the prior conduit that cannulation for RVAD outflow would be nearly impossible. Fourth, does the anatomy demand a particularly creative approach? Although rare, situs inversus totalis unsurprisingly requires significant changes in the location and choice of cannulation, as does dextrocardia, mesocardia, and situs ambiguous. In these cases, the preoperative evaluation with cardiac catheterization, magnetic resonance imaging (MRI), and computed tomography (CT) scan is of utmost importance.

An essential question is also whether the patient would best be served with one of several less traditional options. The most common of these is ECMO, which can often be approached percutaneously and/or peripherally. As with ECMO for any other indication, it will be less effective in the presence of moderate or severe aortic (or neoaortic) valve regurgitation. If ECMO is being pursued in the presence of an intact atrial septum, it must be remembered that this therapy will not completely decompress the systemic ventricle, which is of pertinence if ventricular recovery is being considered. For these patients, a blade septostomy may allow for capture of pulmonary venous return, as may an additional pulmonary artery catheter. However, for those with significant aortopulmonary collaterals, only inflow from a site distal to the left atrium will afford adequate drainage and decompression of the systemic ventricle. Ultimately, however, ECMO requires intubation and sedation, with no realistic hope for extubation or mobilization; for an adult with a projected long waiting time to transplantation, this may not be a viable therapeutic strategy.

A new option that is also for short to medium term (days to weeks) use is represented by new percutaneous support devices. We have used RVAD support with two percutaneous venous cannulae (BioMedicus centrifugal pump, Medtronic Inc, Minneapolis, MN) in the right atrium (via right internal jugular) and main pulmonary artery (via femoral venous access) with a centrifugal pump for RVAD or ECMO support, in concert with an Impella 2.5 (Abiomed, Danvers, MA) device for partial ventricular support in a teenager with fulminant transplant rejection. Here, the risks of hemorrhage and infection from reoperative sternotomy and the potential need for an open chest are obviated, but again the duration of support is somewhat limited. Other devices that have been considered in this realm are the TandemHeart (Cardiac Assist, Pittsburgh, PA) and other percutaneous assist devices under current investigation. The possibility of a full-flow device (e.g., Impella 5.0) for adult sizes may make this particular strategy more appealing in the future.

Finally, the "ultimate" mechanical solution in some patients may be complete cardiac excision and support with either a total artificial heart (TAH) device, or support with "reconstructed" inflow and biventricular assistance. For those with normal atrial situs, and enough pulmonary arterial tissue to cannulate for outflow, the TAH may be feasible. For many adults with congenital heart disease, however, after cardiac excision, the remaining heart tissue may not be amenable for TAH connections. We have previously performed complete cardiac excision in a Fontan patient, where the systemic venous return was recreated with a Dacron tube graft into which an RVAD inflow cannula was secured. The RVAD outflow cannula was then similarly inserted into a Dacron graft sewn end to side to the pulmonary arterial confluence. Reconstruction of the pulmonary veins with a Dacron cuff allowed a small "dumpling-like" chamber for LVAD inflow, and the aortic cannula was placed end to side into the aorta. In this arrangement, a Thoratec (Thoratec, Pleasantville, MA) P-VAD biventricular assist device was used for support as in prior descriptions in the literature for non-congenital patients. While this approach is conceptually appealing because it can remove many anatomic obstacles to inflow and outflow, balancing the compliance of the left atrial reconstructed chamber is not simple, and ongoing hemorrhage can be significant.

In sum, mechanical ventricular assistance of the adult with congenital heart disease can be quite challenging and likely is best done by a congenital surgeon whose experience with modified and unmodified congenital anatomy and physiology is extensive. The techniques for reconstruction at the time of transplantation are covered in the next section, all of which should be kept in mind when planning support as a bridge to transplantation.

Cardiac Transplantation in Congenital Patients

Cardiac transplantation for complex congenital heart disease incorporates aspects of both reparative and replacement surgery. While intracardiac congenital malformations are replaced, and therefore pose few obstacles to the transplant surgeon, extracardiac malformations (be they congenital, acquired, or iatrogenic) present a major challenge to the operative team.

Pre-transplant, a full comprehension of the operative plan for the management of each patient (and his or her lesion), is essential for the donor team so that they may harvest appropriate amounts of donor tissue to allow for adequate reconstruction and potential conduit formation. This understanding extends as well to the perioperative recipient teams—especially in the case of adult congenital patients—where the cardiac anesthesia team in particular may be less familiar with congenital lesions and their perioperative concerns.

Donor Operation

The donor operation proceeds as routine for heart transplantation except for the frequent need for additional donor tissue to be used to reconstruct the recipient. In general, there are three main anatomic concerns for the majority of recipient reconstructive techniques. First, donor procurement for a recipient with a persistent left superior vena cava (LSVC) may require the mobilization and extirpation of the entire donor innominate vein. Second, reconstruction of recipient main pulmonary artery after Rastelli reconstruction, or with branch pulmonary artery stenosis, may mandate harvesting of the donor's entire intrapericardial main and branch pulmonary arteries. Finally, donor procurement for recipients with aortic arch hypoplasia or other arch abnormalities can require full mobilization and removal of the aortic arch, arch vessels, and portions of the descending aorta if necessary.

Recipient Operation

In patients with multiple prior procedures, and for those in whom cardiomegaly and volume overload may significantly complicate reoperative dissection, peripheral cardiopulmonary bypass is often instituted through cannulation of the femoral artery and vein. Once safe entry into the chest has been accomplished and the great vessels and atria dissected, it is not uncommon to recannulate the patient centrally in order to ensure sufficient flow at low line pressure. Aortic cannulation, when performed centrally, naturally must be done sufficiently distally along the aortic arch to allow for appropriate reconstruction in cases requiring aortoplasty for size mismatch. Iatrogenic venous considerations (e.g., Glenn shunt) may also require very proximal cannulation for venous drainage.

The recipient is cooled to 32 °C if a relatively straightforward procedure and short ischemic time are anticipated. However, for complex cases requiring significant reconstruction, and for recipients with increased bronchial venous return, more profound hypothermia, or even deep hypothermic circulatory arrest at 18 °C, may be utilized.

Anomalous Conditions

Anomalies of the Atria

There are essentially three types of anomalies of the atria: (1) those involving size discrepancies between donor and recipient, (2) those created by iatrogenic surgical distortion, and (3) viscero-atrial situs inversus in which the donor and recipient atria are spatially inverted.

For donor–recipient atrial discrepancies, we have employed two techniques (often in concert) to better align the atria. First, the recipient atrium may be reduced in size by oversewing the cephalic atrium, thereby extending the length of the recipient SVC. Second, the donor right atrial incision may be performed in the sinus venosus region of the right atrium, just posterior to the sinoatrial node. This paraseptal incision may then be extended to increase the size of the donor right atrium as needed. Interestingly, in our experience, this second technique has not resulted in an increased incidence of atrial arrhythmias.

Patients who have undergone prior Mustard or Senning atrial inversion procedures often develop significant distortion of their atria. First, in such patients, the right atrium may be abnormally large and the left atrium abnormally small, and the venae cavae are often drawn to the left side. Because of this, after baffle excision, the orifices of the cavae then tend to be aligned in close proximity to the orifices of the pulmonary veins. The size discrepancies of donor and recipient atria may be addressed with the two techniques previously described. The interatrial septum of the donor heart may be used to fashion a new atrial septum in the common atrium of the recipient, or, as has been suggested, the inclusion of a "tongue" of left atrial wall on the right side may allow for the creation of atrial septation when anchored either to the posterior atrial wall (common atrium) or to a septal remnant.

Viscero-atrial situs inversus represents an anatomic variant for which several complicated techniques have been previously described. One method, which may be used in the setting of bilateral superior venae cavae (SVCs) with the LSVC and inferior venae cavae (IVC) entering to the right of the pulmonary veins, allows for the excision of the interatrial septum and creation of a lateral "T" incision in the left atrium. Two baffles may then be created along the back wall of the common atrium to bring the vena caval return rightward and thereby allow for standard left atrial and right atrial anastomoses.

Anomalies of Systemic and Pulmonary Venous Return

We have encountered two types of anomalies of systemic and pulmonary venous connections: (1) left SVC and (2) deficiencies of SVC tissue from prior operations. For those patients with a left SVC, in which the vena cava drains into a coronary sinus *not* in communication with the left atrium, we have found that the recipient cardiectomy may be performed leaving the coronary sinus intact. However, here the middle cardiac vein must be transected and oversewn prior to the completion of the left atrial anastomosis. In addition, in those in whom the coronary sinus is massive, this strategy may predispose to mitral inflow occlusion of the recipient heart when implanted in situ. In contrast, for those patients in whom the coronary sinus is unroofed, the left SVC may either be ligated, divided, and subsequently anastomosed directly to the donor innominate vein or be baffled to the right atrium using additional adjacent recipient left atrial tissue.

Those single-ventricle patients who either have previously undergone cavopulmonary shunts or have bilateral SVC may be reconstructed easily using donor SVC and innominate vein to anastomose the left and right vena cavae, respectively. Naturally, cannulation in these cases must be sufficiently high along the SVC to allow for the necessary dissection, mobilization, and reconstruction of the SVC. If the donor innominate vein is long enough, it can rest in the orthotopic position in front of the aorta; more likely, its more "natural" position will be in the transverse sinus behind the reconstructed great vessels (thus of pertinence to have enough donor pulmonary artery and aorta to allow for a gentle curvature to bring these great vessels anteriorly off the reconstructed innominate).

Anomalies of the Great Arteries

These anatomic variants represent anomalies of position, size, and surgical distortion, in addition to those anomalies produced by aortopulmonary collateral arteries. Simple malposition can be reconstructed easily with harvesting of additional donor great vessels.

Reconstruction of the pulmonary arteries may be necessary because of (1) abnormalities of position, (2) abnormalities of pulmonary outflow obstruction, or (3) previous cavopulmonary, atriopulmonary, or systemic pulmonary shunts. Either or both branch pulmonary arteries may be congenitally atretic or stenotic, or they alternatively may have areas of acquired stenosis or distortion from prior shunt procedures mandating reconstruction. In addition, we have performed transplantation in individuals with only one "functional" pulmonary artery (the other having been rendered nonfunctional by congenital unilateral atresia), a condition which requires "baffling" of the donor pulmonary artery to allow for unobstructed, unilateral pulmonary blood flow. In general, abnormalities of the pulmonary artery may be bypassed completely or augmented via patch angioplasty or with additional donor pulmonary arterial tissue.

For those with L-TGA (congenitally corrected transposition of the great arteries) who have received prior reconstructions with pulmonary artery conduits, the conduit may either be transected distal to the prosthesis (and donor pulmonary artery anastomosed directly end to end to the remaining conduit) or, preferably, the entire conduit tissue may be removed and the pulmonary arteries reconstructed and enlarged (if necessary) with extended donor pulmonary artery tissue.

For those patients with pulmonary outflow obstruction who have undergone prior Waterston shunts or pulmonary artery banding procedures or who have pulmonary stenosis or atresia at baseline, reconstruction of the pulmonary arteries may be performed with band removal, and partial pulmonary arterioplasty may be performed with either bovine pericardium or extended donor pulmonary artery. Alternatively, Waterston shunts may be repaired from within the aorta, and pulmonary artery band tissue may simply be excised and the pulmonary arterial anastomosis performed directly to the pulmonary artery bifurcation. Prior modified Blalock–Taussig shunts may be ligated or oversewn from within the pulmonary artery, and the cavopulmonary shunts may be reconstructed bilaterally, the pulmonary arteries repaired, and the venae cavae reconstructed end to end with extended donor SVC and/or innominate vein.

Additionally, those who have had a right classic Glenn cavopulmonary anastomosis in conjunction with a Fontan to the left or main pulmonary artery can often have a significant gap between the orifice of the right pulmonary artery and the main or left pulmonary artery. This requires reconstruction with donor pulmonary arterial tissue at the time of transplant.

Summary

The most common indications for transplantation in congenital heart disease in adults are post-repair of tetralogy of Fallot, d-transposition of the great vessels after Senning or Mustard procedure (failing systemic right ventricle), and failed Fontan from either poor ventricular function, protein-losing enteropathy, or progressive cyanosis. All of the techniques described above are utilized to reconstruct the great vessels and to account for additional abnormalities of situs. Cannulation of Senning and Mustard patients can be particularly challenging so as to avoid cannulating the systemic venous return outside of the Senning/Mustard baffle. Those with dextrocardia also will require takedown of the left pleural reflection so as to allow space within the mediastinum for the (normal) donor leftward facing apex, and additionally require some reduction of the potential space on the right so as to prevent herniation of the allograft rightward.

Fontan patients require particular note. These always complex patients represent the largest growing population of potential transplant candidates; they also generally require the largest amount of intraoperative reconstruction. The operative mortality nationwide for transplantation for the failing Fontan approaches 25 %. Those with additional risk factors, such as renal insufficiency, poor nutrition and/or albumin from protein-losing enteropathy, and hepatic dysfunction from chronically elevated central venous pressures, will have even high operative risks. It is essential to fully evaluate these compounding risk factors in order to establish transplant candidacy. Surgical planning for likely femoral or axillary cannulation (e.g., ultrasound to determine patency, CT scan to evaluate proximity to the sternum) is essential. While bovine pericardium or other adjunctive exogenous tissue can be used to reconstruct the pulmonary arteriotomy that remains after the recipient cardiectomy, additional donor pulmonary artery provides the best "lie" of the allograft. This limits the donor pool available to such patients to those in whom lungs are not being procured, as the additional pulmonary tissue required is that otherwise used for lung transplantation. Finally, preparing patients for the likely potential scenarios of tracheostomy, gastrostomy, and prolonged hospitalization is ethically appropriate.

Finally, the congenital transplant surgeon must also try to plan preoperatively for those anatomic or physiologic problems that they may not be able to repair immediately, or may require time or additional percutaneous procedures to fix. While transplantation is the most likely treatment for protein-losing enteropathy in the single-ventricle patient, resolution of symptoms may take up to a year or more for conclusion. Control of aortopulmonary collaterals or residual surgical shunts may require deep hypothermic circulatory arrest intraoperatively to maintain a dry operative field but may best be addressed with coil occlusion postoperatively to avoid volume loading and heart failure. Finally, peripheral stenoses in the pulmonary artery are general best addressed with stenting if they are beyond the first bifurcation and even potentially if they are beyond the mid-branch pulmonary artery; choosing not to attempt repair at the time of transplantation may often provide the less morbid approach ("less is more").

Cardiac transplantation for congenital heart disease offers a wide variety of challenges to traditional techniques for heart replacement. Incorporating the reparative methodology of congenital heart surgery, transplantation in this setting often requires reconstruction of extracardiac great vessels as well as intracardiac baffling to ameliorate anomalous systemic and pulmonary venous return. With the advent of therapeutic adjuncts to aid in the perioperative management of these often critically ill patients, many patients with congenital heart disease can anticipate survival comparable to patients with acquired heart disease. Because of the growing cohort of adult congenital patients, this population will certainly become more prominent in the near future.

Index

J.A. Morgan and Y. Naka (eds.), *Surgical Treatment for Advanced Heart Failure*,
DOI 10.1007/978-1-4614-6919-3,

MIX
Papier aus verantwortungsvollen Quellen
Paper from responsible sources
FSC® C105338

If you have any concerns about our products,
you can contact us on
ProductSafety@springernature.com

In case Publisher is established outside the EU,
the EU authorized representative is:
Springer Nature Customer Service Center GmbH
Europaplatz 3, 69115 Heidelberg, Germany

Printed by Libri Plureos GmbH
in Hamburg, Germany